SENSORY
NEUROPHYSIOLOGY

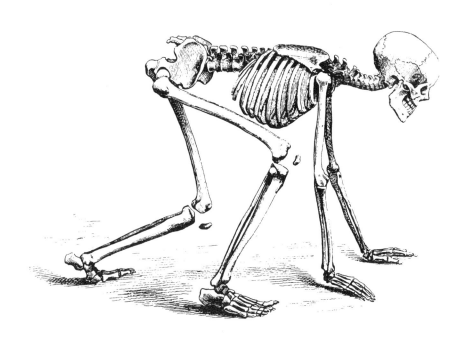

The human skeleton in the position of a cat. (Jayne, 1898)

SENSORY NEUROPHYSIOLOGY

With Special Reference to the Cat

James C. Boudreau

Chiyeko Tsuchitani

VNR **VAN NOSTRAND REINHOLD COMPANY**
New York / Cincinnati / Toronto / London / Melbourne

Van Nostrand Reinhold Company Regional Offices:
New York   Cincinnati   Chicago   Millbrae   Dallas

Van Nostrand Reinhold Company International Offices:
London   Toronto   Melbourne

Copyright © 1973 by Litton Educational Publishing, Inc.

Library of Congress Catalog Card Number: 72-11654
ISBN: 0-442-20935-5

Manufactured in the United States of America

Published by Van Nostrand Reinhold Company
450 West 33rd Street, New York, N.Y. 10001

Published simultaneously in Canada by Van Nostrand Reinhold Ltd.

15 14 13 12 11 10 9 8 7 6 5 4 3 2 1

Library of Congress Cataloging in Publication Data

Boudreau, James C   1936-
  Sensory neurophysiology.

  1. Senses and sensation. 2. Neurophysiology.
I. Tsuchitani, Chiyeko, 1938-   joint author.
II. Title. [DNLM: 1. Nervous system—Anatomy and
histology. 2. Neurophysiology. 3. Sensation.
WL 102 B756s 1973]
QP431.B63   591.1'82   72-11654
ISBN 0-442-20935-5

PREFACE

We describe in *Sensory Neurophysiology* an area of brain research that is currently making rapid advances. Our book examines in detail the structure and function of sensory nervous systems. It concentrates on peripheral neural systems from which pulse signals can be recorded, since these systems are most amenable to study and interpretation.

To keep the subject matter within manageable limits and to focus *Sensory Neurophysiology*, we have organized it around the peripheral nervous system of the cat, an animal depicted in detail in Chapter 2, "The Cat, *Felis Catus*." Unfortunately, by so having to restrict the book, we must forego a great deal of the varied and rich literature on sensory systems. We have tried wherever possible to provide references to work on other species. The peripheral nervous system of the cat may be but a small part of the totality of sensory processes, yet it is nevertheless an area of research so highly developed and rigorous that it affects all other areas of brain research, especially techniques in use and the interpretation of results. A knowledge of sensory neurophysiology is essential for any serious student of the nervous system, for sensory neurophysiology is forming a core foundation for the construction of theoretical models of nervous-system functioning.

Sensory Neurophysiology does not attempt to review all of the literature of the anatomy and physiology of the cat's sensory systems; rather, it is intended to present a conceptual and experimental view of a sensory neurophysiological approach to the analysis of neural mechanisms. Anatomy is extensively introduced only if there exists adequate neurophysiology on a sensory system; neurophysiology is explored in detail only if it is sufficiently developed. In many cases, the available studies on a specific sensory system are difficult or impossible to compare because of the differences in their techniques and measures. To avoid questionable comparisons and excessive detail, we have frequently limited our reportage to one investigator or a small group of investigators.

Sensory Neurophysiology is both elementary and advanced. It is elementary in that it requires little previous knowledge on the part of the reader. A comprehensive grasp of the English language and some familiarity with technical material should be sufficient. To give the reader a background that will enable him to understand the work on sensory systems, we include separate chapters on essential neuroanatomy and essential neurophysiology. These preparatory chapters are "essential" only for an understanding of the material in this book: they do not attempt to review these vast areas of research. Chapter 5, "Theoretical Sensory Neurophysiology," is intended to provide the reader with a simple theoretical framework for the interpretation of sensory neurophysiological data.

In the entire book, the emphasis is on description. Possible mechanisms are rarely mentioned or considered, since current speculation on sensory mechanisms is almost invariably based upon an inadequate understanding of the structural and functional complexities of sensory systems. *Sensory Neurophysiology* explores the basic questions: what are the anatomical elements of sensory systems, how are they connected, and how do they function? On the other hand, our book is advanced in that it offers the reader a systematic interpretation and rationale of the current status of much of the research on the structure and function of mammalian sensory systems. We describe in detail most of the major mammalian sensory systems, and derive our illustrations and data from the current work in these areas of workers using the most sophisticated techniques. We have written *Sensory Neurophysiology* so that it can be used for individual study; as a text for a course in neural sciences; or as a reference book for a critical reading of current research on sensory systems.

Because of the structural and functional complexity of the nervous system, a great amount of detail is inherent in the description of sensory neural systems. To understand the nervous system, however, an appreciation for detail is necessary. This appreciation for detail can be acquired. To aid in its acquisition, we have included many illustrations from the abundant anatomical and neurophysiological literature on sensory systems. We suggest that the serious reader involve himself in a project of construction in which he will put together, piece by piece, a cat. It will also help to have a pet cat available for visual inspection.

N. Crawford and P. R. Bierer have assisted us with most aspects of our work. We thank D. S. Ferrera and J. M. Utzman for the photography for this book; M. Berman for the art work; M. Petruska and K. Dignazio for secretarial assistance; and S. Kruger, N. Alev, B. Whitsel, P. R. Burgess, H. Scalzi, G. Werner, and J. Sechrist for reading and commenting on sections of the book. We are grateful also to the many investigators who took the time to answer our letters concerning their work.

We appreciate the help of the following librarians and their staffs: J. E. Bandemer and L. Eakin of the Falk Library; J. Reilley of the Leech Farm V. A. Medical Library; C. M. Brosky of the WP/RMP Library System; and A. Tauber of the Carnegie Museum Library. We thank also the many library workers who obtained papers for us via inter-library loan services, and the many publishers who granted us permission to reproduce copyrighted material.

Our work was aided by United States Public Health research grants and by the University of Pittsburgh Computer Center.

J. C. Boudreau
C. Tsuchitani

Pittsburgh, Pennsylvania

CONTENTS

1
INTRODUCTION TO SENSORY NEUROPHYSIOLOGY

The universe as we know it comprises a multitude of objects. These objects are composed of subcomponents put together in certain proportions and in certain configurations. They vary tremendously in complexity, from atoms to molecules to self-reproducing living cells to large organisms consisting of many multicellular subsystems. The scientific study of an organism includes the classification of that organism with respect to other organisms and the investigation of whole organism properties. Such studies involve the general scientific fields of biology, zoology, and psychology. A description of the properties of an organism is not exhausted, however, when the activities of the whole organism have been described. Within any organism are separate functional subsystems that unite to form that whole organism although separately they perform specialized tasks. It is the task of anatomy to depict the structure and interconnection of these subsystems, and that of physiology to account for their function.

The subsystem that has proved most difficult to analyze scientifically is the nervous system, the subsystem that controls all other subsystems. The difficulties we encounter in analyzing the nervous system are many. The nervous system does not perform any single unitary bodily function; rather, its duties are multiple. In agreement with the multiple functional duties of the nervous system is the division of the nervous system into a multitude of anatomically distinguishable subsystems. Unlike other bodily systems such as the respiratory or digestive systems, the nervous system does not process substances such as oxygen or proteins but rather information, and thus the nervous system — like a computer — is an information-processing system. The computerlike properties of the nervous system delayed its study since it is only recently that computer science and communication theory have developed to the degree that they can provide some of the conceptual tools essential to this study. Another obstacle to our study of the nervous system has been the complex task of taking measurements from the nervous system and assembling these measurements within a logical framework. The study of the nervous system was delayed until the age of electronics, which produced such invaluable instruments as oscilloscopes and high-impedance preamplifiers. More recently computers have been brought into the laboratory to both control an experiment and analyze the enormous quantities of data compiled in the process. Despite these difficulties, progress has occurred in the analysis of the function of the nervous system, a progress that has been most conspicuous in the area of research known as sensory neurophysiology.

Sensory neurophysiology can be defined as the quantitative study of the structure and function of sensory neural systems. Although the first experiment in sensory neurophysiology was performed as long ago as 1926 by Adrian and Zotterman, marked progress in this science has occurred only in the last few years. Sensory neurophysiology is the method of choice in the study of the nervous system, and the only approach with a sophistication akin to that of the nervous system itself. Sensory neurophysiology reveals the identity, number, location, and connections of the individual cellular elements that are the structure of the sensory system. The function of sensory systems is studied with quantitative neuroelectric measures taken from individual neural elements.

Ours is an exact science. It deals with a set of physically definable objects (cells) and a set of physically measurable events (neural pulses), which are used to measure the activities of the neural cells. The electrical pulses produced by nerve cells are interpreted in terms of the stimuli that elicit them; the stimuli themselves are usually described by the measures of classical physics.

The field of sensory neurophysiology as laid out in this book has three attributes that make it the preferred method for analyzing all kinds of neural systems. These attributes are: (1) simplicity; (2) precision; and (3) power. Sensory neurophysiology is simple in that it makes few assumptions as to the meaning of its measures. In approaching the analysis of anything as complex as the nervous system, we must work within a context that is as unambiguous as possible and one in which the empirical measures themselves have validity. In much research on the nervous system, the measures taken by various investigators are often given meaning by interpreting them with respect to an imaginary nervous system, i.e., one possessing certain hypothesized properties. It is often difficult to extricate fact from fancy, so inextricably interwoven into the experiments are the conceptualizations of the researchers. In sensory neurophysiology, the neural measures stand by themselves. The only assumptions made about the nervous system are those that relate pulse production to nerve cells (see Chapter 4). Because of this simplicity, someone other than the investigator can interpret an experiment in sensory neurophysiology, and in the chapters that follow, the results of experiments are presented so that the reader can examine some of the basic measures and interpret them himself.

The second attribute of sensory neurophysiology rendering it the method of choice in studying the nervous system is its precision. Sensory neurophysiology is exact in the measures it utilizes. The response from a neural system is measured in terms of discrete pulses. The stimuli used to elicit the neural pulse trains are usually physical variables such as sound waves or linear displacements, measured in terms of Hz (cycles/sec) or microns respectively. The neural pulse trains elicited by the stimuli can often be measured from one stimulus presentation to another with an accuracy of plus- or minus-one pulse. The relationships between stimulus parameters and the neural pulse response can also be precisely quantified, and these relationships can be utilized to distinguish between different neural elements and to establish the nature of the pulse-encoded neural message. So invariant are the properties of the nervous system that the quantitative relationships established by a properly conducted experiment become the principal factors for the formulation of a theoretical model of the sensory systems.

The last point leads us into the third attribute of sensory neurophysiology, its power, which makes it such an appealing area of neurophysiological investigation. Because sensory neurophysiology refers neural events to external events, it offers a means by which one can interpret the nature of the pulse train. Detailed quantitative observational studies form the foundation for any worthwhile theory of neural functioning. The quantitative relationships between stimulus-response measures form the basis for any theory of the nervous system, and any theory that ignores them is building on sand.

Sensory neurophysiology is also powerful in the sense that the techniques used to study one sensory system are to a great extent applicable to other sensory systems. Thus, if one learns about one sensory system, the knowledge and techniques acquired are relevant to the study of other sensory systems. Although it is common to think of sensory systems as limited to the classical ones of vision, hearing, taste, smell, and touch, the body contains a multitude of sensory systems measuring every aspect of bodily functioning. The domain of sensory neurophysiology extends far beyond those few neural systems currently considered as sensory. Because the nervous system is involved in the control and regulation of practically all bodily functions, the techniques of sensory neurophysiology seem to be applicable to probably every area of physiology. The application of sensory neurophysiological principles to the study of blood chemistry is just getting under way in the study of the sensory systems of the carotid body. We expect that future sensory neurophysiological research will have much to offer traditional physiology in its study of such organ systems as the kidney, the heart, and the intestine where our present knowledge of neural control is minimal.

The power of sensory neurophysiology is not limited to the analysis of peripheral sensory systems or even to the central neural structures that directly receive this peripheral input. Indeed, the function of the central nervous system can be studied only if the inputs are known and can be systematically varied. Sensory systems constitute the major form of input (the other major pathway is the blood stream) to the central nervous system. If the response of neurons within peripheral sensory systems to certain stimuli is known, then by producing identical stimulus conditions, known neural inputs can be sent to those nerve cells that receive the projections of the peripheral neurons. In many cases, the centrally located neurons combine one kind of sensory information with another or utilize some aspect of the incoming neural message to perform some particular bodily function (such as contracting a muscle or secreting a substance). Thus, by a technique of systematically advancing from nerve center to nerve center, one enters the brain and prepares the groundwork for the analysis of central mechanisms.

INFLUENCES ON SENSORY NEUROPHYSIOLOGY

Sensory neurophysiology has reached a maturity whereby it can stand on its own. Certain areas of investigation, however, have influenced its development, and others have proven so essential to its core that they must be mentioned, at least in passing. They are clinical neurology and psychophysics, and the physical and engineering sciences and anatomy respectively.

Anatomy, as the study of the structure of living organisms, is involved in any experiment in sensory neurophysiology. One of our primary concerns is the elucidation of the type of cellular elements comprising the sensory systems we study with neurophysiological techniques. Any neural unit has anatomical identity and is located within a structurally organized neural population. Furthermore, the neural unit has peripheral and central connections specific to that unit and the neural group of which it is a member. For example, if one measures the response of a sensory ganglion cell, this ganglion cell may be distinguished from other ganglion cells by its position within an organized neural group, and the cells in this group will be structurally and chemically different from other ganglion-cell groups. The cell will peripherally innervate a specific type of receptor and will send a specific type of information from this receptor to specific types of cells in the central nervous system. Thus, the neuroanatomical characteristics of any sensory system is one of the essential properties we can study in sensory neurophysiology.

Sensory neuroanatomy and sensory neurophysiology are two ways of looking at the same object. We shall see in the chapters to follow that frequently sensory neurophysiological research has been directed toward the discovery of the functional difference between elements that have been distinguished on anatomical grounds. In many cases, however, we shall observe that it is not neuroanatomy that is leading and directing the neurophysiology but rather the opposite. Sensory neurophysiological experiments, especially those involving the skin, may demand structural distinctions that the anatomists have not made. In this sense neurophysiology forms a natural complement to neuroanatomy, since much of neuroanatomy is directed toward the distinction of differences between neural elements, and frequently the validity of these distinctions cannot be resolved on anatomical grounds alone. Sensory neurophysiology provides us with a means to make quantitative functional distinctions between neural elements. Early neuroanatomists established that the single cell is the fundamental structural unit in the nervous system; neurophysiology has established that the fundamental functional unit is the neuron.

How predominately anatomy looms in the study of sensory systems will be made apparent in our separate chapter on essential neuroanatomy; and each of the chapters dealing with the sensory systems describes the structure of that system in detail.

The physical sciences provide us with the tools necessary for an analysis of sensory systems. The stimulus is usually measurable in physical units whether one is working in vision or with mechanoreceptive skin systems. Thus, if a unit is measuring the position of, say, a hair, the position of that hair can be stated in physical units as can the various physical parameters of movement such as direction, rate, and acceleration. The stimulus for chemoreceptors must be identified and quantified in terms of known chemical measurements. Similarly, the study of the senses for receiving light and sound involves the presentation of stimuli exactly quantifiable in established physical units. The relation of physical sciences to sensory neurophysiology is probably closer than that of any other biological science. Different physical sciences are needed for the study of different senses, however.

The recent impact of the engineering and computer sciences upon sensory neurophysiology has been tremendous. The effect has been practical and conceptual, for they have provided a framework within which we can interpret the functioning of sensory systems. The engineering and computer sciences have in the last decade or two advanced rapidly in the construction, design and theory of sensory elements, communication theory, control systems and computer processing of information. Many of the problems of construction and analysis faced by a computer are similar to those faced by a brain. Engineers and mathematicians have worked out some of the possible solutions to problems faced by computing systems.

Clinical neurology and psychophysics are two areas of investigation that have directed a great deal of research in our field. We grouped them together because both sciences rely primarily on behavioral measurements in their studies of the nervous system. In clinical neurology, the function of a nerve or nucleus is interpreted on the basis of the behavioral disruption produced by a lesion in the neural structure. Thus the role of the chorda tympani in the chemical senses of the tongue was determined by observing that damage to the nerve is followed by unilateral loss of taste on the front two thirds of the tongue. Clinical neurology has provided us with much of our knowledge concerning the composition of sensory and motor nerves and their central connections. Because the techniques in clinical neurology are not quantitative, however, the functional neural interpretations are necessarily crude and inexact.

Psychophysics is the study of the behavioral responses of an organism to physical stimuli. By means of these behavioral responses, an investigator determines what stimulus variables are effective in eliciting distinctive responses. In most cases, the behavioral responses are in the form of verbal reports from humans, but other types of behavioral responses — bar pressing, for example — can be utilized from both humans and other animals. By these means, the psychophysicist can determine the nature of the physical continuum to which a sensory system is responsive, and the ability of the organism to make distinctions within this physical continuum. Thus, it is possible to determine the threshold at which different sound frequencies are effective, or the rate at which a flickering light fuses. Much of our knowledge about the functioning of certain sensory systems has been obtained with psychophysics. It is wise for any sensory neurophysiological investigator to examine closely the psychophysical literature in his own area both for techniques and for some estimate as to the limitations and capabilities of his sensory system. Without strong psychophysics, there is a tendency to underestimate the capabilities of a sensory system. We believe that the advancements in auditory neurophysiology can be in large part attributed to the extensive human psychophysical literature, which presented the sensory neurophysiologists with a functioning system endowed with qualities they could not ignore.

Psychophysics can only be used as a tool, however, and not as the guiding force in sensory neurophysiology. Since most experiments on neural recording are done on animals, human psychophysics is often of doubtful applicability. Most of the neurophysiological work on the skin senses has been performed on the cat, which has quite a different organization of the skin senses. In addition, the cat's visual system and oral chemoreception systems seem different in many ways from these human sensory systems. Many investigators are aware of the differences between animals and are attempting to examine behavioral capacities. Often, however, the interpretation of nerve responses is done in human psychophysical terms, a most unfortunate state of affairs; psychophysical responses are an end product of neural-data processing and are only indirectly related to neural-discharge measures.

In many cases no psychophysical data exist for a sensory system simply because relatively little of the activity of a sensory system is accessible to the "consciousness" of a behaving organism. For example, the vestibular system has an extremely complex set of receptor end organs innervated by 10-20,000 fibers; and yet what does an organism know about the functioning of this system other than an awareness of where its head is (i.e., in the traditional sense)? The carotid body monitors the chemistry of the blood, and there are sensory systems in the lungs, stomach, liver, and intestines; yet there exists little in the way of psychophysics for these systems. It has been said that the innervation of the anal exit of the digestive tract is as massive as that of the oral cavity, and yet there exists no anal psychophysics to speak of. The activities of many of these sensory systems are not even indirectly accessible to psychophysical experimentation. Yet, they are all amenable to sensory neurophysiological investigation.

THE SELECTION OF AN EXPERIMENTAL ANIMAL

Much thought must be given to the selection of the species of animal employed for sensory neurophysiological research, for each species is unique in some ways. The types of sensory systems an animal has depend to a great extent upon the kind of animal it is and the particular mode of life for which it is adapted. Although the various types of sensory systems are related to the evolutionary scale of development of the animal, the structure and function of different sensory systems cannot always be predicted from a knowledge of the family or even genus under which a species is subsumed. The cat has a vibrissalike sensory system on the back of its forelegs known as the carpal hairs, but the tiger, another member of the *Felidae,* does not. There are even differences between species that appear in sensory systems one might expect to be highly similar; e.g., there are anatomical differences in the types of joint receptors among closely related species. Differences in the arrangement of receptors in the vestibular organs can also occur. If distinctions between species in peripheral sensory systems exist, central nervous-system differences will surely follow; the structure of central sensory mechanisms is dependent upon the structure of peripheral sensory mechanisms.

The selection of an animal for study is, therefore, a serious problem. As we shall see, the elucidation of either the anatomical structure of a sensory system or the neurophysiological analysis of function requires the labors of many workers over an extended period of time. We would even go so far as to say that the first year or two of an anatomical or neurophysiological investigation should be devoted to the perfection of techniques and the formulation of the problems. In most cases, it is not clear just what the relevant variables to measure are, and a long period of development time may elapse before the investigators can ask pertinent questions. The researchers who have enlightened us most about the structure and function of sensory systems are those who have painstakingly isolated some of the major sources of variability and have quantitatively described the elements of the system. An investigator who bounces around from one nerve or nucleus to another every six months or year is certain to discover little about any of them.

Because of the immense labors involved, the proper choice of animals is crucial. Extensive neuroanatomical studies are most profitably undertaken when there is a promise that extensive neurophysiological studies will also be undertaken on the same structures. Anatomical studies frequently include the subdivision of cells into groups on the basis of subtle anatomical distinctions. The validation of these subdivisions can be established with neurophysiological techniques. Similarly, extensive neurophysiological investigations require an anatomical interpretive substrate. Electrical recordings from an exotic animal are meaningless if no neuroanatomy exists on the animal. Properly, extensive anatomical and neurophysiological studies should be conducted on the same species. The species chosen should be one receiving intensive investigations on other sensory systems, since different types of information from separate peripheral sensory systems may be fed into the same group of centrally located neurons with the responsibility for the simultaneous processing of the two different types of sensory inputs. Thus, if the anatomy and neurophysiology of the different peripheral sensory systems have been worked out on different animals, the studies must all be repeated for the same animal. Conservation of research effort demands that one or more animals be designated the official animals of sensory neurophysiology.

Because of the complexity of the mammalian nervous system, some investigators have suggested that simpler nervous systems, such as those of invertebrates, should be studied first since there are fewer elements in these nervous systems. The difficulty with this selection is that the nerve cells composing invertebrate nervous systems are dissimilar from those of mammalian nervous systems; thus, one ends up studying maybe a simpler nervous system but certainly a different nervous system. And whereas one tends to generalize to a certain degree from one mammal to another or from one vertebrate to another, partly on the basis of similarity of structural units, it is rarely possible to generalize from vertebrates to invertebrates, since there are few if any structural comparisons. There is the additional difficulty that, as the invertebrate sensory systems are so anatomically dissimilar from mammalian systems, one is not able to utilize the substantial accumulation of psychophysical and behavioral information available on vertebrates. Thus, it is not known what the function of the well-studied Limulus eye is; it is not even known whether it is used for form perception. Suppose the eye of an invertebrate is used to regulate molting or seasonal migration or something similar. What type of information would it then extract from the light world?

In many respects the best candidate for a standard sensory neurophysiological animal would be the human. The structure and function of the human nervous system is naturally of prime concern to us. By using the human, one can also directly utilize much of the psychophysical and clinical neurological findings that have accrued on this species. In addition, more is known about the neuroanatomy of the human sensory systems than that of any other animal, save perhaps the cat's. Indeed, some experiments in sensory neurophysiology have been performed on humans. Whole nerve recordings have been taken from the aforementioned chorda tympani, the nerve that innervates the taste buds on the fungiform papillae of the tongue (Borg et al, 1967). Electrical recordings have also been taken from single fibers innervating the skin (Hensel and Boman, 1960). In most cases, however, the neural structures supplying sensory systems are inaccessible to superficial surgery. In addition, the present state of development of most sensory research is too crude to even specify the types of questions to ask, let alone understand the neural answer. Also much information is required to describe the structure of sensory systems, information that can be obtained only by sacrificing the animal in a preordained manner, often after surgically interrupting a part of the nervous system. At the present time, human sensory systems can be studied only piecemeal or indirectly.

The prime candidate for an official sensory neurophysiological animal is the cat. Actually, the cat has long been the standard animal used in the study of the neuroanatomy of peripheral and central sensory structures. Cat brains are fairly uniform with respect to neural structures and vary little in size. Much of the detailed quantitative neuroanatomical work required to unravel the anatomical complexity of the sensory systems has already been performed on cats. More is known about the anatomy of cat sensory systems—e.g., the skin, joint, muscle, and auditory senses — than those of any other animal. The neurophysiologists have not been laggard in the study of cat sensory systems. Most of the neurophysiological work in audition, skin, muscle, joint, and some chemical senses has been performed on cats. No other animal has been studied in such detailed fashion. Rodents have been but cursorily studied and dogs not at all. The studies on primates are scattered about on a half-dozen species. Sensory neurophysiology as it is today is largely cat sensory neurophysiology.

We have made it a policy to utilize anatomical and neurophysiological material derived from the cat wherever available. Examples from other animals are used only when material on the cat is not available and when the structural relationships between cat sensory systems and other animals do not seem to invalidate the comparison. In some cases, we also summarize briefly work on other animals and compare structures.

Sensory neurophysiology is the study of the functioning of the parts of an animal. The sensory systems of the cat are designed to assist the cat in his day-to-day activities. The accumulation of knowledge of sensory systems apart from a familiarity with the animal possessing them is a futile occupation. We have, therefore, included an extensive chapter on the behavior of the cat and his place in the world of living organisms. Although we must dissect the cat to study his sensory systems, we must in the end put him together again as a living, functioning entity.

2

THE CAT
FELIS CATUS

INTRODUCTION

As we mentioned before, sensory systems cannot be discussed independently of the type of animal they invest. Each species of animal inhabits a particular environmental niche and its sensory systems may be specially designed to function within its own unique surroundings. Any species of animal has certain properties that we can to a certain extent predict if we know that the animal is a vertebrate, a mammal or, say, a primate; but any particular sensory system may be specifically redesigned for that species, and thus the sensory system may in many respects be peculiar to that species.

The animal about which we know the most, both neuroanatomically and neurophysiologically, is the cat. In many anatomical and physiological aspects, the cat is representative of the other *Felidae*, other mammals, and other vertebrates, but he has a number of characteristics peculiar to himself. Only by a thorough understanding of the structure and function of the cat can we evaluate and compare these features.

A single living organism undergoes various changes during its development from a single cell to birth, to adulthood, and to senescence. The organism in these various developmental stages possesses different structures, different whole-organism properties, and different physiological functions. The embryological development of the cat has been described by Hill and Tribe (1924); and the fetal behavior of the cat by Langworthy (1929) and Coronios (1933). In our description of the various structures and functions of the cat, we will focus on the fully developed or the almost fully developed cat, although some of the anatomical studies were performed on kittens.

THE CAT, FELIS CATUS

Cats are small carnivores of the family *Felidae*, and the most numerous members of any of the species of this family. This ubiquitous occurrence is

11

due to both the generalized carnivoral habits of small *Felidae* and to their close association with their host primate species, man. Although only one species of cat, *Felis catus*, is generally recognized, cats occur in the widest varieties of any recognized species of *Felidae*. Some individual cats resemble distinct wild species more than they may some other strains of cats (Fig. 2-1, see color insert). This marked variation in cat appearance is due to both the diverse origins of the cat and the selective pressure from humans who prefer variety in the appearance of their domestic animals. The cat is also capable of interbreeding with many of the other small species of *Felidae* and producing viable offspring.

There are several different varieties or breeds of cats (Simpson, 1903), breeds maintained by selective-breeding pressures exerted by humans. The Siamese, Persian, Manx, and Abyssinian are among the recognized breeds of cats. Most cats, however, come from a common breeding pool to which these recognized breeds also contribute. They are known as mixed breeds or alley cats and, unlike wild species of *Felidae*, are endowed with a wide variety of colors and patterns. There are two varieties of the common tabby cat, blotched and striped; the latter resembles patterns found in wildcats (Pocock, 1907). There are black cats, black-and-white cats, white cats, yellow cats, and tortoise-shell or calico cats, which are almost always female cats (Robinson, 1971). These are just the more common types of cats known to us; many other varieties can be described. These cats are the same in most respects since all of them exhibit cat species behaviors and possess similar anatomical structures. Some of the breeds have distinctive anatomical and behavioral features that set them off from other cats, however. The Siamese cats, for example, have blue eyes and sleek, dense, and distinctively marked coats, and are typically nosier and more aggressive than the run-of-the-mill cat. Although current measurements seem to indicate that there is a great deal of uniformity among cats in the anatomy and physiology of their sense organs, the genetic diversity among different strains could be an influential factor in the outcome of any investigation.

The cat is referred to as a domestic animal and often by the name *Felis domesticus*. As a domesticated animal, the cat is frequently equated with others of that type, such as pigs, goats, and chickens. As Darwin remarked in 1896, however, "The cat lives a freer life than other domestic animals." Although the cat is actively promoted as a pet object and as a companion to man, cats readily revert in part or wholly to an outdoor life with other cats and other animals. Anyone familiar with a fair number of relationships between cats and humans knows of many cases in which the cat associates but little with the people who feed it. Most adult uncastrated tomcats, given the opportunity and the proper environment, will spend most of their time away from the human dwelling, scarcely bothering with those who raised him. An adult tom will often drop by only for food or to rest up from his nocturnal activities. In this sense the cat is using the human as a stable (and often not sole) source of food and the house as a warm, safe den. Many, if not all, of the present-day breeds of cats possess all the skills of their wild ancestors and will, if need be, ply their ancestral craft. Forced to it, cats can adapt to life in the wild, where they become known as feral cats.

The cat lives to a great extent under the control of man and as such is subject to selective pressure in much the same way that an environmental condition on earth selects certain individuals most amenable to the prevailing conditions. Man changes domestic animals according to his desires. Thus, turkeys are bred to produce dry, tasteless breast meat and cattle are bred to produce tender, tasteless steaks. In the process of an animal's transformation into end products for human utilization some of its anatomical and physiological systems may change from those that were valuable in the normal wild state it enjoyed before association with man. It is therefore necessary to ask to what degree the cat may differ from those in the wild. Our occasional comparison of cats and other members of the *Felidae* (as well as other mammals) can be invalidated by the changes induced by the domestication process. This question has been examined in some detail by Zeuner (1963) who thinks that there may be some change toward shorter jaws, and by Pocock (1907) who finds that colorations include coat patterns other than those found in the wild. The general conclusion of these and other investigators — and indeed, anyone who has seriously considered the problem — is that most cats could fend for themselves in the wild, given suitable game and the proper experience during their first year or so of life. That many do is evidenced by the many feral cats that exist throughout the world. In terms of the species behaviors described in this chapter, all cats are cats.

Despite human pressures for genetic diversity and genetic diversity introduced by the proclivity of cats to interbreed with other small species of wild *Felidae*, the breeds of cats are far less variable than the existing breeds of dogs, another domesticated carnivore. The major differences among cats are in body-hair color, hair length, and hair patterning, although the Manx cat is tailless. Cats are generally of the same shape, size, form, and behavior. Male cats or tomcats weigh 8 to 15 lbs. when adult, and measure about two and one half to three feet from nose to tail. Female cats tend to be smaller and daintier and average 6 to 10 lbs. in weight. Under domestication, cats will breed two to four times a year, producing litters of two to six kittens. Cats manifest a variety of behaviors, which we will examine in greater detail later in this chapter.

THE *FELIDAE*

As we mentioned before, the cat is classified in the family *Felidae* within the order *Carnivora*. Altogether there are about 36 species of *Felidae* (Pocock,

1917; 1951; Denis, 1964; Walker, 1964). The animals considered to be of that family are usually fairly standard, although occasionally the Madagascan fossa, *Cryptoprocta ferox*, is classified as a member (most recently by Thenius, 1967). Pocock (1951) considers it a heresy to so classify the Madagascan fossa because, except for tooth structure, the fossa is quite "uncatlike" with respect to various structural features of the head, feet, anus, and genitalia. Of the existing *Felidae* the cheetah with its distinctive features is usually put into a separate genus, *Acinonyx jubatus*. The larger species of *Felidae* are usually placed in the genus *Panthera* (also sometimes called *Leo*) and include the lion, *Panthera leo*; the tiger, *Panthera tigris*, the leopard, *Panthera pardus*; and the jaguar, *Panthera onca*. All of the small *Felidae*, including the cat, are usually placed within the genus *Felis*. Some of the members of the genus *Felis* are the European wildcat, *Felis sylvestris*; the jungle cat, *Felis chaus*; the caracal, *Felis caracal*; the lynx, *Felis lynx*; the

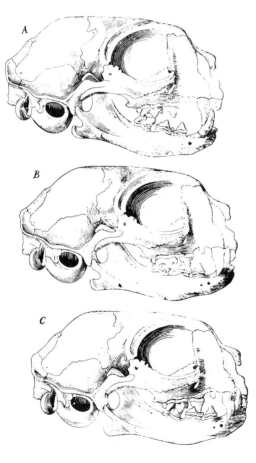

Fig. 2-2. Cat. Skull of the cat. The large front side teeth, the canines, are used for killing; the specialized back teeth, the carnassials, are used to slice up the carcass. A, jaws opened; B, jaws almost closed; C, jaws closed. (Jayne, 1898)

bobcat, *Felis rufus;* the serval, *Felis serval;* the ocelot, *Felis pardalis;* the jaguarundi, *Felis yagouarundi;* and the large puma, *Felis concolor.*

There exist numerous disagreements about the number of genera and which *Felidae* to classify where. Linnaeus put all *Felidae* within a single genus called *Felis.* Indeed, an inspection of most of the species of *Felidae* reveals more similarities than differences. They seem to vary primarily in size; most of the species has much the same body build and behaviors. All of the *Felidae* have distinctive teeth, one of the primary characteristics use to classify animals. The types of teeth that an animal has indicate to a great extent the kind of animal it is.

The teeth of the cat can be seen in Fig. 2-2. This characteristic tooth pattern of the *Felidae* demonstrates the total dependence of these animals on the carnivorous way of life for survival. The side teeth, the large and sharply pointed canines, are used like daggers to kill their prey. The *Felidae* do not have teeth for cutting off vegetation or grinding food, nor can they move their jaws laterally. Their premolar and molar teeth have developed into specialized shearing teeth known as carnassials. With these, the *Felidae* slice pieces of meat off the prey. The small incisor teeth in the front of the mouth are used for grooming.

All of the *Felidae*, except the cheetah, are characterized by retractable claws (Fig. 2-3). When the animal is walking, the claws are withdrawn. By these means the *Felidae* can preserve their surgically sharp points until they require them. The cheetah makes use of its running ability to a greater extent than the other *Felidae* in pursuit of its prey. The cheetah, the fastest land animal alive, has been clocked at over sixty m.p.h.

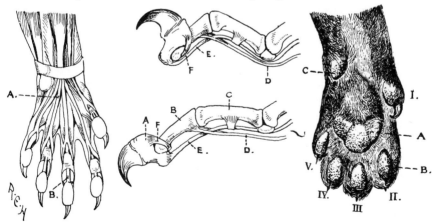

Fig. 2-3. Cat. Left: Superficial flexor tendons of the cat's left forefoot. A, perforatus or flexor subdigitorum; B, perforans or flexor profundus digitorum. Center: Bones and principal ligaments of a cat's toe, showing mechanism of retractile claw. A, distal or terminal phalanx; B, middle; C. proximal; D, perforatus tendon; E, perforans tendon; F, elastic ligament. Right: Pads of left forefoot. A, plantar pad; B, digital pad; C, pisiform pad. (Simpson, 1903)

The classification of animals as *Felidae* is based primarily upon bone and tooth structure (Pocock, 1917). Divisions within the *Felidae* are also based on anatomical features. Thus, the lion and the tiger are put into the genus *Panthera* primarily on the basis of the hyoid bone structure of the larynx. On the basis of other characteristics, however, the lion and the tiger might be classified separately. The behavior of the tiger is, in most ways, more like the cat's than the lion's. The lion is the only social species; i.e., the only one with a social organization — a pride. Presumably because of his social orientation, the lion has a marked visual sex distinction and many behavioral habits unlike those of the other *Felidae* (Guggisberg, 1962). Consequently, classification by bone structure can be misleading. It is, however, the only means by which existent species can be compared to extinct species.

The life styles of most of the species of *Felidae* are quite similar, at least as far as is known. Most of the species lead solitary lives, hunting alone and often over large territories. The hunting behaviors of all of the *Felidae*, including the cheetah, are quite similar. The prey is approached stealthily and captured with a final quick lunge or attacked from ambush. The food of the *Felidae*, unlike that of herbivores, is not usually available in large quantities, but consists of other animals who have survived in part because of their abilities to elude the *Felidae*. To obtain regular sustenance, the *Felidae* must rely on stealth, patience, and athletic abilities. Life in the wild is undoubtedly a risky existence for the species.

Members of the Felidae are widely distributed throughout the world except in the polar regions, Australia, and some islands. The largest varieties of *Felidae* (twenty-one species) are found in Asia. Some species of *Felidae* are scattered over extremely wide geographical ranges. The range of the puma, for instance, extends from Canada to the southern tip of South America; and that of the leopard extends from the southern portion of Africa to northern Asia. Others, such as the black-footed cat *(Felis negripes)*, the sand cat *(Felis margarita)*, the Pampas cat *(Felis colocolo)*, and the snow leopard *(Panthera uncia)* have quite limited distributions (Ronnefeld, 1969; Boorer, 1970). The existence of many species of *Felidae* is being threatened by the activities of humans who have reduced the number of animals upon which the *Felidae* prey. In addition, the predilection of humans for the skins of the *Felidae* has put some of the more sparsely distributed species on the list of animals threatened with extinction (Sitwell, 1970). Only the cat, *Felis catus*, has benefited by the proliferation of the species *Homo sapiens*.

The *Felidae* are members of the fissiped (cleft-footed) carnivores, as distinguished from the pinniped (fin-footed) carnivores such as walruses, seals, and sea lions. Other members of the fissiped carnivores are hyenas, genets, weasels, dogs, bears, and raccoons (Fig. 2-4). The fissiped carnivores and the pinniped carnivores are believed to have developed from early mammals known as creodonts, especially the miacid group.

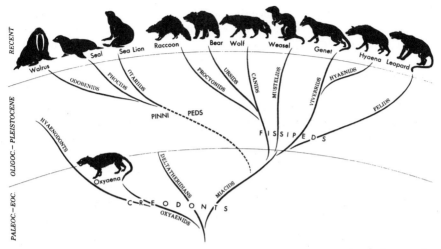

Fig. 2-4. The evolution and relationship of the major groups of carnivorous placental mammals. From *Evolution of the Vertebrates* by E.H. Colbert. Illustrated by Lois Darling.

PALEONTOLOGY OF THE *FELIDAE*

The existent species of animals classified as *Felidae* represent but a small number of the many types of *Felidae* that have inhabited the earth in the past. The science of paleontology studies the fossil remains of dead animals. The fossils studied are, in most cases, bones — particularly skulls and teeth — although other fossil remains are available; footprints and other imprints, and sometimes even whole animals have been preserved in amber or in ice. By comparing the bones of fossils with those of existent species, it is often possible to obtain a historical record of development and evolutionary changes in the past. The more complete the fossil record, the more precisely the historical record of the development of a species can be reconstructed. The greater the abundance of the animals in the past, the more likely and the more numerous are their fossil remains. Thus, the paleontological record of some herbivores is quite complete (Romer, 1966; Colbert, 1969).

Members of the *Felidae*, because they are in general solitary hunters and flesh-eating creatures, are usually sparsely distributed. There exist some large accumulations of fossil remains of the *Felidae*, however, notably the La Brea tar-pit dig (Merriam and Stock, 1932) where about 35 percent of the large animal bones (mostly saber tooths) are the remains of members of the *Felidae*.

Fossil remains of small wild *Felidae* have been discovered in a fair number of digs of Pleistocene age. These remains have been referred to wild species of *Felidae* such as *Felis sylvestris*, *Felis ocreata*, or *Felis manul*; although apparently one cannot distinguish between these species (or *Felis catus*) on the basis of bone structure (Pocock, 1907; Zeuner, 1950; 1963). As a result, the earliest representatives of the cat, *Felis catus*, are established on the basis of archeological finds. The history of the cat is inextricably bound up with that of man; such historical remnants as footprints in tile and pictorial representations are used to establish the cat's existence (Zeuner, 1963).

The further back in time the fossils are, the more unlike modern *Felidae* they are. As we have seen, the most common feature we use to distinguish the modern *Felidae* is the shape and size of the teeth. The earliest skull with features characteristic of modern Felidae dates back to the early Pliocene period (about ten million years ago).

Paleontological studies have shown that animals with skulls similar to that of the modern *Felidae* were widespread throughout both hemispheres. Large *Felidae* of several types roamed throughout North America and Europe. Among these were the cave lion of Europe, which was much larger than any current species; and *Felis atrox*, a lion-sized species of *Felidae* that used to roam around the environs of southern California.

Contemporaries of these large *Felidae* (and of some species of *Felidae* still in existence) were *Felidae* known collectively as the Macherodonts or saber tooths. The saber tooths are sometimes referred to as the "stabbing cats" as opposed to the "biting cats" or *Felinae*. The saber-tooth *Felidae* can be characterized by tooth pattern; the upper canines are much larger than the bottom canines. All fossil skulls of the *Felidae* that existed more than about ten million years ago are classified as Macherodonts, although they are frequently separated into the saber tooths and false saber tooths, the latter possessing less well-developed upper canines (Fig. 2-5).

The saber-tooth cats were apparently heavier and slower moving than the *Felinae*. The general consensus of paleontological speculation is that they preyed upon large slowly moving prey such as mastodon and other large, thick-skinned creatures. Presumably they dispatched their victims by downward thrusts of their saberlike weapons. Matthew (1910) has shown that they were capable of opening their mouths far wider than the *Felinae* and had different muscle structures for opening the jaw. As the mastodons and other large mammals disappeared in the spectacular Pleistocene die-off (Martin and Wright, 1967), the saber tooths became extinct also, apparently unable to compete with the *Felinae* in pursuit of the modern fast-moving herbivores. Modern elephants and rhinoceroses are rarely preyed upon by modern *Felidae* (Guggisberg, 1962).

CAT BEHAVIOR

An organism can be characterized in terms of measurements taken on whole-organism activities, or by the activities of subsystems of the organism. From measurements taken on whole-organism activities, we derive proper-

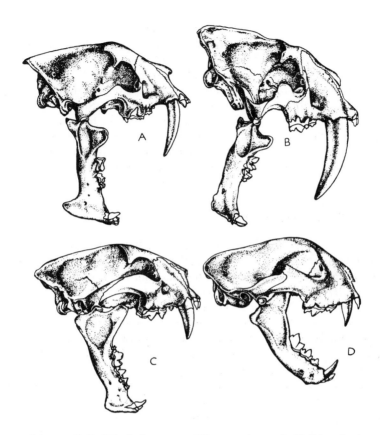

Fig. 2-5. Felidae. A: Skull of Hoplophoneus, an Oligocene saber tooth. Skull length, about 6.25 inches. B: Smilodon, a Pleistocene saber tooth. Skull length, about 12 inches. C: Dinictis, an Oligocene form with small sabers. Skull length, about 6.12 inches. D: Pseudaelurus minor, a Pliocene feline with teeth similar to those of modern members of the *Felidae*. Skull length, about 5.75 inches. (Romer, 1966. From *Vertebrate Paleontology* by A.S. Romer. Copyright © by the University of Chicago 1933, 1945, 1966)

ties that we use to describe and typify the whole animal and the species to which it belongs. These whole-organism properties, called "behaviors," involve the activities of many neural subsystems, some of which are partially described in other chapters of this book. These behaviors are important properties of the organism and are involved in the survival of the individual and the species.

Behaviors may be classified into two types, individual behaviors and species behaviors. Species behaviors tend to appear in every individual in a highly stereotyped manner. Every member of the species shows them and they tend to appear in an orderly sequence in time in accordance with the growth and maturation of the animal. Individual behaviors tend to be capricious in their appearance, difficult to classify, and subject to alterations with experience. Of the two, species behaviors are the most amenable to scientific investigations, since measurements and observations on different individuals tend to be reproducible. The performance of both individual and species behaviors involves the functioning and interaction of many sensory systems such as those we describe in this book. In addition, many neural effector systems are involved in the performance of behaviors, as well as complex central neural coordination-and-command systems. An analysis of these systems in the rigorous manner prescribed for peripheral sensory systems is not possible with the present techniques and level of understanding.

SPECIES BEHAVIORS

The cat has a number of highly characteristic behaviors that can be used to define the species. Some of these behaviors — hunting, for example — require a vast assembly of individual skills, plus extensive experience in the field. Others, such as excretory behavior and scent marking come close to the stereotyped behaviors described by ethologists for fish and birds. Many of the behaviors of the cat are shared with other members of the family *Felidae*, although our knowledge of the behaviors of most of the existent species of *Felidae* is fragmentary. The description of cat behaviors we include here is based upon reports in the literature (e. g., Ewer, 1968; Lessing, 1967; Wilson and Weston, 1946) and close personal observations over the last four years. During this time we shared living quarters with a colony of cats in an urban environment in a manner similar to the habit of humans and cats throughout history. This colony of cats varied in size from one male to several adults and many kittens. It almost always included one adult tomcat and one breeding female. The cats were allowed free access to the outside world through a window opening into an alley. The colony included five generations of permanent members as well as an occasional stray tomcat seeking shelter, food, or female companionship. Although this human-and-cat living arrangement is not without its drawbacks, it permits long-term observations on a freely ranging group of cats.

Unlike most animals, the cat can inhabit two quite distinct environments. In one, they are widely dispersed and probably spend most of their time in solitary hunting; in the other, they dwell with humans and spend most of their time either sleeping or on social activities that would probably occupy only a small proportion of their time in the wild. The behaviors we describe here are those that would occur in both wild strains of cats (feral cats) and domesticated cats; although it is possible that some of the details would differ in the two environments.

EXCRETORY BEHAVIOR

The behavior of the cat during the elimination of bodily wastes is highly characteristic of the species. The general procedure is as follows: Faced with the necessity of defecating or urinating, the cat will search out suitable latrine facilities at a distance from his usual sleeping quarters. He first digs a hole in the dirt with his front feet. He then positions himself over the hole and defecates or urinates in the hole by positioning his hind quarters above the hole. He then covers the excrement by scraping dirt over it with his front feet.

This complicated series of behavior appears right after the kitten begins to walk. It is apparently elicited by the texture of the ground on which the animal is walking. Kittens will not show this behavior on hard floors but will go into the excretory behavior sequence if placed in a box of dirt or sand. Snow will also elicit excretory behavior.

SCENTS AND SCENT-MARKING BEHAVIOR

Like most mammals, cats are equipped with special glands that produce odorous substances used by members of the species to communicate with one another. Scents are often deposited on surfaces such as trees, bushes, houses, etc. The act of depositing scent is known as scent marking. The roles of these scents in the activities of the animal are not well understood (Mykytowycz, 1970; Ralls, 1971), but they seem important in distinguishing individuals, the sex and sexual receptivity of the individual, and in delineating territory.

Cats seem to have at least three different sources of scents. One of these is located near the anus and is associated with a special gland. The scent from this gland is apparently deposited with feces. A second source of scent is either saliva or a specialized scent gland in the mouth. Cats mark with this scent by spreading their lips and rubbing their gums against head-high objects. This scent-marking behavior is known as "chinning." The third source of cat scents is the genitals. The genital scent is deposited with urine or a special fluid. Here the female behavior differs from the male. Apparently female cats only mark with this scent when they are sexually receptive. However it is done, the odor, though imperceptible to humans, can entice all the male cats in the neighborhood, even though the female cat is not allowed outside the house. Tomcats will routinely mark with scent trees, walls, shrubs, buildings, cars, and in fact any large stationary object with a particularly odorous and adhesive fluid. This marking is accomplished by the tomcat pointing his hind quarters in the direction of the surface to be marked and, with his tail held high, emitting a jet of viscous fluid from his penis (Ewer, 1968) that adheres to the surface. The tail is vibrated during the ejection procedure. *Other Felidae* such as lions, tigers, pumas, and bobcats spray also. Scent marking is apparently part of the territorial behavior in *Felidae* (Hornocker, 1969). In our experience it is also associated with mating behavior in the cat. A female cat in heat will induce indiscriminate spraying from male cats. A house with an estrous female can often be detected half a block away. Female cats will also act out the male spraying behavior during estrus and at other times but will not usually eject any fluid. Cats smelling the spray will adopt a dopey-eyed expression with their mouths hanging open and the upper lip curled. This characteristic behavior is known as flehmen and is thought to facilitate access of the odor to the vomeronasal organ (Ewer, 1968).

The cat may utilize these scents in a different manner from that of other species of animals. Anyone who has observed cats for an extended period of time realizes that cats cannot readily identify one another by sight. If a new cat comes into view, the other cats are often alarmed and do not calm down until the new cat is thoroughly sniffed over. This sniffing behavior is focused on two areas: the mouth and the anus. A cat's behavior toward another cat is based more upon the smell of the other cat than on his appearance.

PLAY

Many animals engage in activities that have been termed "play." In the young animal, these activities are engaged in for their own intrinsic benefits, but in adult animals these behaviors or modifications of them may become associated with various adult behaviors. Cats engage in play activities of obvious relevance to mature behaviors. Because of the close relationship between most of the cat's play behavior and his hunting behavior, we have designated this play behavior as "kill play." Kill play is actually a complex of games that we have subdivided into three games — mouse, bird, and rabbit. These games can be played alone, with a real or imaginary object, or with another cat. They are played universally by all young cats and by many active adult cats. Adult females seem to engage in them more than adult toms, who often tend to get involved with sexual and social activities. The cat will engage in these behaviors by the hour and to the point of exhaustion. These games involve an assemblage of a vast complex of sensory, central, and motor neural mechanisms. They are furthermore subject to modification by experience and individual behaviors. But because of their ubiquitous occurrence and general constancy of form, they may be truly designated species behaviors.

Mouse

The game of mouse is played with a small object, usually one that is moving or capable of movement. Thus, a cat will play mouse with a feather, small

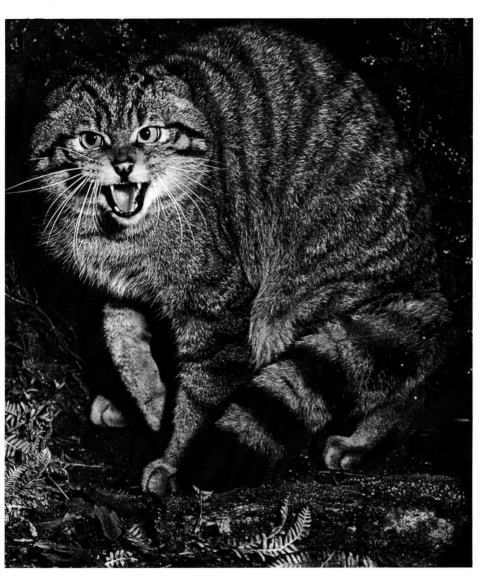

Fig. 2-1.   The European wildcat, *Felis sylvestris*. This and similar wild species of *Felidae* are believed to be the ancestors of the cat.
Reprinted with permission of Geoffrey Kinns / A. F. A. Ltd.

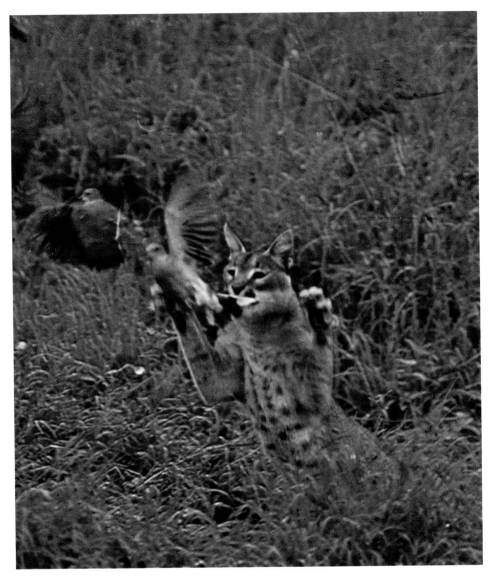

Fig. 2-6.   *Caracal, Felis caracal.* A member of the *Felidae,* utilizing some of its sensory systems. (Figure by permission of J. Dominis and Time-Life, Inc.)

ball, or some other object. Mouse is also played by a cat with his tail or another cat's tail. Mouse in most of its varieties is best observed when a human mimics in some way the part of the "mouse" by putting his hand (or a small stick) under paper or a blanket and making small twitchy movements. The cat will attack this mouse by leaping on it and securing it with its forepaws, pouncing on it, or engaging in a series of foreclaw hooking actions accompanied by an acrobatic series of body movements. Cats especially enjoy reaching under blankets or newspapers to hook the mouse with their fully extended claws. As long as there is a moving object of little danger to themselves (the mouse is not supposed to attack), most cats will play this game by the hour. Mouse is played by cats of all ages, although as toms get older, they tend to lose interest. Cats with gentle dispositions may prefer mouse to the other more boisterous games. Naturally, mouse can be played with insects or even real mice; and, no doubt, a cat would prefer it so.

Bird

Bird involves the interception of a flying object. This flying object can be the end of a string, a small furry ball attached to the end of a string, or some similar object. One of the most effective objects we have found for eliciting the game of bird from the cat is a toy bird with feathers of the type that is sold in circuses. This bird is on the end of a string, and when it is pulled through the air, the tail twirls and the bird emits a squeaky sound. To intercept the bird, the cat must invoke a number of complex acrobatic skills. The cat plays the game of bird in its simplest form by sitting on its hind quarters and engaging in a series of hooking motions with the extended claws of the forefeet. Objects are often hooked with the claws and then brought into the mouth, which then fastens onto the object. In its more complex form, the game of bird involves the cat projecting himself into the air to intercept the moving object. The object is grabbed with the front claws and drawn down toward the mouth. A cat will play bird by the hour but tires of it if the flying object is presented in the same manner all the time. It particularly enjoys intercepting flying objects that are taking off from the ground or flying from one surface to another (jumping). The game of bird can also be played with insects or real birds. Once intercepted, these living objects may or may not be killed. Once killed, they may or may not be eaten. Bird, like the other games in kill play, has intrinsic satisfaction although its relationship to the hunting behavior of the cat and of other members of the *Felidae* (Dominis and Edey, 1968) is easy to see (Fig. 2-6, see color insert).

Rabbit

Rabbit is the cat's favorite game. Kittens engage in rabbit almost constantly. Young cats play it by the hour. Even adult cats engage in rabbit. The game of rabbit requires a number of skills far more complex than those utilized in mouse or bird. In addition, rabbit entails an element of danger to the cat not found in either bird or mouse. Rabbit involves the interception and capture of a large moving object. As this large moving object is usually another cat of the same age group, we shall describe the game as such. In rabbit, one cat intercepts and mock-kills another cat. One cat will ambush another with an attack often directed toward bringing the other animal to the ground. To do so, the attacker either pins the other cat to the ground with its forelegs while it bites at the neck, or it embraces the other cat around the body and brings it down, all the while seeking the throat with its teeth. Often two cats will stalk one another or will alternate in chasing each other. There are many varieties to the game of rabbit and two or more cats will play it endlessly from the time they are kittens. Cats also like to play rabbit with cats younger or weaker than they are, thus placing the other cat in the position of being the rabbit all the time. Cats are always fairly serious about the game and often forget themselves at times, biting and scratching one another quite hard and frequently causing squabbles. Because of the risk of injury, most cats are forced to discontinue the game as they get older because no one will play with them. A cat will also play rabbit with humans if there is no suitable cat-rabbit around.

FIGHTING

Fighting is a behavior exhibited almost entirely by mature tomcats. Young cats will rarely fight. A mature female cat will usually engage in fighting only to protect her home and often only then when she has kittens or is expecting them. In a situation where a tomcat has access to an outdoors populated with other tomcats, many adult male cats will engage frequently in nocturnal battles. Young male cats and adult female cats are not singled out for attack; fighting is an occupation between two mature toms. Fighting can be to the kill. Although cats have various signs of submission (rolling over, etc.), these do not seem to be sufficient to stop an attack, and fleeing is often the only means of survival. Fighting seems to be intermixed with sexual behavior and perhaps territory rites. Some adult toms, especially large older cats, engage in fighting behavior weekly and sometimes almost nightly. As a result of these battles, many older cats have scars about their head and shoulders. Raw or festering wounds can often be seen on the heads of toms, and their ears often have large sections torn out of them. Cats castrated before puberty will not usually fight; and castrating a fully adult tom with years of fighting behind him is sometimes sufficient to eliminate this behavior.

CATNIP EATING

Although cats will sometimes eat grass and other vegetation (presumably for purgative reasons), there is one plant they consume avidly for a definitely nonpurgative purpose. This plant is catnip, *Nepeta cataria* (McElvain et al, 1941; 1942). The leaves of this plant are tremendously stimulating to members of the *Felidae*, including lions, tigers, pumas, and bobcats. House cats will eat the leaves of this plant in both fresh and dried form. An adult tomcat can consume about a tablespoonful or so a day at one or two sittings.

The cat's response to catnip depends upon the individual cat, his age, and his experience with the plant. In general, kittens and cats below the age of about one year will not consume any of the plant or will do so only occasionally. This refusal seems to be based in part on experience, since young cats will frequently consume catnip when they are first offered it but will refuse further offerings until they are older. In our experience tomcats consume more of the plant and more often than females. When being fed catnip upon demand, a tom will decide upon a catnip-feeding schedule of once or twice a day, at which time it will consume a fair quantity of the dried leaves (which it prefers dampened down with water to cut the dust).

The behavior of the cat while eating catnip or just after eating it varies with the cat. Young cats will often roll around in the leaves. This reaction to catnip is also sometimes exhibited by older cats, too, but more experienced catnip eaters often do not show this type of behavior. Usually, they just sit around quietly after eating catnip and often go to sleep; at other times, they play, eat food, or engage in other activities.

GROOMING

Cats spend a great deal of their time keeping their body in immaculate condition. Grooming develops along with other motor abilities in the kitten, first appearing when the cat is about two to three weeks old. Not only is the body fur cleaned but also the face, ears, anus, and feet. This cleansing is accomplished by the use of the tongue, the small front teeth, and some sort of detergent cleansing fluid that, unlike normal saliva, leaves the fur clean and fresh smelling. Most of the cleaning is accomplished by the use of the animal's rough tongue, which is covered with sharp filiform papilla. To clean the head, the cat covers the backs of the paws with cleaning fluid and then rubs the paw over the head. After excretory behavior and after sexual activity, the besmirched parts are licked clean, and a walk in the mud is followed by a foot cleansing. Upon meeting, two cats will frequently groom one another's fur, usually the head, ears, and the anus, which is also smelled. If a mother cat does not groom her kittens, they will not survive.

CLAW SHARPENING

An examination of the claws of the cat reveals that the claws of the front feet are extremely sharp and dangerous ripping weapons. The claws on the hind feet, although still of formidable appearance, are quite a bit duller and often have the points broken off. The cat keeps the claws on the front feet in surgical condition by retracting them into the cutaneous covering during walking (the claws in the hind feet are frequently extruded during movements that involve leaping from one surface to another), and by a process of claw sharpening. Claw sharpening is accomplished by sinking the fore claws into a tree or some other stiff but penetrable suface and exerting force on the claws with a stretching motion (frequently after napping). This procedure removes an outer covering from the claw such as would a pencil sharpener (Wynne-Edwards, 1962).

SEX BEHAVIOR

The female cat's sex behavior is known as estrus and can be induced hormonally (Colby, 1970), but she will normally go into estrus two to four times a year. This high frequency of estrus is undoubtedly an adaptation of the cat to domestication, since in the wild the young must stay with the female cat until they have achieved some degree of self-sufficiency. Female cheetahs and lions in the wild apparently only go into estrus every year and a half to two years (Adamson, 1960; 1961; 1969; Guggisberg, 1962). It is possible that under wild conditions cats would not go into heat more often than once a year, as the arrival of a new litter will cause the female to reject her previous litter. Cats under a year in age would be unlikely to survive without their mother in a wild environment. In the wild, the initial period of separation from the mother is undoubtedly a traumatic experience and is doubtless a time of great mortality for the less able members of a litter.

At the age of about ten months, the female cat will go into an estrus that lasts two to five days, providing conception occurs (Manolson, 1970; Michael, 1961). During estrus the female cat will spend most of her time engaging in sexual activity, scarcely stopping to eat or sleep. A day or two prior to the actual estrous behavior, tomcats will begin to converge on the dwelling of the estrous female, apparently lured there by an odor in the urine of the female. When the female is in estrus, she will mate every twenty minutes to an hour. More than one tomcat is accepted. We have seen an estrous female refuse the attentions of one tom with whom she has already mated and then present herself to another tom. Sometimes a female mating with one tom will be surrounded by a circle of others waiting their turn. The more aggressive toms will usually scare off the younger male cats, although if the latter wait around long enough, their opportunity for mating will sometimes arise.

The estrous behavior of the female cat is quite stereotyped. She will actively search out male cats; even timid female cats who before estrus studiously avoided the presence of other cats will do so. The female cat presents herself to the male by adapting a low crouched position and

Table 2-1. Synchronization of Male and Female Courtship, Copulation and Postcopulatory Reactions (Rosenblatt, 1965)

Time	Male	Female
	COURTSHIP	
10 seconds to 5 minutes	orients toward	crouches
	trails	rubs nose and mouth
	sniffs genitalia	rolls
	circles	vocalizes
	runs toward	treads
	COPULATION	
1 to 3 minutes	takes neck grip	stands
	mounts with front legs	crouches
	at angle to female	
	mounts with hind legs;	
	places himself above	
	and parallel to female	
	rubs with forepaws	treads
	steps	
	penile erection	
	arches back	
	pelvic thrusts	swings tail to one side
	pelvic lunge	vaginal dilation
5 to 10 seconds	intromission	copulatory cry
	ejaculation	pulls forward
	penis withdrawn	turns on male
	POSTCOPULATORY REACTIONS	
♂ less than 1 minute	licks penis and forepaws	licks genitalia
	sits near female	rolls
		rubs nose and mouth
		licks paws
♀ about 5 minutes		watches male
		paws male

frequently will call to the tom. She keeps her body quite low, elevates her hind quarters, and displaces her tail to the side to allow access to her genitals. The tomcat positions himself over her body and grabs the skin at the back of her neck with his teeth. The tomat and the female both engage in a series of in-place leg movements (treading) accompanied by a continuous series of howls. The male cat effects intromission by a series of pelvic movements. Actual ejaculation is greeted by a series of screeches from both partners and is followed by abrupt disengagement, often with the female hissing and spitting and scratching at the tom. Following disengagement, the female engages in a series of rolling motions in which she may roll over and over; the period is often referred to as the "after reaction." During the rolling movements the tomcat watches her or cleans his genitals. Ovulation in the cat apparently occurs during the intromission of the penis, which is covered with a series of rough protuberances (Chapter 9), into the vagina (Longley, 1910). Rosenblatt and Aronson (1958) have broken premating behavior (terming it courtship) and mating behavior into a series of actions (Table 2-1).

The period of heat is as hard for a male cat as the female's is for her and is termed male rutting behavior. During rut the behavior of the tomcat is as dominated by the sex act as is that of the female cat. Tomcats will often go for days without food or sleep and during this time will attempt to be the constant companion of the estrous female. He will constantly be in her attendance and will call for her if she slips away. During rut, the tom will often behave quite abnormally and will even spray humans. In addition, at this time he will often engage in bloody battles with other tomcats. The performance of the sex behaviors of both male and female cats can best be typified as the enactment of a ritual compulsory performance.

KITTEN REARING

An adult female cat will spend practically all of her time rearing kittens. Following estrous behavior, approximately sixty-two days (Schneirla et al, 1963; Manolson, 1970) elapse before the delivery of the young. The delivery of the young occurs in some sheltered place or den that the female has selected during her pregnancy; a hidden corner or box is usually preferred. Like all the other *Felidae*, cats do not form breeding pairs; rather, the female cat does all the rearing by herself. Two to six kittens are usually born although there may be as many as eight (Hall and Pierce, 1934). The kittens are usually born one after another over a period of an hour or two. As each kitten arrives, the female licks it clean of membranes.

The rearing of kittens is a complex of integrated behaviors on the part of the mother cat. Over a period of several months the mother must feed, clean, protect, and otherwise care for the young from infancy to adulthood. Scott (1968) reports that in captivity cats lose weight while lactating, even with the best of diets. In the wild a female cat must also train the young cats in the arts of hunting. The magnitude of the tasks of kitten rearing in the wild can be partially appreciated by the accounts of Adamson, who introduced a tame female lion and a female cheetah to life in the wild (Adamson, 1961; 1963; 1969).

Kittens are born blind with their eyelids closed. They spend most of the first few weeks of life sleeping or nursing. At first the female cat will initiate nursing by calling her kittens, licking them, and then presenting her nipples to them. The kittens locate the nipples (six to eight per female) by nuzzling the mother's body with their snouts. Having found a nipple, a kitten proceeds to suckle vigorously. During nursing both the mother and her kittens purr and the kittens knead the mother with their front paws. This purring and kneading behavior continues over into adult life. Many adult cats of both sexes can be observed to knead soft or furry objects while they purr. Frequently cats will bite buttons or other objects, and knead and purr while they are being petted. As the kittens get older, they will often initiate nursing. The amount of time the female cat spends nursing depends upon the age of the kittens and the size of the litter (Schneirla et al, 1963).

While the kittens are being nursed or just after feeding, the female cat will groom them and ingest their waste products. Urination and defecation are apparently initiated in kittens by the mother licking the anus and genitals. During this cleaning procedure, the kitten lies on its back with its legs wide apart. The consumption of the kittens' waste products by the mother keeps the living quarters clean.

HUNTING

To survive in the wild, a cat must be quicker and more agile than the small animals upon which it feeds. The cat requires large quantities of proteinaceous food and must therefore be consistently more capable of killing than the other animals are of escaping being killed. Successful hunting requires a vast assemblage of skills (such as those described in play behavior) and a long period of experience.

The methods of hunting used by all Felidae are apparently much the same. In obtaining prey on the ground, the cat locates it by scent, sight, and sound, and stealthily approaches it by crawling, slinking, and making use of every bit of cover. When within leaping distance, the cat makes a final dash or leap, the prey is grabbed by the claws, and the death blow is delivered to the neck by the teeth. In approaching the prey, the cat brings into play its remarkably supple body and its capacity to move in discontinuous motions and then freeze in any position for long periods of time. Alternatively, the cat will lie in wait for an animal to unwarily pass by its camouflaged position. The cat is one of the few land animals able to climb trees. Most Felidae, even some of the larger ones, are adept at climbing trees to obtain birds and other animal inhabitants.

There are reports (Forbush, 1916) of feral cats killing rabbits and chickens. Probably nothing under 10 to 20 pounds, especially if young, is safe from the cat's depredations. One need only feed a large active tom or a lactating female to realize that a large amount of material is required to satisfy a cat's natural appetite, an appetite that does not result in obesity. The largest part of a feral cat's diet is composed of rodents and small rabbits; birds are taken when available. Cats are capable of leaping six feet straight up from a crouching position; many birds are slow in getting under way and may therefore be caught in mid-air. Further aspects of this subject are discussed under Eating Behavior.

EATING BEHAVIOR

The cat is totally committed to the carnivorous way of life (Scott, 1968). Not only are the cat's teeth inadequate for consuming nonanimal materials, but it cannot digest most uncooked carbohydrates and sugars may cause diarrhea. The cat is unable to utilize Vitamin A in the form of carotene but relies instead on fat-soluble forms found in the bodies of other animals. At least one third of the dry weight of a cat's diet must be in the form of animal protein. Scott (1968) has prepared a table illustrating the meat requirements of the cat and other members of the *Felidae* (Table 2-2). Meat alone is an inadequate diet, however, and must be supplemented with vitamins and minerals.

Cats have two types of diet, the one that they would obtain in the wild and the other that they obtain as the result of domestication. The diet of the wild has been explored by examining the contents of the stomachs of feral cats (usually cats killed by cars). Several stomach-content studies have been conducted in different parts of the United States (Eberhard, 1954). The cat devours about anything that moves, although small rodents and rabbits predominate in the diet. Lizards form a fair part of the diet of Oklahoma cats (McMurray and Sperry, 1941) at certain times of the year. Insects are also occasionally taken. Birds are usually but a small part of a feral cat's diet, no doubt because of their small size and the difficulty in capturing them. In a study on California cats though, Hubbs (1951) found that 25.2 percent of the volume of the stomach contents were birds, principally adult female pheasants and ducks. Under the proper conditions, cats will catch and eat frogs, salamanders, toads, snakes, and fish (Forbush, 1916).

Table 2-2. Meat requirements of Some Species of Felidae Based on Four Weeks Observation of Food Intake (Scott, 1968)

Species	Meat required per week (lb./stone° body wt.)	Average body wt. (stones)
Lions (10)	1.59	23
Tigers (5)	1.9	20
Jaguar (1)	1.5	14
Puma (1)	1.6	12
Domestic cat (4) adult,	6.1	0.57
Domestic cat (3) Kittens half grown.	6.4	0.27

° 1 stone = 14 lbs.

A cat will eat a whole small animal from the head on back, slicing it into swallowable pieces like a sausage. In eating a mouse, only a bit of the tail may remain; from a bird, only a few large feathers. When eating from a large carcass, the cat will slice off protruding pieces with his carnassial teeth or first rip one end free with its canines and then use its carnassials.

Cats can frequently be seen to eat grass, no mean feat with their tooth structure. Grass is also occasionally found in the stomachs of feral cats (Eberhard, 1954) and in the stomach or feces of bobcats (Young, 1958) and pumas (Young and Goldman, 1946). Schaller (1967) reports that he found grass in much of the feces of wild tigers he examined. He thought that most of it may have been inadvertently consumed along with its normal prey, but he found that 2.3 percent of the tiger scats he examined consisted of 50 percent grass, or more. These findings suggest that small quantities of grass or similar substances may be essential for the cat.

We have offered domesticated cats a choice of a large variety of foodstuffs, including fresh animal products of many types — fish, shellfish, etc. A cat's initial selection is based upon odor; if the proffered food does not smell right, he will show no further interest in the food. If the food smells right, the cat then hits it with the front part of its tongue, which is loaded with chemoreceptors (see Chapter 12). Experience plays a part in food acceptance also. A cat, in general, will not eat foods of vegetable origin; a cat's preference for canned cat food can be predicted from the price on the can, since lower-priced cat foods have more vegetable material in them. Both raw and cooked meats are eaten, the preference depending on flavor. We find that older cats prefer raw pork liver or raw pork kidney to most other types of food. In general, the cat's preference for cooked meats and meat dishes parallels that of humans. The addition of anything of vegetable origin to meat dishes is usually not tolerated unless the sauces are spicy like chili or spaghetti sauce. A cat will attempt to cover food it does not like (i.e., low-priced canned cat food) by scraping the floor with its claws and raking imaginary debris atop the offending food.

Cats apparently have no rules as to who will eat first from a carcass or a plate of food. Which cat will eat or how many cats will eat from a plate depends upon the individual differences among the cats; it cannot be predicted on the basis of age or sex. An aggressive kitten will often drive the adult cats from a plate loaded with food because of his growls, which intimidate the others. Since cats don't know how to behave toward one another while eating from the same plate, they will often wait their turns to eat, preferring the possibility of no food to the uncertainties and anxieties of communal feeding. Similar behavior has been reported for tigers (Schaller, 1967); but lions, the social Felidae, have rigid rules concerning the protocol of the order of eating and death may be the outcome for those who disobey the rules (Guggisberg, 1962).

SLEEPING

When not engaged in the foregoing species behaviors, a cat will spend most of its time sleeping. A cat will usually sleep for one or two long periods a day and then take an occasional nap. The long sleeping periods may occur during the day or night, depending upon the social schedule of the particular cat. Apparently the sleeping behavior of the cat is similar to that of most mammals in that it can be subdivided into different stages on the basis of EEG recording and eye movements. A sleeping cat often can be observed to make rapid eye movements frequently accompanied by whisker twitches and forepaw movements. In humans, rapid eye movements have been associated with dreams.

Cats prefer sleeping on elevated surfaces such as chairs, beds, etc., and on soft, warm surfaces rather than those that are hard and cold. Cats will sleep on things that rest on other things. If a newspaper is put on a bed, the cat will often sleep on the newspaper. In our experience, a cat will sleep in different places on different days. It may sleep in one place for weeks and then start sleeping in another place. Clean bedding is preferred. One cat will frequently take another cat's sleeping place by pestering the sleeping cat until it leaves.

PETTING BEHAVIOR

Petting behavior involves a human and a cat. The human is supposed to rub the neck, head, and shoulder region with a series of gentle stroking motions. The preferred petting area is on the back and sides of the neck, the same region of the body where the mother cat grabs a kitten to pick it up and where a tomcat bites a female cat during mating. Other areas can be rubbed during petting, sometimes even the ears, which normally elicit an aversive response. During the petting procedure, the cat will frequently purr and knead with its forepaws, and often try to bite on buttons or cloth. Some cats will lie down during petting and present different parts of the body for rubbing; some will walk around; still others will get excited or drool.

CAT SOUNDS

Like other species of *Felidae* (Tembrock, 1970) cats use sounds for communicating with one another and with other animals. In the main, these sounds are highly stereotyped from cat to cat. Moelk (1944) identified in an adult female cat 16 different phonetic patterns, 13 of which were observed in other cats. These sounds fell into three classes: (1) murmurs made with the mouth closed; (2) sounds generated with the mouth initially opened and then closed; and (3) sounds produced when the mouth is held tensely open in a fixed position. Examples of the murmur pattern are purrs and greetings. The second type of sounds is exemplified by the meows used in demands, anger, and complaints. The third pattern of strained intensity is the growl, snarl, cry of pain, and spitting. Nine sounds can be identified in kittens who produce sounds on their first day. Wilson and Weston (1946) report that explosive hissing appears early in kittens. Moelk describes eight different sounds characteristic of mating and fighting. Another period of active vocalization occurs during kittening; the mother cat sounds a special come-hither murmur call that all her kittens heed immediately.

INDIVIDUAL BEHAVIORS

According to our description of species behaviors, all cats are the same. Yet, as is well known by anyone who has closely observed the activities of a large number of cats, each cat is different. Each cat has behaviors that are peculiar to this one animal and that can be used to distinguish the cat from others. These behaviors we shall call "individual behaviors." Individual behaviors are extremely difficult to typify, for they are most capricious in their appearance and frequently change or disappear with age. Individual behaviors are also strongly influenced by experience. Because of this lability and great variability, individual behaviors cannot be used to typify a species and are least amenable to scientific study.

Tentatively, individual behaviors may be broken down into specific individual behaviors and general behavioral tendencies. Thus, we can list under specific individual behaviors such actions as toe sucking or carrying a water bowl in the mouth — two behaviors we have observed in different cats. The cat that used to suck her toe daily by the hour discontinued this practice after her first litter. Examples of general behavioral tendencies are timidity or social aggressiveness. Some cats are afraid of everything. Other cats dominate the food dish or a preferred sleeping place. In our experience, neither sex nor age is important in many social situations; the behavior of the cats is almost entirely determined by the natures of the animals involved. General tendencies may show up at a very early age and continue into adulthood, and they can be entirely over-ridden by species behaviors. Thus, an extremely timid female cat who ordinarily would avoid all other cats will brazenly seek adult toms during estrus. General tendencies may also change as a cat grows older, has a litter or two, and learns how to deal with some of the problems and responsibilities involved in being a cat.

INTEGRATIVE BEHAVIOR

Our discussion of the different types of species behaviors and individual behaviors tended to view them singly and in isolation. Species behaviors do not appear in a fixed unvarying manner however but are often modified to fit the circumstances. In many cases of species behaviors, there seem to exist only general guidelines; in maternal behavior, for example, the mother must carry out the guidelines as best she can, depending upon local conditions. To perform many of these species behaviors, the cat must execute a complex plan of action by way of preparation for various exigencies. Frequently, several factors must be taken into consideration by the cat, some of these relevant for species survival and others relevant to individual survival or individual inclination. When everything is put together, it becomes integrative behavior.

THE SOCIOLOGY OF THE CAT

Although adult cats (especially toms) seem to prefer solitude to the company of other cats, there are times when they come in contact with other cats. Usually these meetings are for the survival of the species and the enactment of species behaviors, but there are other occasions, too. Leyhausen (1963) has described some examples in farm and town cats. We have devised a set of social rules for adult cats based upon our observation of social behavior in cats for several years. This set of rules, which constitutes the main basis for cat interactions, differs for males and females; and the rules do not apply to castrates.

    A. Social Rules for adult male cats:
      1. To fight adult males smaller, less agile, and less powerful than oneself.
      2. To mate with female cats in estrus.
      3. To stay away from kittens.
    B. Social Rules for adult female cats:
      1. To mate with tomcats when in estrus.
      2. To care for kittens.
      3. To keep other cats away from the kitten den.

There do not seem to be any other rules as far as we can determine; in all other aspects of social behavior, the cat is on its own. The instructions received by the cat for most of the preceding rules are almost certainly odorous in nature; i.e., a cat knows how to behave toward another cat on the basis of how the other cat smells. Female rule no. 2 is actually composed of a whole subset of rules, as are the other rules to a more limited degree. All the rules, however, apply to strange cats. They may not hold true for cats in the same house where close association and human interference may modify these rules to some degree.

A consequence of the above rules is that an adult tom is almost always responding according to instructions (i.e., mating and fighting). Furthermore, tomcats can't make friends with one another and thus can't play rabbit. A female cat is not so relentlessly driven to perform strenuous actions as the tom, since she is in estrus only a few days a year when rule no. 1 is in action. On the other hand, she is always pregnant or rearing kittens. A cat, therefore, constantly enacts its predetermined behavior patterns to produce more cats who will do so in turn.

CAT CULTURE

Culture can be defined as a body of acquired information that is carried over from generation to generation. Although it is common to consider culture as an exclusive attribute of the human species, reports on wild species of *Felidae* indicate that in wild conditions cats would possess a culture. A long period of training is required for a member of the *Felidae* to acquire the skills it needs to support itself by independent hunting. Studies on lions, cheetahs, and tigers reveal that this period of training may take as long as one and a half to 2 years. Schaller (1967), for instance, reports that tiger cubs about a year old were inept in killing a bullock that was tied to a stake. The Indian maharajas who imported African cheetahs for coursing preferred adult animals because they were trained in hunting (Pocock, 1939). The first year or two of life of the *Felidae* is spent acquiring the necessary hunting skills through experience and learning from the mother.

Guggisberg (1962) reports that lions in different parts of Africa hunt quite distinct types of game. Lions in one part may hunt zebras almost exclusively, whereas lions in another part hunt buffalo, avoided by the other group. Lions apparently hunt what their mother hunted. Cubs of a female maneater develop a taste for humans. Similarly Young (1958) reports that bobcats (*Felis rufa*) in one section of the United States will feed almost exclusively on deer, whereas bobcats in another section rarely touch venison.

It seems likely that wild cats would develop a similar type of culture. Presumably, the mother cat acquires a set of skills that she finds adequate for survival under the existent conditions. These skills are learned by the young through the experience of hunting with the mother during the first year of life. Cat culture is thus passed from mother to offspring. Should one culture prove superior to another in terms of survival, eventually most of the cats in a given area will have a similar culture. We can presume also that this culture will not be static but will be added to and enriched by successive generations of cats.

CATS AND HUMANS

It is impossible to discuss cats independently of humans. Not only do the large majority of cats dwell with humans, but their history is inextricably intermixed with that of man. The association of cat and man is almost as old as civilization itself. The cat has been authenticated to have lived with Egyptians from at least 1500 B.C.; and Zeuner (1963) is of the opinion that, given the Egyptians' proclivity for domesticating animals, the cat was probably tamed many centuries earlier. Although there is some evidence that the Greeks and certainly the early Romans had cats, they did not spread throughout Europe in any number until early Christian times. Cats lived with people in India in at least the second century B.C. and in China from about 400 B.C. Cats are only found in stable, sedentary human cultures that have a large agricultural foundation. Few cats are found in the many human nomadic societies, hunting and gathering societies, or in primitive agricultural societies.

The cat was domesticated by man at a much later period in time than the dog or even the goat and the sheep. There are many reasons why animals are domesticated by humans. Some of these are discussed at length by Zeuner (1963), who is of the opinion that domestication is a natural development arising out of the needs and practices of the two species of animals. Dogs, the first domesticated animals, were probably utilized by man in hunting, which required the dog to do what he did naturally, anyway, and in a social situation similar to that found in a dog pack; the major difference was that the leader of the pack was a different species of animal. Similarly, herbivores that run in herds could have progressed from a casual association in which man first follows the herd and then, dispatching the natural leaders, takes command.

Although the precise reasons for the initial domestication of the cat are forever lost in antiquity, it is still possible to discuss some of the factors that may have played a role in forming the association. Early man and cats were hunters, but they apparently did not get together on a permanent basis until humans settled down and became hewers of wood and toilers of the field. It has been noted that agricultural societies based upon vegetable grains tend to attract a lot of rodents and birds who feed upon this large accumulation of foodstuffs. Cats feed upon birds and rodents and therefore would probably have been enticed out of the surrounding forests. No doubt, farmers observed that the activities of the cats were beneficial to both species and welcomed them. Once the female cat had moved her den from the woods to the farms, the association of cats and man became closer and more permanent.

It is relevant to remark here that the female cheetah and the female lion raised by Adamson from cubs turned to the wild, rather than human civilization, to deliver and rear their young. Female cats often prefer to have humans in attendance during parturition (Chandoha, 1963).

Throughout recorded history cats have provided all or part of their own food and at certain times there have existed official ratters. There is more to the human-and-cat association than the cat's ability to exterminate vermin, however. Humans have much to offer cats: A safe den and an occasional meal would go far toward relieving the rigors and hazards of the carnivorous life. In addition, cats like to sit on warm laps and near warm fires. Besides their utilitarian aspects, cats provide humans with a means of observing the behavior of another animal — one that is clean and neat, looks after itself in the main, and is a soft and purry object to pet, a procedure that both humans and cats seem to enjoy.

Man's treatment of cats has varied throughout the history of the association of these two animals (Simpson, 1903). In Egyptian times the cat was revered and mistreatment of a cat was a punishable offense. In later Christian periods of time in Europe, the cat was thought to be an emissary of evil and there were often public burnings of living cats. Even today, there are ambivalent attitudes about cats and superstitions are often associated with cats, although cats are treated by many as objects of beauty and exhibited at cat shows. Bird and other wildlife enthusiasts are likely to look askance at the predatory cat wandering through the woods. Forbush (1916) states that in the middle of winter, in the wilds of Maine many miles from human dwellings, there were more cat tracks in the snow than tracks from any other animal. Feral cats and their near relatives, the bobcats and pumas, are often hunted relentlessly with dogs, traps, and poisons.

The association of the cat with man has been quite successful in that it has enabled the cat to spread throughout the world and inhabit places seldom occupied by *Felidae*. Although many other members of the *Felidae* are imperiled by the spread of man and forced into more and more restricted environments, cats increase in numbers yearly and surely must be considered one of the most successful of the carnivores. Matheson (1944) estimated the number of cats in Cardiff and Newport as about 13 percent of the human population, with about 10.5 percent house-kept cats and 2 to 3 percent strays. Ralston Purina, a cat-food company, estimates the current cat population of the United States to be about 38 million, with 11 million of them strays (Kramer, 1970).

The existence of such a large population of prolifically breeding carnivores has produced a surplus of cats that cannot be fed by humans or by their own means. Few countries make use of cat carcasses, which are not considered suitable for eating. Humane societies were organized largely to deal with the excess of cats and dogs produced in civilized countries (Forbush, 1916). Smith (1971) estimates that humane societies kill 14 million cats a year and that another 14 million cats are killed by automobiles, or starve. According to Kramer (1970), humane societies kill cats by asphyxiation by withdrawing air from a chamber or by introducing CO_2 into the chamber.

One use for the surplus of cats produced in this country is scientific research, which disposed of about 165,000 cats in 1969 (Kramer, 1970). Cats have long been a favored animal for research. They are of a fair size and take readily to caging, and until recently, they were freely available and cheap.

One primary reason for the considerable work done on cats is the continuous large number of excess cats. Many scientific studies, particularly those in anatomy, result in a carcass unfit to eat, so most anatomy is done on small rodents or cats that no one wants. With the recent passage of new laws, cats have become more expensive and more difficult to obtain. Professional cat-killing organizations are usually loath to provide animals for scientific research. The New York A.S.P.C.A., for example, killed sixty-two thousand cats in 1969 but yielded only nine hundred for laboratory use.

Humane societies and biological science are often at loggerheads over the treatment of cats; although, as far as the cats are concerned, the activities of these two organizations produce the same consequences, namely dead cats. As we have observed, cat killing is at present a socially approved human activity and is even considered to be in the best interest of the cats. The main bone of contention seems to be the method of dispatching the cat. It is possible to conduct scientific experiments in which little or no pain is produced in the cat. In most of the neurophysiological experiments described in this book, the cats are killed at the end of the experiment.

3
ESSENTIAL
NEUROANATOMY

In the analysis of an organism, it is customary to divide the organism into anatomically and functionally distinct parts. One part that has been identified is the nervous system. The nervous system is of special construction and is concerned with the coordination, control, and regulation of the other parts and of whole organism activities. Inspection of the nervous system reveals that it is composed of a myriad of subcomponents, each with a different organization and function. These parts can be described crudely, as in gross anatomy, or in fine detail, as in microscopic anatomy. The single neural cell is the basic anatomical and functional unit of the nervous system. Thus, though the description of a part of the nervous system may start out with large systems such as nuclei or nerves, complete and exact description is achieved only when it includes the basic structural and functional units of the nervous system—the individual nerve cells and their connections. The goal of neuroanatomy in sensory neurophysiology is the complete description of the cells constituting a sensory system; a description that would include identifiable cell types, their number, arrangement, and central and peripheral connections.

Any experiment in sensory neurophysiology is automatically an experiment in neuroanatomy. In sensory neurophysiology, we measure the function of individual elements in an organized subsystem of the nervous system. The neurophysiological investigations we describe cannot be appreciated without a knowledge of the neuroanatomical substrate upon which they are performed. The neuroanatomy of sensory systems cannot be evaluated without some background in neuroanatomy.

TERMINOLOGY

Certain terms are used to denote the direction and orientation of body parts when describing the anatomical relationships of body structures. We define

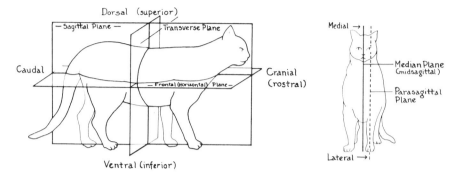

Fig. 3-1. Anatomical terminology.

these terms with respect to a body-axis running longitudinally from the head to the buttocks of an animal, or with respect to body posture. Difficulties arise because those terms based upon body posture have different meanings when they are applied to man—who has an erect, biped posture—from their use in describing quadrupled animals (Fig. 3-1). Although terms based upon body-axis are preferred, both types of terms will be defined because they are often used interchangeably in the description of human anatomy.

Rostral, cephalad, and cranial refer to positions toward the head, while caudal refers to positions in the direction of the buttocks. The terms anterior for quadrupeds and superior for bipeds are often used in place of the term rostral. However, they both have different meanings when applied to animals with different body postures. The anterior surface of man is his belly surface, while the superior surface of a quadruped is the back surface (Fig. 3-1). The median or midline refers to a line that divides the body into symmetrical right and left halves. A medial structure is located toward the midline; a lateral one, away from the midline. The terms proximal and distal indicate a direction toward or away from the attached end of a limb, the origin of a structure, or the center of the body. The dorsal or back surface of a quadruped corresponds to the posterior surface of bipeds, while the ventral or abdominal surface of a quadruped corresponds to the anterior surface of bipeds. The terms dorsal and posterior and the terms ventral and anterior are often used interchangeably in the descriptive neuroanatomy of man.

An animal is described as being intersected by three planes of reference: sagittal, frontal, and transverse. The sagittal plane divides the animal rostrocaudally into right and left parts. The midsagittal plane falls along the midline and divides the animal into right and left halves. All other planes parallel to the midsagittal plane are parasagittal and divide the animal into unequal right and left parts. The frontal plane also extends from the rostral to caudal limits of an animal. However, it is perpendicular to the sagittal plane and divides the animal into a dorsal or an anterior and a ventral or a posterior part. Originally, the term frontal referred to a relation to the front or face of humans. Often, in describing quadripeds, the term horizontal is used in place of frontal because this plane is parallel to the horizon for quadrupeds. The transverse plane is at right angles to the sagittal and frontal planes and divides an animal into a rostral and a caudal part. Often a section taken in the transverse plane is termed a cross section, since it is taken across the longitudinal axis of a structure. Although the transverse plane of bipeds is parallel to the horizon, the term horizontal plane is used only in describing a transverse section through the cerebral hemispheres of man.

GENERAL METHODS

There are many different ways we can study the structure of the nervous system. We can describe the structures that are visible to the naked eye, in which case we become involved with gross anatomy, or we can describe the microscopic structure of the nervous system. The various ways we may observe the structure of the inner ear are depicted in Fig. 3-2. As this figure shows, the description of the components and the cellular organization of sensory systems can proceed on many levels—from gross structure to cellular organization to the subcellular composition of a single cell. To enable an investigator to achieve a perceptual view of a sensory system, the description must proceed from a gross level to finer levels. Each level of description is necessary for an understanding of the structural organization of a sensory system.

Many different techniques are used to prepare the nervous system for anatomical studies. Since most parts of the nervous system have a jellylike consistency and are achromatic, the tissues of the nervous system are usually fixed and stained. The methods of fixation are fairly standard and involve perfusing the tissues with formalin, alcohol, glutaraldehyde, or some other fixative. The methods of staining or coloring the tissues vary widely and depend most critically upon the microscopical techniques in use, the structure under study, and the part of the nerve cell to be visualized (Brodal, 1969). Some of the more commonly used stains will be discussed in the section on microscopic anatomy that follows.

As Fig. 3-2 indicates, there are several different techniques for studying cellular structure, depending upon the size of the parts we are studying. With the light microscope, structures of a micron or two in diameter can be distinguished. In light microscopy, the image is magnified through a series of lenses. Light microscopy, however, is inadequate for a visualization of the components of cells, and the anatomist must turn to the electron microscope. With the electron microscope, he can resolve structures on the order of about 10 angstroms. Even more powerful microscopes have been devised to resolve

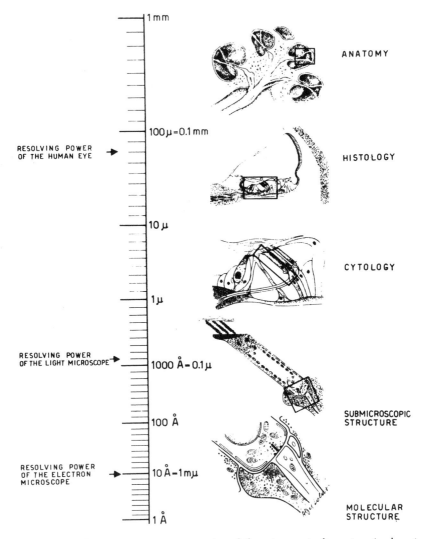

Fig. 3-2. Mammal. Diagrammatic representation of the microscopic dimensions (each main division represents a dimension ten times greater than the one below). The figure shows also the cochlear duct and the organ of Corti at progressively higher magnifications. In each figure the outlined area corresponds to the figure represented below at a higher magnification (Iurato *et al.*, 1967).

molecules and atoms. A recent tool for anatomical investigations, the scanning electron microscope, yields an in-depth picture of the surface of a structure.

THE BASIC DIVISIONS OF THE NERVOUS SYSTEM

For descriptive purposes, the nervous system is divided into two major divisions: the central nervous system and the peripheral nervous system. The central nervous system (CNS) or neuraxis consists of the brain, which is located in the cranial cavity, and the spinal cord, which is located in the vertebral canal. The peripheral nervous system is composed of all nervous tissue located outside the brain and spinal cord, and serves to keep other body tissues in communication with the central nervous system.

The peripheral nervous system is divided on the basis of the direction of the conduction of nerve impulses into sensory and motor systems. Peripherally located nervous tissues conducting nerve impulses toward the CNS are classified as part of the peripheral afferent or sensory nervous system. In most cases peripheral sensory nervous tissue is associated with specialized cell systems called sensory receptors that have the capacity to react to internally or externally applied physical or chemical agents. Stimulation of these receptors with an adequate stimulus is believed to initiate the nerve impulses that are conducted centrally by the peripheral sensory nervous system. Thus, the peripheral sensory nervous system supplies the CNS with most information concerning internal body state, the motion and position of the body parts, and the nature of the external forces impinging upon the body surfaces.

The peripheral efferent or motor nervous system is composed of peripherally located nervous tissues that conduct nerve impulses away from the CNS. The peripheral motor nervous system is connected with peripheral effector organs such as the muscles and secretory organs of the body. Nerve impulses conducted peripherally by elements of the peripheral motor system produce contraction of muscular tissue or secretion by glandular tissue. A small part of the peripheral motor system is connected to sensory receptors or the afferent neurons innervating them. The peripheral motor system is often divided into two components on the basis of the type of body tissue associated with it. The peripheral autonomic nervous system is associated with body viscera, such as the heart, lungs, digestive tract, kidneys, etc., and with smooth muscles, blood vessels, and sweat glands. The peripheral somatic motor system is associated with the striated musculature of the body skeleton.

NEUROHISTOLOGY

The basic unit of the nervous system is the neuron or nerve cell. Each neuron is composed of a cell body containing the cell nucleus and cytoplasmic extensions forming neural processes. Neurons are not in protoplasmic continuity but are separated entirely by membrane walls. The absence of cytoplasmic continuity between neurons forms the basis for the neuron doctrine, which maintains that each neuron is morphologically separate from, and trophically independent of, other neurons (Ramón y Cajal, 1954). The trophic center of a neuron is its cell body and nucleus. The sectioning of a neural process from its cell body usually results in degeneration of that process. In most cases, if a neuron is damaged, adjoining neurons are not affected. Exceptions do occur—as in the case of the neurons of the eye, destruction of which results in the transneural degeneration of neurons in the CNS that normally make contact with neural processes that arise from the retina.

Essentially, the nervous system consists of complex chains of neurons that are anatomically and functionally interrelated at points of contact called "synapses." Nerve impulses are transmitted from one neuron to another at the synapse. Neurons also make anatomical and functional contacts with receptors, muscular and glandular cells.

THE NEURON

Each neuron has a cell body, soma, or perikaryon consisting of a nucleus and the surrounding cytoplasm (Fig. 3-3). Within the CNS, an isolated cluster of neuron bodies is called a "nucleus" if the cluster is surrounded by a zone of nervous tissue devoid of neural bodies; or a "cortex" if the aggregate forms a distinct layer along the surface of the CNS. Outside the CNS, an aggregate of neuron cell bodies is called a "ganglion." Ganglia of the peripheral sensory nervous system are primarily located within the cranial cavity (the cranial sensory ganglia) or within the vertebral column (the spinal sensory ganglia). The ganglia of the peripheral autonomic nervous system, the autonomic ganglia, are found close to the vertebrae or close to the organs they innervate.

Two types of cytoplasmic processes arise from the cell body of a neuron: the dendrites, which conduct information toward the cell body, and the axon, which conducts information away from the cell body. Typically, neurons within the CNS have several short cytoplasmic expansions radiating from the cell body called "dendrites" and a single long process known as either the "axon" or "axon cylinder." The point at which the axon arises from the neuron cell body is sometimes referred to as the "axon hillock." The dendrites of CNS neurons typically do not extend beyond the limits of the nucleus or cortex that their cell bodies form. Axons of many CNS neurons do leave the confines of the nucleus or cortex, often to travel great distances before terminating. Neurons located in sensory ganglia give rise to two long processes that arise either directly from the cell body (bipolar cells), or from a single process that arises from the cell body (unipolar cells as illustrated in Fig. 3-3, far left). The term for the neural process of a sensory ganglion cell

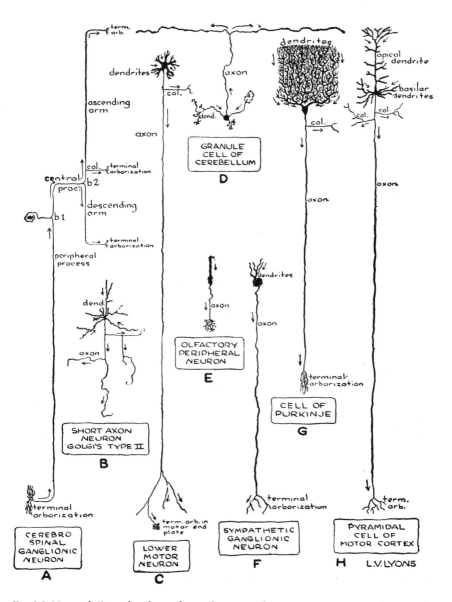

Fig. 3-3. Mammal. Examples of some forms of neurons. The axons, except in B, are shown much shorter in proportion to the size of the neuron cell body and dendrites than they actually are. The direction of conduction of the nerve impulse is shown by the arrows. Col, collateral branch; proc, process; term. arb., terminal arborization. From Copenhaver, W.M. and Johnson, D.D. (1958) *Bailey's Textbook of Histology*, Fourteenth edition. ® 1958, The Williams & Wilkins Co., Baltimore.

conducting impulses away from the cell body and toward the CNS is the "axon" or "central process," while the process conducting impulses toward the cell body is called the "dendrite" or "peripheral process." "Tracts" are bundles of long neural processes located within the CNS; those compact bundles of neural processes located outside the CNS are the "roots," if they are located within the cranial cavity or vertebral canal, and "trunks" or "nerves," if they are located outside the cranial cavity or vertebral canal.

In most cases, a single neuron makes synaptic contact with a number of neurons both at its input or dendritic end and at its output or axonal end. The axon of a nerve cell usually branches repeatedly near its terminus to produce a number of axon terminals, thus expanding its output capacity. Usually, the terminal branches of an axon spread out and make contact with a number of neurons, although they may in some cases only make contact with a single neuron. In turn, a single neuron may receive axon terminals from a number of neurons or from a single neuron. Usually, the dendrites and often the cell body of a neuron are covered by numerous small axon terminals. The peripheral process of a sensory ganglion cell often branches extensively with the ramifications contacting more than one receptor, and occasionally contacting morphologically different types of receptors. Conversely, a single receptor may receive terminals of a single sensory ganglion cell or of numerous sensory ganglion cells.

Axon terminals make synaptic contact with the cell bodies (axosomatic), dendrites (axodendritic), or, less frequently, with the axons (axoaxonic) of other neurons. These nerve terminals take an infinite variety of forms. Most commonly the terminals end in small bulblike expansions, the "end feet" or "boutons." Others may be delicate terminal twigs that form rings or loose baskets around the cell body and dendrites of another neuron. A few form large cuplike endings known as "calyces" that envelop the cell body of another neuron.

SUPPORTING TISSUE

Neurons located within the CNS are surrounded by neuroglial or glial cells that outnumber the neurons tenfold. Glial cells invest neuron cell bodies and processes and help isolate their synapses. In the CNS, axons may be myelinated or unmyelinated. The myelinated axon possesses a sheath of thin concentric sheets of protein alternating with layers of lipids called "myelin." The myelin sheath appears a short distance from the cell body and surrounds the axon up to its proximal portion. The myelin sheath is not continuous but is interrupted at regular intervals. The areas of the axon free from myelin appear as constrictions known as "the nodes of Ranvier" (Fig. 3-4). Numerous unmyelinated axons occur in the white and gray matter of the CNS; they appear as fine naked axons embedded in glial cell processes.

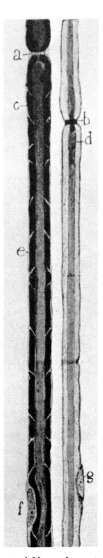

Fig. 3-4. Rabbit. Myelinated fibers of a peripheral (the sciatic) nerve. The fiber on the left is stained with osmic acid, a myelin stain: the fiber on the right with silver nitrate, a neurofibril stain. a, node; b, cementing disc; c, myelin sheath; d, axon; e, membrane of Schwann; f, g, nuclei. Notice the Schmidt-Lantermann clefts in the fiber on the left, which appear as a series of light oblique lines in the darkly stained myelin sheath (Ramón y Cajal, 1928).

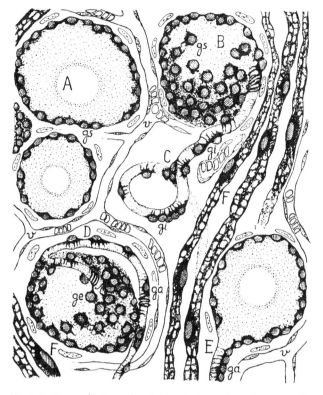

Fig. 3-5. Mammal. Neuroglia of the spinal ganglion of a mammal (semi-schematic drawing). Nerve cells focused through their equator (A); superficially focused (B), surrounded by endocapsular satellite elements: perisomatic gliocytes (gs) may be distinguished, partially associated forming a syncytium, and periaxonic gliocytes (ga and ge) whose cytoplasmic appendages embrace a sector of the neurite or twist themselves spirally on it; gi, interstitial gliocytes intimately attached to the neurite in its extracapsular course (C) enveloping it with fine cytoplasmic appendage. F, myelinated nerve fibers covered by a syncytium of schwannic elements; v vascular net of pericapsular capillaries. (Ortiz-Picón, 1955)

The cell bodies of ganglion neurons are covered by supporting tissue, the "satellite cells" (Fig. 3-5) that some consider to be of neuroglial origin (Ortiz-Picón, 1955). The cell bodies of two of the cranial sensory ganglia are invested by a myelin sheath (Ballantyne and Engström, 1969). Peripherally located long neural processes are invested by Schwann cells that form a Schwann sheath around the process. A number of unmyelinated neural processes indent the surface of a Schwann cell and become imbedded by a portion of the cell; thus a single Schwann cell may ensheath a number of unmyelinated neural processes. The Schwann sheath is formed by a chain of Schwann cells surrounding the neural processes. Myelinated neural processes are also ensheathed by a series of Schwann cells, but a single Schwann cell invests only one myelinated process. The Schwann cell forms the myelin sheath; and the nodes of Ranvier demark the boundaries between successive Schwann cells along the length of the nerve fiber. Thus, the myelin sheath appears as a series of tubes surrounding the neural process that is interrupted at regular intervals by the nodes of Ranvier (Fig. 3-4). Within any internode segment of the myelin sheath of peripheral nerve fibers, there appear several oblique incisures in the myelin, the "Schmidt-Lantermann clefts." These clefts represent areas of the myelin sheath where the myelin layers are separated by cytoplasm of the Schwann sheath.

STAINING METHODS

In order to visualize nervous tissue, which is in most cases achromatic and semitransparent, special dyes must be used to color it. Two constituents of the neuron cytoplasm that are often stained are neurofibrils and Nissl or chromatin substance. Neurofibrils are found throughout the neuron down to its finest terminal processes, and can be impregnated with silver stains that color the entire extent of the neuron. Nissl granules or bodies are abundant in the neuroplasm of the cell body, cell nucleus, and the base of dendrites, but are absent from the most peripheral region of the cell body, the axon hillock, fine dendrites, and the axon. The central and peripheral processes of sensory ganglion cells are both devoid of Nissl substance and therefore are similar to axons of CNS neurons. Nissl bodies are best demonstrated by staining with the basic aniline dyes. Such stains color only the cell body, its nucleus, and the base of dendrites of a neuron. The myelin sheath of myelinated neurons can also be selectively stained when properly fixed. The myelin sheath is formed by concentric layers of lipid substance that appear white in color in fresh tissue.

Whole neuron-staining methods such as the Golgi method of silver staining (Nauta and Ebbesson, 1970) and the methylene blue method (Polyak, 1941) color the entire neuron, often down to its finest ramifications. These staining methods result in the coloring of only a fraction of the total of neural elements in the specimen treated. Because only a few neurons are stained, relatively thick sections or whole mount specimens can be utilized to examine the entire extent of a neuron. Neurons can be identified and classified on the basis of the shape and size of the cell body, the arrangement, the size and course of the neural processes, and the shape and site of termination of the terminal expansions. One difficulty encountered with whole neuron stains is their selectivity, since the small fraction of cells colored by these stains may represent only a small portion of the cell types present in the specimen. Also, these stains either completely mask or blur the inner structure of the neuron and, as in the case of Golgi-treated material, present a dark silhouette of the entire cell.

The Nissl method of staining is often utilized to examine the cytoarchitecture of various cell groups within nuclei, cortices, or ganglia. This staining process is based upon the special chemical affinity of Nissl granules in the neuron cell body, nucleus, and dendrites to certain basic dyes. The use of these staining methods allows selective coloring of the cell bodies and the bases of large dendrites of all neurons in a given specimen, while axons and non-neural elements remain unstained or stained only lightly. With Nissl-staining methods, neurons may be identified and classified on the basis of the shape and size of the cell body, the position of the nucleus within the cell body; and on the basis of the appearance of the Nissl substance itself. However, with the Nissl method the size, shape, and course of axons, axon terminals, and fine dendrites cannot be examined. Also, fairly thin sections must be used with Nissl-stained tissue because the cell bodies of all neurons within the specimen are colored, and the greater the density of neurons, the thinner the section must be to permit visualization of the individual neurons within a section.

Myelin and special neurofibril stains are often used to trace the course and termination of nerve fibers. Myelin-staining methods result in the selective staining of normal lipids of the myelin sheath. The disadvantage of the myelin stains is that the myelin and not the neural process is stained, and therefore only the myelinated parts of the fiber are visible. Unmyelinated fibers and the terminal processes of myelinated fibers, as well as cell bodies and CNS dendrites, are not visible in myelin-stained tissue. Modified silver staining methods have been developed to selectively stain the neural processes of myelinated and unmyelinated fibers down to their finest terminals. Because most silver stains color the entire nerve cell, the terminals of nerve fibers cannot be distinguished upon cell body or dendrites. Special silver-staining methods that color only the terminals permit visualization of the terminals upon cell body and dendrites.

Myelin and special neurofibril stains are often used to measure the diameters of nerve fibers within a nerve or tract (Fig. 3-6). However, there are various factors that may affect the actual and measured diameters of fibers. Stacey (1969) has demonstrated that the techniques used to stain the fibers may influence the measurements. According to Sunderland and Roche (1958), fairly marked variations may occur in the diameter of a single fiber.

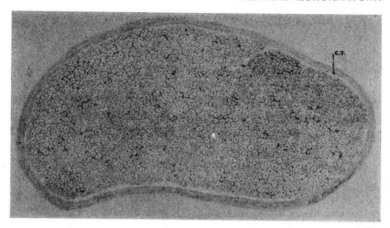

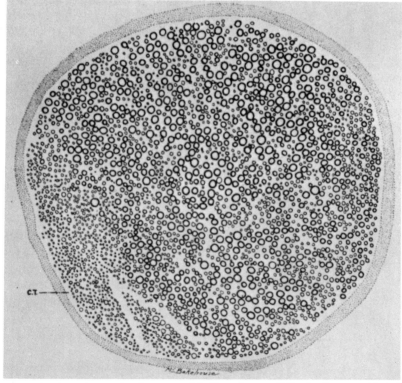

Fig. 3-6. Cat. Top: Camera-lucida tracing of the lingual nerve. C.T., chorda tympani branch of the seventh cranial nerve. Neurofibrils stained with pyridine-silver. Bottom: Camera-lucida tracing of the lingual nerve. C.T., chorda tympani nerve. Myelin stained with osmic-acid. (Windle, 1926)

These variations are most prominent at the nodes of Ranvier and at the clefts of Schmidt-Lantermann, but may also occur at other parts of the nerve fiber such as at points of bifurcation. In one myelinated fiber inner diameter measurements varied from 3.25 to 11.75 microns, while the outer diameter (including the myelin sheath) varied from 6.5 to 16.0 microns (Sunderland and Roche, 1958).

A technique used in conjunction with special stains is that of neural degeneration. If a neural process is severed from its cell body, the neural process and its myelin usually disintegrate completely (secondary or Wallerian degeneration). Certain staining techniques permit the selective impregnation of degenerating nerve processes (the Nauta-Gygax method), of degenerating nerve terminals (the Glees method), or of degenerating myelin (the Marchi method). Because the Nissl substance in the cell bodies of injured neurons undergoes a dissolution process called chromatolysis, the cells of origin of a sectioned nerve or tract can be identified on the basis of the appearance of the cell-body Nissl substance. A combination of Nissl stain and special stains for degenerating nerve fibers is often used to trace the course of a tract or nerve from its distal end to its cell of origin.

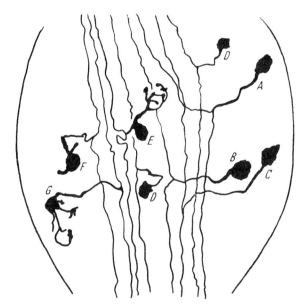

Fig. 3-7. Cat. Neurons of the spinal ganglion. Above: Cells in the spinal ganglion of a fetal cat A, B, C; simple pseudounipolar cells. D, small pseudounipolar cell. E, F, G; cells with dendriticlike appendages, Golgi silver impregnation. (Ramón y Cajal, 1909). Right: Typical and atypical spinal ganglion cells. A, A´, B; unipolar large and small cells. C, bipolar cell. D, multipolar cell. h, neurites branching to form peripheral (p) and central (c) processes; k collaterals. (Dogiel, 1897)

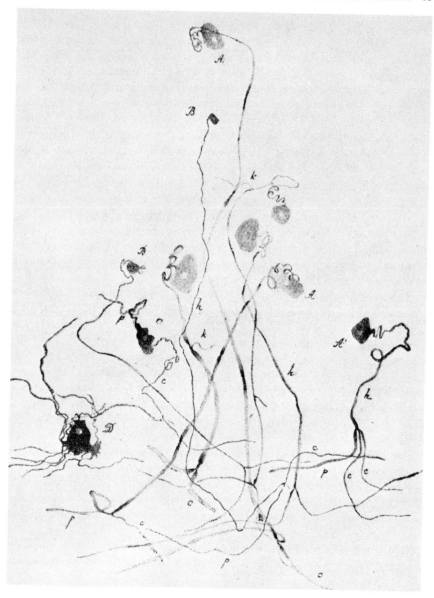

Fig. 3-7 *(contd.)*

VARIETIES OF NEURONS

Neurons can be classified on the basis of the shape and size of the cell body; the position of the nucleus within the cell body; the form, size, and distribution of the Nissl substance within the cell body; or in terms of the number, length, thickness, and mode of branching of neural processes. The shape of the neuron cell body is variable: It may be spherical, ovoid, fusiform, or multiangular. Cell body size ranges from a minimum diameter of 4 microns to a maximum of 150 microns. The cell nucleus may be centrally placed within the cell or eccentrically placed near the cell membrane. The Nissl bodies may take the form of a fine granular substance or may form large, coarse clumps. The Nissl bodies may be abundant or scarce, evenly distributed within the cell body, or may form a ring around the cell nucleus. A single process may extend from a pear-shaped cell body (unipolar cell), two processes may extend from opposite ends of a fusiform-shaped cell body (bipolar cell), or numerous processes may arise from a cell body of variable shape (multipolar cell). The shape of a multipolar neuron, which represents the majority of neurons, is determined by the number and arrangement of its neural processes. Some neurons give rise to long axons that form tracts within the CNS and nerves peripherally (Golgi type I neurons). Others give rise to short axons that do not leave the confines of the gray matter where their cell bodies are located (Golgi type II neurons).

The central nervous system is formed of billions of neurons organized into thousands of nuclei and hundreds of cytologically distinct cortical areas. CNS neurons appear in a wide variety of shapes and have an infinite variety of arrangements of their neural processes. Although attempts at classifying neurons in selected nuclei or cortical areas on the basis of cell morphology have been successful, no standard scheme of classification of all CNS neurons exists. Ramón-Moliner (1968) has attempted to classify CNS neurons on the basis of the arrangement of their dendrites. In Golgi preparations three general groups of neurons were observed: those with relatively straight dendrites that radiate in all directions; those with dendrites that are asymmetrically distributed; and those with dendritic patterns that are unique to the neurons within a specific nucleus or cortical area.

Neurons of the peripheral nervous system are less numerous than those in the CNS and are less variable in appearance. The ganglion cells of the peripheral autonomic nervous system are generally small and multipolar. Some give rise to dendrites and axons that are clearly distinguishable, but others give rise to processes showing no obvious differences. On the basis of investigations by Dogiel and by Ramón y Cajal, who both used whole-neuron staining methods, de Castro (1932) has classified autonomic ganglion neurons into five types: (1) neurons with long neural processes; (2) neurons with dendrites that form dense glomeruli; (3) neurons with short or accessory dendrites; (4) fenestrated (windowed) neurons; and (5) small neurons with few dendrites.

The majority of neurons in the peripheral sensory nervous system appear to fall into two major categories, bipolar or unipolar, on the basis of appearance in whole-neuron stained material. The bipolar neuron has an oval or round-shaped body that gives rise to two opposing neural processes. The unipolar neuron gives rise to a single process that divides to produce two neural processes. This neuron is often called a pseudounipolar cell because, first, during embryological development the neuron is bipolar, and later, during further development the two opposing processes are brought together to form a single neural process. The single process may be short or may run a considerable distance before bifurcating. Other sensory-ganglion cell types have been described by Ramón y Cajal (1907) and by Dogiel (1908), who used Golgi silver and methylene blue staining methods (Fig. 3-7). Ramón y Cajal (1928) later reported that he considered all but the bipolar and unipolar types to be atypical and possibly pathological.

Sensory ganglion cells have also been classified on the basis of morphological differences observed in Nissl-stained sections of sensory ganglia (Scharf, 1958). Sensory ganglion neurons stained with basic dyes differ with respect to cell body size and with respect to the appearance of the Nissl substance. Warrington and Griffith (1904) classified the spinal sensory-ganglion cells of the cat into four types on the basis of size and appearance of the Nissl substance. In a more recent study utilizing rapidly preserved sensory ganglia, differences were not observed in the size and dispersion of Nissl substance within the ganglion cell bodies (Pineda et al., 1967). It has been suggested that the staining variations observed in earlier studies might reflect differences in the cell life cycle or in cell metabolism at the time of fixation (Ranson, 1909).

GROSS ANATOMY OF THE NERVOUS SYSTEM

As was mentioned previously, for the convenience of description the nervous system is subdivided into the central nervous system (brain and spinal cord) and the peripheral nervous system (roots, trunks, ganglia, and nerves). This division is arbitrary since these parts do not function separately, but work together to integrate bodily functions. The rostral portion of the CNS is composed of the brain, which occupies and nearly fills the cranial cavity of the skull. The brain is continuous through the foramen magnum with the spinal cord, which is enclosed within the vertebral canal of the backbone. In the cranial portion of the peripheral nervous system, twelve pairs of cranial nerves emerge from the ventral surface of the brain (Fig. 3-8) and travel through various foramina of the skull to supply muscles, integument, cranial autonomic ganglia, and receptor organs of the facial region of the head, and in one case, the autonomic ganglia of the body. As part of the spinal portion of the peripheral nervous system, 38 pairs of spinal nerves take origin from the spinal cord of the cat and pass through the intervertebral foramina to be

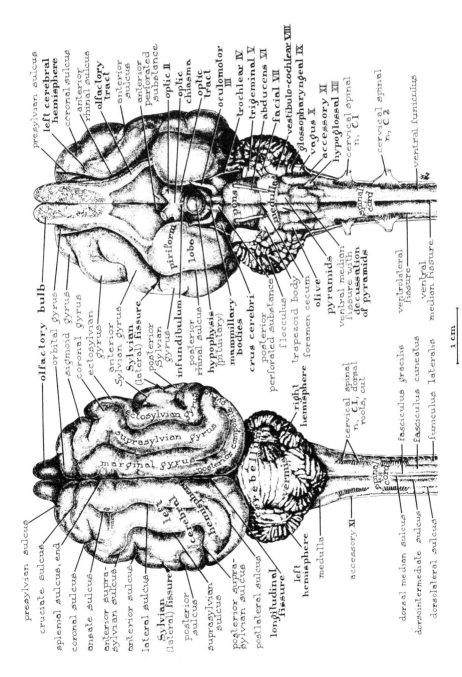

Fig. 3-8. Cat. Left: Dorsal aspect of the brain. Right: Ventral aspect of the brain. (Crouch, 1969)

distributed to the back of the head, the neck, and the rest of the body. The peripheral autonomic nervous system consists of nerves and ganglia that are involved in carrying nerve impulses to body viscera, smooth muscles, and glands throughout the body.

THE CNS: SPINAL CORD

The spinal cord is a cylindric-shaped structure located within the vertebral canal (Fig. 3-9). For descriptive purposes the spinal cord is divided into five general longitudinal areas: cervical, thoracic, lumbar, sacral, and caudal. The diameter of the spinal cord is not uniform throughout its length, being less in the thoracic, sacral, and caudal portions than in the cervical and lumbar portions (Fig. 3-9). The cervical and lumbar enlargements represent those areas of the spinal cord associated with the extremities of the body. Below the level of the lumbar enlargement the spinal cord decreases in size and at its caudal extremity forms a cone-shaped termination, the conus medullaris. On the dorsal surface of the spinal cord, a shallow longitudinal groove, the dorsal median sulcus, appears along the midline. In Fig. 3-9, 38 pairs of dorsal roots can be seen entering the spinal cord laterally at the dorsolateral sulcus (Reighard and Jennings, 1929). On the ventral surface of the spinal cord, a deep longitudinal groove, the ventral median fissure, appears along the midline of the cord. Lateral to it, irregular groups of filaments of the ventral root emerge from the ventrolateral sulcus of the spinal cord.

The internal structure of the spinal cord is fairly uniform throughout its longitudinal extent. In transverse section the spinal cord can be observed by the unaided eye to consist of centrally placed gray matter surrounded by a mantle of white matter. The gray matter consists primarily of neuron cell bodies, the white matter of myelinated nerve fibers. The centrally located gray matter takes the form of an "H" when viewed in cross section. The vertical bars on the H form the gray horns or gray columns of the spinal cord and the cross bar of the H, the gray commissure. In each half of the spinal cord, the gray extending dorsal to the gray commissure forms the dorsal horns, while the gray extending ventrally forms the ventral horns. Many of the fibers of a dorsal root enter the dorsal horn of the spinal cord and terminate upon cells within it. Most of the ventral root fibers arise from neurons whose cell bodies are located in the ventral horn of the spinal cord. The mantle of white matter is divided by filaments of the dorsal and ventral roots into three main fiber groups. The dorsal funiculus is located between the dorsal median sulcus and the filaments of the dorsal root; the lateral funiculus between the filaments of the dorsal and ventral roots; and the ventral funiculus between the filaments of the ventral root and the ventral median fissure. Just anterior to the gray commissure fibers crossing the midline form the anterior white commissure.

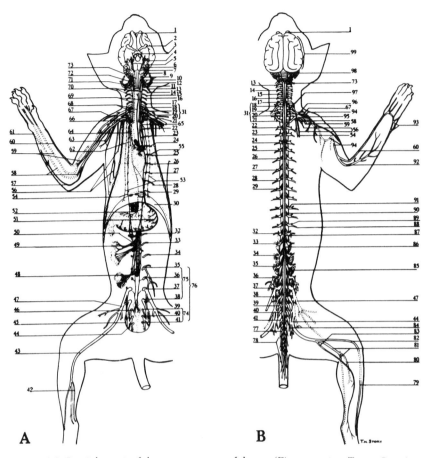

A   B

Fig. 3-9. Cat. Schematic of the nervous system of the cat. (Figure courtesy Turtox Corp.)

A. Ventral view
B. Dorsal view
1. First cranial nerve
   (Olfactory)
2. Second cranial nerve
   (Optic)
3. Third cranial nerve
   (Oculomotor)
4. Fourth cranial nerve
   (Trochlear)
5. Fifth cranial nerve
   (Trigeminal)
6. Sixth cranial nerve
   (Abducens)
7. Seventh cranial nerve
   (Facial)
8. Eighth cranial nerve
   (Vestibulocochlear)
9. Ninth cranial nerve
   (Glossopharyngeal)

10. Tenth cranial nerve
    (Vagus)
11. Eleventh cranial nerve
    (Accessory)
12. Twelfth cranial nerve
    (Hypoglossal)
13. First cervical nerve
14. Second cervical nerve
15. Third cervical nerve
16. Fourth cervical nerve
17. Fifth cervical nerve
18. Sixth cervical nerve
19. Seventh cervical nerve
20. Eighth cervical nerve
21. First thoracic nerve
    (the diaphragm conceals thoracic nerves 10, 11, 12,
    and 13)
22. Second thoracic nerve
23. Third thoracic nerve
24. Fourth thoracic nerve

THE CNS: BRAIN

The brain is the larger and more rostral portion of the CNS. It is continuous with the spinal cord but differs considerably in shape and internal structure. The brain consists of a tubular portion called the brain stem and of two irregularly convoluted eminences, the cerebrum and the cerebellum (Fig. 3-8). The cerebrum and cerebellum cover almost the entire dorsal surface of the brain stem (Fig. 3-8, left). Only a small portion of the dorsal surface of the caudalmost segment of the brain stem, the medulla, can be seen caudal to the cerebellum. The cerebellum is divided by fissures into three parts: an unpaired median portion called the "vermis" and two large lateral masses known as the "cerebellar hemispheres." The surface of the cerebellum is folded into numerous long slender convolutions or folia, that are separated by

25. Fifth thoracic nerve
26. Sixth thoracic nerve
27. Seventh thoracic nerve
28. Eighth thoracic nerve
29. Ninth thoracic nerve
30. Diaphragm
31. Brachial plexus
32. First lumbar nerve
33. Second lumbar nerve
34. Third lumbar nerve
35. Fourth lumbar nerve
36. Fifth lumbar nerve
37. Sixth lumbar nerve
38. Seventh lumbar nerve
39. First sacral nerve
40. Second sacral nerve
41. Third sacral nerve
42. Tibial nerve
43. Saphenous nerve
44. Great sciatic nerve
45. Obturator nerve
46. Sympathetic plexus of urinary bladder
47. Femoral or anterior crural nerve
48. Inferior mesenteric plexus of the sympathetic system
49. Superior mesenteric plexus of the sympathetic system
50. Coelic ganglion (or semilunar) of the sympathetic system
51. Posterior gastric plexus (formed by the dorsal esophageal branch of the vagus nerve)
52. Anterior gastric plexus (formed by ventral esophageal branch of the vagus nerve)
53. Phrenic nerve to diaphragm
54. Right sympathetic trunk and ganglia
55. Ramus communicans between sympathetic ganglion and the fifth thoracic nerve
56. Anterior and posterior thoracic nerves
57. Cutaneous medalis nerve
58. Ulnar nerve
59. Median nerve
60. Superficial radial nerve
61. Palmar branch of the ulnar nerve
62. Pulmonary nerve
63. Subscapular nerves
64. Cardiac nerve
65. Inferior cervical ganglion (Stellate ganglion)
66. Middle cervical ganglion of sympathetic trunk
67. Suprascapular nerve
68. Right inferior laryngeal nerve
69. Right and left sympathetic trunk
70. Right and left vagus nerves
71. Nodose ganglion of vagus nerve
72. Superior cervical ganglion of sympathetic trunk
73. Medulla oblongata
74. Sacral plexus
75. Sciatic plexus
76. Lumbosacral plexus
77. Cauda equina
78. Filum terminale
79. Superficial peroneal nerve (external peroneal)
80. Branch of tibial nerve to lateral head of gastronemius muscle
81. Tibial nerve
82. Common peroneal nerve
83. Suralis nerve
84. Lessor sciatic nerve
85. Lumbar enlargement
86. Dorsal median sulcus
87. Dorsolateral sulcus
88. Ventral ramus of the thirteenth thoracic nerve
89. Dorsal ramus of thirteenth thoracic nerve
90. Dorsal roots of twelfth thoracic nerve
91. Dorsal root ganglion of the eleventh thoracic nerve
92. Dorsal or posterior interosseal nerve
93. Dorsal cutaneous branch of ulnar nerve
94. Radial nerve or musculospiral nerve
95. Axillary or circumflex nerve
96. Nerve to deltoid muscle
97. Brachial enlargement
98. Cerebellum
99. Right cerebral hemisphere

parallel sulci. The cat's cerebellum is normally separated from the cerebrum by a bony partition, the "tentorium." The cerebrum or telencephalon forms the larger part of the brain, and is divided by a deep longitudinal fissure into two cerebral hemispheres. The surface of the cerebrum is also folded into convolutions or gyri separated by sulci or fissures. Rostrally an extension of the cerebrum forms a pair of gray masses referred to as the "olfactory bulbs."

A ventral view of the brain (Fig. 3-8, right) illustrates the brain stem to greater advantage. The brain stem is subdivided into the medulla, pons, midbrain, and diencephalon for descriptive purposes. The medulla or myelencephalon has the shape of a truncated cone, the smaller end of which is continuous with the spinal cord. A transverse bulge formed by the trapezoid body called the "trapezium" marks the rostral limit of the medulla. Rostral to the trapezium a massive band of transverse fibers delimits the entire ventral extent of the pons or metencephalon. Partially hidden by the cerebral hemispheres are the crus cerebri of the midbrain, eminences formed by large fiber tracts traveling in a longitudinal direction. Surrounded laterally by the pyriform lobes of the cerebral hemispheres, a small portion of the diencephalon can be seen where it attaches to the hypophysis. The olfactory bulbs extend rostrally from the cerebral hemispheres.

Internally the brain stem is composed of groups of neuron cell bodies called "nuclei" and of groups of nerve fibers referred to as tracts, lemnisci, peduncles, or brachia. While the internal structure of the spinal cord is fairly uniform in its longitudinal extent, the internal structure of the brain stem varies from level to level. The masses of gray and white matter are also more difficult to distinguish in unstained sections of the brain stem. Certain of the brain-stem nuclei give rise to efferent fibers that leave the brain in the cranial nerve roots, while others receive terminals of the central processes of sensory cranial fibers. The remaining nuclei form the greater part of the brain stem, along with numerous ascending and descending tracts. The cerebellum is composed of the cerebellar cortex, a superficial sheet of gray matter, that encloses an internal mass of white matter and the cerebellar nuclei. The cerebral cortex of the cerebrum encloses an internal mass of white matter and nuclear matter known as "basal ganglia."

THE PERIPHERAL NERVOUS SYSTEM: SPINAL PORTION

The spinal cord of the cat gives rise to 38 pairs of spinal nerves that connect the spinal cord with the rest of the body. Each spinal nerve is formed by the nerve fibers of a single dorsal root and its corresponding ventral root (Fig. 3-11). A dorsal root arises from the dorsolateral aspect of the spinal cord, passes laterally, and enters a dorsal root ganglion. The dorsal root ganglia, most of which are located within the vertebral canal or in the intervertebral foramen, contain the cell bodies of sensory neurons innervating the viscera, muscles, and integument of the body. The fibers of the dorsal root that connect the spinal cord to the dorsal root ganglion are the central processes of dorsal root ganglion cells. The peripheral processes of the dorsal root ganglion cells emerge from the ganglion as a compact bundle and join the ventral root to form a spinal nerve. Nerve filaments emerging from the ventrolateral surface of the spinal cord are motor fibers that converge to form a ventral root. The ventral root passes laterally and joins the dorsal root as it emerges from the dorsal root ganglion. The resulting spinal nerve emerges from the vertebral column by way of an intervertebral foramen. The level of exit of the nerve is used to name the nerve and the roots and ganglion giving rise to the nerve, as well as to the spinal-cord segment connected to the dorsal and ventral roots. Thus, in the cat there are eight cervical, thirteen thoracic, seven lumbar, three sacral, and seven or eight caudal spinal nerves, dorsal and ventral roots, and spinal-cord segments. The most rostral spinal-cord segment, the first cervical, gives rise to the first cervical dorsal and ventral roots, which join to form the first cervical spinal nerve.

After leaving the intervertebral foramen, a spinal nerve divides into two main branches, a small dorsal ramus and a larger ventral ramus. Each of the rami gives off branches forming the peripheral nerves that travel to the body organs. Each of the peripheral nerves is composed of motor (ventral root) and/or sensory (dorsal root) fibers. In most cases the branches of the dorsal rami are distributed to the muscles and integument of the back. Most of the branches of the ventral ramus are distributed to the muscles and integument of the ventral or belly portion of the body and to the limbs. A small branch of the ventral ramus, the ramus communicans, connects the spinal cord with the peripheral autonomic nervous system.

THE PERIPHERAL NERVOUS SYSTEM: AUTONOMIC PORTION

Those parts of the peripheral nervous system concerned with the motor control of the body viscera, smooth muscles, blood vessels, and glandular tissue are grouped into a system called the autonomic nervous system. This system consists of the sympathetic trunks and autonomic ganglia, and of the nerves that connect them to the CNS and to the peripheral effector organs. The sympathetic trunks are two long nerve cords located symmetrically along the ventrolateral aspect of the vertebral column from the base of the skull to the tail (Fig. 3-9, item no. 69). Each trunk consists of a large bundle of nerve fibers along which a series of autonomic chain ganglia occur. The sympathetic trunks are connected to the cervical, thoracic, first four lumbar, last lumbar, and sacral spinal nerves by communicating rami. Nerves pass peripherally from the sympathetic trunk to collateral autonomic ganglia that lie along the abdominal aorta. There are also terminal autonomic ganglia located in or near body viscera that are connected with the brain and spinal cord, but are not directly connected with the sympathetic trunks.

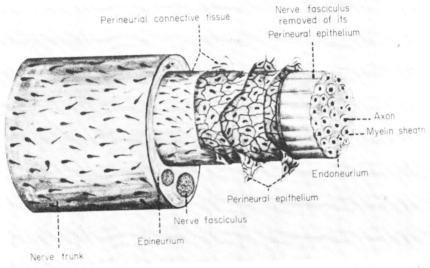

Fig. 3-10. Mammal. Diagram of the connective tissue sheaths about a peripheral nerve. The epineurium covers the entire nerve trunk, the perineurium divides the fibers into groups called fasciculi, and the endoneurium surrounds each individual myelinated nerve fiber. (Shantha and Bourne, 1968)

THE PERIPHERAL NERVOUS SYSTEM: CRANIAL PORTION

Twelve pairs of cranial nerves arise from the brain to innervate the facial region of the head and parts of the peripheral autonomic nervous system. The cranial nerves are not formed as systematically as are the spinal nerves of sensory and motor roots. Some cranial nerves are formed by cranial roots containing only sensory or only motor fibers. Those cranial nerves containing both sensory and motor fibers are not necessarily formed by a convergence of separate motor and sensory roots. In some cases the motor and sensory fibers emerge from the brain to form a common cranial root. The cranial nerve ganglia are composed of the cell bodies of sensory neurons and therefore are only found along cranial roots that contain sensory fibers. Each of the cranial nerves is uniquely formed and the peripheral course of cranial nerves does not form a common pattern. In this chapter only the sensory portions of the cranial nerves will be described.

COVERINGS OF THE NERVOUS SYSTEM

The brain and spinal cord are invested by three connective tissue coverings called collectively the "meninges." The pia mater is a delicate tissue that adheres to the surface of the CNS. The arachnoid is a spider-weblike tissue that connects the pia mater with the tough outer covering of the CNS, the dura mater. Nerve roots, upon emerging from the CNS, receive an investment of connective tissue as they pass through the pia. This tissue is further reinforced by additional connective tissue as the roots pass through the arachnoid and dura. The ganglion of a nerve root is surrounded by a connective-tissue capsule that is continuous with the outer connective-tissue covering of the root and nerve. Each nerve is invested by a thick covering called the epineurium (Fig. 3-10). Within a given nerve, the fibers are divided into bundles or fascicles of varying size, each of which is surrounded by a sheath of perineurium. Within each fascicle, connective tissue called "endoneurium" separates the fibers into smaller and smaller bundles and ultimately invests each nerve fiber as a delicate tubular membrane (Shantha and Bourne, 1968).

PERIPHERAL SENSORY SYSTEMS

A peripheral sensory system consists of sensory receptors and the peripheral afferent neurons that connect the receptors to the central nervous system (Fig. 3-11). Sensory receptors are designed to measure some aspect of the internal environment or of the external world. The receptors encode and send these measures to the CNS by initiating nerve impulses in the peripheral afferent neurons innervating them. A sensory receptor may take the form of a specialized neuron (olfactory receptors) or of a specialized neuroepithelial cell (visual, auditory, vestibular, and gustatory receptors). Receptors in the skin, joints, and viscera take the form of free nerve endings or of a complex of specialized epithelial cells and sensory nerve endings. The muscle spindle receptor is a complex of specialized mesodermal cells and sensory and efferent nerve endings. Sensory receptors are located within a receptor organ that optimizes the conditions for reception of the signal the receptor is designed to receive. Receptors may be localized in specialized receptor organs that function only to deliver the signal to the receptors—for example, the photoreceptors in the eye. Other receptors are located in special areas of the body where contact with the signal normally occurs, such as the chemoreceptors in the tongue and the olfactory receptors in the nose. Most receptors are located in generalized body areas, but within specific portions of these areas, such as the muscle spindle receptors in the striated muscles of the body. For descriptive purposes we have divided the peripheral sensory system on the basis of location of the sensory receptors into the skin (skin, exposed mucous membranes, and subcutaneous tissue), joint, muscle (muscle and tendons), visceral, vestibular, visual, and auditory systems. We combine the olfactory and gustatory systems of the nose and tongue and the chemosensory system of the blood vessels in the chapter on the chemical sensory systems.

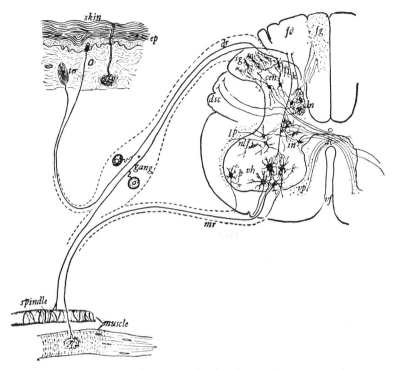

Fig. 3-11. Mammal. Diagram of some peripheral and central connections of sensory spinal ganglion cells. Also shown are efferent motor fibers to the muscle. (Papez, 1929)

cen: central nucleus of dorsal horn	k: collateral
dn: dorsal nucleus of cord	lp: lateral fasciculus proprius
dr: dorsal root	mr: motor or ventral root
dsc: dorsal spinal cerebellar tract	nlf: nucleus of lateral fasciculus
ep: epithelium	sg: substantia gelatinosa
fc: fasciculus cuneatus	ter: nerve terminal
fg: fasciculus gracilis	vf: ventral fissure
in: intermediate nucleus	vh: ventral horn
	vp: ventral fasciculus proprius

The peripheral sensory nervous system serves as a line of communication between the sensory receptors and the CNS. In most peripheral sensory systems — i.e., the skin system of the face and body, the joint and muscle systems of the body, and the auditory, vestibular, and gustatory systems — sensory ganglion neurons connect the receptors directly with the CNS. In a few sensory systems, i.e., the visual and olfactory systems and the muscle and joint systems of the face, the cell bodies of the neurons connecting the receptors to the CNS are not located in sensory ganglia. In one system, the visual system, a chain of at least two neurons is interposed between the receptors and the CNS.

All of the dorsal root ganglia contain the cell bodies of neurons whose peripheral processes innervate skin, joint, muscle, or visceral receptors. The types of sensory receptors innervated by the cranial ganglia vary markedly from ganglion to ganglion. The semilunar ganglion of the trigeminal nerve contains the cell bodies of afferents innervating receptors in the skin of the face, the mucous membranes of the eye, nose, sinuses, and oral cavity, and in the teeth and cranial dura. The geniculate ganglion of the facial nerve contains the cell bodies of neurons that supply the chemoreceptors and some skin receptors of the anterior two thirds of the tongue, the skin receptors of the outer ear, and the receptors in the soft palate of the oral cavity. The spiral ganglion of the cochlear nerve contains neurons that innervate only the auditory receptors of the inner ear, while the cells of Scarpa's ganglion of the vestibular nerve innervate only the vestibular receptors of the inner ear. The inferior ganglion of the glossopharyngeal nerve contains afferents that innervate receptors in the skin of the outer ear; also the cells of the inferior (petrosal) ganglion of the glossopharyngeal nerve innervate chemoreceptors in the posterior one third of the tongue and receptors in the carotid body and sinus of the vascular system. The afferents of the jugular (superior) ganglion of the vagus nerve also innervate receptors in the skin of the outer ear. The afferents of the nodose (inferior) ganglion of the vagus nerve innervate chemoreceptors in the epiglottis and receptors in the viscera of the throat, thorax, and abdomen. The afferents of the inconstant ganglion of the accessory nerve are believed to supply receptors in the muscles of the neck and shoulder.

In most cases each sensory ganglion is covered by a thick connective tissue capsule that is continuous with the dura of the CNS and the epineurium of the nerves. Within most sensory ganglia the neuron cell bodies are located around a central core of nerve fibers. While most of the cell bodies of the spiral ganglion and of Scarpa's ganglion are bipolar and myelinated, the majority of the cell bodies in the rest of the cranial ganglia and in all the dorsal root ganglia are unipolar and unmyelinated. The most consistent observations of unipolar cell differences are related to cell body size. A small unipolar cell usually gives rise to a single initial process that takes a fairly straight course before bifurcating into a peripheral and a central process a short distance from the cell body. The processes of most small cells are unmyelinated and appear to differ with respect to diameter. The peripheral processes of small dorsal root ganglion cells are approximately six times greater in diameter than the central processes (Ha, 1970). A large ganglion cell often gives rise to a long single process that, before bifurcating, coils around the cell body forming a glomerulus. In cat dorsal root ganglia, large

Table 3-1 Numbers of Nerve Cells and Fibers in the Dorsal Roots of Cat (Holmes and Davenport, 1940)

Cat No. and Sex		Seg-ment	Side	Cells in D. R. Gang.	Fibers in D.R.	% Less F. than C.
5	F	C1	R	---	---	-
5	F	C1	L	3,800	3,800	0
6	F	C2	R	32,400	23,400	28
8	F	C2	L	27,000	23,500	13
5	F	C3	L	31,000	30,100	3
6	F	C3	L	27,900	29,400	5 more
8	F	C3	L	29,200	27,000	8
7	F	C4	L	19,500	17,000	13
8	F	C4	R	17,700	16,900	5
6	F	C5	L	26,400	25,700	3
8	F	C6	L	25,200	24,100	4
8	F	C7	L	33,400	32,800	2
8	F	C8	L	27,900	26,400	5
8	F	T1	L	22,500	21,500	4
10	M	T2	R	15,300	14,400	6
4	F	T3	L	10,500	9,800	7
1	F	T4	R	9,300	8,200	12
4	F	T4	R	12,200	10,700	12
4	F	T5	R	8,800	8,400	5
4	F	T6	R	7,600	6,800	11
9	M	T7	L	11,000	9,500	14
9	M	T8	L	10,700	9,800	8
9	M	T9	R	8,000	11,000	38 more
9	M	T10	L	11,000	10,500	5
9	M	T11	L	9,000	9,100	1 more
9	M	T12	L	10,500	10,500	0
9	M	T13	L	11,000	10,500	5
11	M	L1	R	10,000	10,000	0
12	M	L2	L	12,100	12,100	0
11	M	L3	R	14,000	14,000	0
12	M	L4	L	18,000	17,600	2
12	M	L5	L	25,800	22,300	14
12	M	L6	R	27,000	25,000	7
6	F	L7	R	32,000	29,600	8
12	M	S1	L	17,500	17,500	0
2	F	S2	-	15,000	16,500	10 more
3	F	S3	L	9,200	8,800	4
12	M	Cc1	R	5,850	6,450	10 more
12	M	Cc2	R	4,650	4,650	0
13	M	Cc3	L	2,300	2,250	2
12	M	Cc4	R	2,100	2,550	18 more
Totals, high a				543,200	515,200	5
Totals, low a				530,000	509,400	4

Ratio of dorsal to ventral roots, 4,3:1.
a Where more than one nerve of a segment was counted, only one nerve per segment is included in each total.

Table 3-2. Comparative Fiber Counts from the Peripheral Branches of the Trigeminal Nerve. Fiber Size Classification: Small, less than 5 microns in Diameter; Medium, Between 5 & 9 Microns, Large, 9 Microns or Greater in Diameter (Windle, 1926)

NERVE COUNTED	Osmic acid — Number counted: Large	Medium	Small	Osmic acid — % of myelinated: Large	Medium	Small	Pyridine silver — Number counted: Large	Medium	Small	Pyridine silver — % of myelinated: Large	Medium	Small	Unmyelinated (Pyridine silver) — % of myelinated	fibers
Lacrimal....	0	20	160	0	11.12-	88.88+	0	18	146	0	10.98-	89.02+	59.41-	240
Frontal....	70	116	141	21.41-	35.47+	43.12-	106	189	198	21.50+	33.34-	40.16+	20.36-	126
Nasociliary: Type I....	65	122	182	17.84-	32.97+	49.19-	63	107	178	18.10+	30.75-	51.15-	39.05+	223
Type II....	0	32	430	0	6.93-	93.07+	0	32	398	0	7.44+	92.56-	36.86-	251
Zygomatic....	94	240	311	14.57+	37.21-	48.22-	111	217	293	17.88-	34.94+	47.18-	25.27+	210
Infraorbital and Superior alveolar	166	160	199	31.62-	30.40-	37.90+	175	186	212	30.54-	32.46+	37.00-	18.14+	127
Lingual....	133	162	163	29.04-	35.37+	35.59-	93	105	122	29.06+	32.81+	38.13-	27.11-	119
Auriculotemporal	97	121	155	26.01-	32.44-	41.55+	138	184	260	23.71+	31.62-	44.67+	54.57-	699
Inferioralveolar	163	164	158	33.61-	33.81+	32.58-	253	248	231	35.01-	33.65-	31.34+	17.39-	155
Nerves to muscle of mastication	111	58	26	56.92+	29.74+	13.34-	220	121	67	53.92+	29.66-	16.42+	4.89+	21
Nerve to Myelohyoid	106	107	65	38.13-	38.49-	23.38+	120	133	67	37.50-	41.56+	20.94-	38.40-	167

ganglion cells produce central and peripheral processes that are usually myelinated and of equal diameter (Ha, 1970). The cell body and initial process of unipolar neurons are usually invested in a capsule formed by a single layer of satellite cells. The sheath of satellite cells extends over the initial process as it leaves the cell body and is replaced by a Schwann sheath more distally. Neural processes with diameters greater than one to two microns are generally myelinated, while those with smaller diameters are usually unmyelinated. The cell bodies of most bipolar cells in the spiral and Scarpa's ganglia are invested in a myelin sheath and a satellite cell capsule (Ballantine and Engstrom, 1969). Most of the fibers of the cochlear and vestibular nerves have diameters greater than two microns and are myelinated (Gacek and Rasmussen, 1961).

Altogether there are about 535,000 cells in the dorsal root ganglia of the cat (Holmes and Davenport, 1940). The number of cells in each dorsal root ganglion varies from a low of around 2,100 cells in the caudalmost ganglion to a high of about 32,800 cells in the seventh cervical ganglion (Table 3-1). The diameters of dorsal root ganglion cell bodies vary from 10 to 100 microns (Warrington and Griffth, 1904). In most dorsal roots, the number of unmyelinated fibers outnumber the myelinated fibers (Duncan and Keyser, 1938). The percentage of unmyelinated fibers in any dorsal root varies from approximately 3 percent in the first cervical to approximately 78 percent in the eleventh thoracic root.

The number of cells in the cranial ganglia varies considerably from ganglion to ganglion. The semilunar ganglion of the trigeminal nerve has been estimated to contain approximately 44,700 cells (Windle, 1926). Approximately 27,200 myelinated fibers, 2 to 12 microns in diameter, and 17,500 unmyelinated fibers arise from the semilunar ganglion. Table 3-2 presents the comparative fiber counts from the peripheral branches of the trigeminal nerve.

The geniculate ganglion of the facial nerve has been reported to contain an average of 1,711 cells according to Bruesch (1944), or 1,776 cells according to von Buskirk (1945), or 1,819 cells according to Foley, Pepper, and Kessler (1946). The cell bodies vary in size from 5 to 50 microns in diameter, with 50 percent from 20 to 30 microns, 25 percent from 30 to 50 microns, and 25 percent from 5 to 20 microns in diameter (Foley and DuBois, 1943). The geniculate ganglion gives rise to approximately 2,000 fibers of which 81 percent are myelinated (Foley, 1960). The greater superficial petrosal nerve takes origin from the apex of the triangular-shaped ganglion and contains from 33 to 40 percent of the peripheral processes of geniculate ganglion neurons. This nerve contains both sensory and motor fibers and has been estimated to contain an average of 2,193 fibers, of which 597 are sensory (Foley, 1947). Approximately 77 percent of the sensory fibers in the greater superficial petrosal nerve are myelinated (Foley, 1947) and have diameters ranging from 3 to 4 microns (Foley and DuBois, 1943). Peripherally, as the greater superficial petrosal nerve joins the sphenopalatine ganglion, the sensory fibers pass through the ganglion into the palatine nerves, probably to innervate receptors in the soft palate. Just before the facial nerve trunk leaves the facial canal, it gives rise to the chorda tympani nerve, which contains 45 to 55 percent of the peripheral processes of geniculate ganglion cells. The chorda tympani nerve is predominantly sensory and contains an average of 1,955 nerve fibers (Foley, 1945). An average of 1,157 of the fibers are sensory and approximately 82 percent of these sensory fibers are myelinated (Foley, 1945) with diameters from 2 to 4 microns (Foley and DuBois, 1943). The chorda tympani joins the lingual nerve peripherally and sends branches into the mucous membranes of the tongue, primarily. The sensory fibers of the chorda tympani innervate the taste buds and skin receptors on the anterior two thirds of the tongue and possibly receptors in the lingual mucosa (Foley, 1945). The facial nerve distal to the origin of the chorda tympani contains approximately 23 percent of the peripheral processes of geniculate ganglion cells (Foley, 1960). At or slightly proximal to the origin of the chorda tympani, the auricular branch of the vagus nerve joins the facial nerve trunk. The auricular nerve contains from 6,000 to 8,000 fibers, which originate from the jugular ganglion of the vagus nerve (DuBois and Foley, 1936). The facial nerve trunk and the auricular nerve together contain approximately 18,900 to 28,500 fibers (Foley and DuBois, 1943) of which an average of 490 are of geniculate ganglion origin (Foley, 1960). These geniculate ganglion fibers range in diameter from 1.5 to 6.5 microns and appear to be predominantly myelinated (Foley and DuBois, 1943). These fibers are distributed to the skin of the outer ear along with the fibers of the auricular nerve (Foley and DuBois, 1943; Bruesch, 1944; Boudreau et al., 1971).

Scarpa's ganglion of the vestibular nerve has been reported to contain over 12,000 cells (Gacek, 1969). The cell bodies of Scarpa's ganglion cells are bipolar and myelinated (Ballantine and Engström, 1969). The cells of Scarpa's ganglion give rise to approximately 12,400 myelinated fibers, the majority of which are 2 to 4 microns in diameter (Gacek and Rasmussen, 1961). The spiral ganglion of the cochlear nerve contains approximately 40,000 cells according to Schuknecht and Woellner (1953) or approximately 50,000 cells according to Howe (1935). The cell bodies of spiral ganglion neurons are also bipolar and myelinated (Ballantine and Engstrom, 1969). Approximately 51,700 myelinated fibers arise from the spiral ganglion and are 1 to 8 microns in diameter, with most between 3 to 6 microns (Gacek and Rasmussen, 1961).

The glossopharyngeal nerve root contains approximately 4,500 fibers (Foley and Sackett, 1950), most of which are myelinated fibers, 3 to 6 microns in diameter (Koch, 1914). The superior ganglion of the glosso-pharyngeal nerve has been reported to contain an average of 1,445 cells

(DuBois and Foley, 1937) or 1,258 cells (Foley and Sackett, 1950). The petrosal ganglion reportedly contains an average of 2,724 cells (Foley and Sackett, 1950). According to Foley and DuBois (1937), 90 percent of the fibers in the glossopharyngeal nerve are sensory. According to textbooks on human neuroanatomy, a branch from the petrosal ganglion of the glosso-pharyngeal nerve joins the auricular nerve of the vagus; however, DuBois and Foley (1937) report that they did not observe such a contribution in the cat. The main glossopharyngeal nerve descends to the base of the tongue, where it splits into its terminal branches. Its lingual branch contains sensory fibers that innervate taste buds and receptors in the mucous membrane of the posterior one third of the tongue, and its pharyngeal branch contains sensory fibers innervating receptors in the mucosa of the pharynx.

The jugular ganglion of the vagus nerve has been estimated to contain an average of 8,723 neurons (DuBois and Foley, 1937). The auricular branch of the vagus nerve arises from the jugular ganglion and contains approximately 73 percent of the peripheral processes of jugular ganglion neurons. According to DuBois and Foley (1937), the auricular nerve is primarily sensory and contains approximately 8,400 fibers, of which 75 percent are unmyelinated. According to Bruesch (1944), myelinated sensory fibers have diameters that range from 1 or 1.5 to 20 microns. The auricular nerve leaves the jugular ganglion in the jugular foramen, passes through the floor of the tympanic bulla to the facial canal, and leaves the skull with the facial nerve by way of the stylomastoid foramen (Foley and DuBois, 1934). Most of the fibers of the auricular nerve are distributed to the skin of the outer ear (Foley and DuBois, 1943). Approximately 15 percent of the jugular ganglion fibers join the vagus nerve trunk (DuBois and Foley, 1937).

The nodose ganglion of the vagus nerve contains an average of 29,600 neurons (Jones, 1937). The superior laryngeal nerve arises from the middle of the nodose ganglion and contains from 2,400 to 2,900 fibers (DuBois and Foley, 1936). The fibers range in diameter from 1.5 to 8 microns, with the majority of small diameter (1.5 to 5 microns). Most of the sensory fibers of the superior laryngeal nerve appear to be myelinated and appear to innervate the mucosa of the larynx. The vagus nerve trunk distal to the nodose ganglion contains approximately 35,000 fibers (Jones, 1937) of which approximately 31,000 are sensory. Two thirds of the fibers are unmyelinated and the myelinated fibers range in diameter from less than 1 micron to 14 microns (Hoffman and Kuntz, 1957). The recurrent laryngeal nerve arises from the vagus nerve trunk in the thoracic cavity and ascends to the level of the throat. This nerve contains a total of from 900 to 1,400 fibers, of which 600 to 1,000 are sensory. These sensory fibers are small and thinly myelinated (2 to 3 microns in diameter) and are believed to arise from the nodose ganglion of the vagus nerve (DuBois and Foley, 1936). These fibers are believed to be distributed primarily to the mucosa of the trachea and esophagus. The remaining sensory fibers of the vagus nerve trunk are distributed to the mucosa of the digestive and respiratory tracts and to the heart (Jones, 1937).

The inconstant ganglion of the accessory nerve appears as scattered cells numbering from 12 to 20 and as small ganglia containing from 40 to 80 neurons (Windle, 1931). According to DuBois and Foley (1936), most of the sensory fibers in the accessory nerve are myelinated and have diameters ranging from 2 to 17 microns. These sensory fibers are believed to innervate sensory receptors in the neck and shoulder muscles innervated by the motor component of the accessory nerve.

The joint and muscle systems of the jaw and the olfactory and visual systems do not have peripheral afferent cell bodies located in cranial ganglia. The joint and muscle receptors of the jaw are innervated by peripheral nerve fibers that have cell bodies located within the CNS. The peripheral processes of these afferent fibers travel in the ventral root of the trigeminal nerve and the mandibular division of that nerve to the receptors in the jaw joints and muscles. The peripheral neuron of the olfactory system forms both the receptor and the afferent component of this system. The cell bodies and peripheral processes of the peripheral olfactory system are located within the olfactory mucosa and form the olfactory receptors, while the central processes of these neurons form the olfactory nerve. The peripheral visual nervous system is the most complex of all the peripheral sensory systems. It consists of at least four types of neurons, all located within the retina of the eye. The bipolar neurons connect the receptor to a second neuron, the ganglion cell, which sends its central process out the eye in the optic nerve.

A more detailed description of the sensory receptors, the sensory receptor organ and the peripheral afferents will be given in the chapters covering the different sensory systems.

4

ESSENTIAL NEUROPHYSIOLOGY

As stated in our Introduction, sensory neurophysiology is the quantitative study of the structure and function of sensory systems. The previous chapter reviewed some of the neuroanatomical distinctions, terminology, and techniques relevant to the study of sensory systems. Neuroanatomical studies identify and enumerate the different parts composing different sensory systems. With neuroanatomy the elements of a sensory system are given identity, location, and peripheral and central connections. With all the wonders of modern microscopy, however, neuroanatomy cannot determine what the different parts of a sensory system do. To determine what a sensory-system neuron does, we must measure its actions with neurophysiological techniques.

Neurophysiology then is the study of the functions of the parts of the nervous system. The way the function of a part of the nervous system is studied is similar to how the function of non-nervous tissue is studied: its function is described in terms of its actions upon known inputs. To study the digestive function of the stomach, known substances are placed into the stomach and the changes that occur in these substances after processing by the stomach are used to describe the digestive functions of the stomach. Thus, the function of the stomach is described in terms of input-output measures: its function is to change ABC to XYZ.

The function of a sensory system is determined in a similar way. Known things are put into the system and the neural output is then examined. The difference between the nervous system and other body parts is that the nervous system does not deal with substances but rather with information. The things we put into the nervous system become transformed into neural representations. The inputs may be definable in such physical quantities as cycles/sec or grams/mm, but the neural output is in terms of pulses emitted over a period of time. None of the physical elements of the input carry over to the neural output; but they may be represented there and the neural output may be described in terms of these physical elements, since it represents some transformed aspect of them.

The nature of the neural output complicates the study of the function of the nervous system because the output not only has none of the physical elements of the input but also this input is encoded (i.e., represented) in an unknown language. The cells of the nervous system speak to one another with a number of "pulse codes." It is the goal of sensory neurophysiology to interpret these pulse codes and determine the nature of the conversation. The description of the function of a sensory system is only as good as the techniques used to measure neural outputs. In sensory neurophysiology, the most reliable and unambiguous measure of neural activity is desired. We will discuss in this chapter some of the different neurophysiological measures of neural activity and their reliability.

The function of nervous tissue is presently studied at two levels, the molecular-cellular level and the systems level. Cellular neurophysiology or "neuron physiology" is the study of the function of parts of single cells, usually in terms of "mechanisms" that affect the chemical and electrical permiability of nerve cell membranes. The transport of molecules across membranes is a basic mechanism involved in providing nutrients to and removing waste products from a cell. More importantly, in the neuron it is a basic mechanism involved in the generation and transmission of nerve impulses. Sensory neurophysiology is the study of the function of sensory systems, where the function is defined in terms of the encoding and transmission of sensory information along a chain of neurons that constitute the system. Although neuron physiology plays a supporting role to sensory neurophysiology, it is not a major province in its domain. Studies in neuron physiology have, to our way of thinking, contributed little toward the elucidation of the functional properties of sensory systems. Therefore, we will not be discussing in detail speculation concerning cellular phenomena involved in synaptic transmission, initiation, and conduction of nerve impulses.

ELECTRICAL MEASURES OF NEURAL ACTIVITY

The function of a neuron is to process and transmit information from one region of the organism to another, whether from one neuron to another, or from a neuron to an effector organ, or from a receptor organ to another neuron. Although the mechanisms whereby information is transmitted are not fully understood, certain electrical events appear to accompany the transmission of information in nerve cells. Nerve cells, like other living cells, are electrically polarized; i.e., there is a potential difference between the inside and outside of a nerve cell or a nerve fiber (Ochs, 1965). Nerve cells are unique, however, since they have the characteristics of being capable of conducting or transmitting a change in this state. These electrical changes can be picked up with an electrode placed inside or outside the cell. Although a few measures have been taken of the temperature changes and the magnetic fields induced by neural activity, electrical measures are the only ones refined enough to study neural outputs. To obtain an electrical potential measure of neural activity, an electrode is placed in or near the neural structure under study and voltage fluctuations (relative to an indifferent point) are recorded.

GROUP ACTIVITY

One type of electrical activity commonly measured is the population or group potential. Group potentials are recorded from large numbers of cells or fibers with large macroelectrodes. Group potentials are of wide variety. They may be produced by electrical activity in receptors, dendrites, or axons. Examples of group potentials include EEG activity, evoked potentials, and summed multiunit spike activity. Electroencephalogram (EEG) activity consists of slow waves of varying complexity recordable from cortical or subcortical structures (Freeman, 1963). The frequencies of EEG potentials vary from d.c. shifts to waves of about 50Hz. Evoked potentials are wave-potential changes measured from a population of cells or fibers excited with a stimulus. Evoked potentials recorded from a sensory surface are often named according to that structure. Thus, there is the cochlear microphonic, from the cochlea of the ear (Stevens and Davis, 1938); the electro-olfactogram, from the olfactory mucosa of the nose (Ottoson, 1956); and the electro-retinogram, from the retina of the eye (Granit, 1962). Summated spike-activity measures involve the recording of spike activity from a large and unknown number of units that is summed electrically to produce a smooth measure.

These group potentials have one thing in common: The activity of individual neural elements is submerged in the group measure. Individual unit behavior cannot be predicted from knowledge of the group measures since the group response measure results from an unknown contribution of elements in an unknown population. The cells or fibers from which one commonly records group potentials rarely constitute a uniform population, and therefore group potentials represent the activity of a population of units of unknown heterogeneity. The contribution of any single unit depends upon the structure of that unit and its proximity to the large recording electrode. In recording summed spike activity from whole nerves, for instance, the contribution of any unit depends upon the size of the fiber, since large fibers produce larger potentials than small fibers (Zotterman, 1939), and upon the distance of the resistive path between the fiber and the electrode.

Because of these inherent limitations, group potentials cannot be used in sensory neurophysiology to describe the quantitative relationship between neural input and neural output. For example, Nagaki *et al* (1964) demonstrated that the response of the whole chorda tympani nerve to tongue applications of stimuli of different temperature resembled the response of few individual fibers and was the reverse of some.

Group potentials have their uses, however. They have been used as crude indices of effective stimuli. Used in this manner, investigators can sometimes determine within what limits stimuli are effective. Thus, Wever (1965) has compared lizard cochleas by comparing the cochlear microphonics recordable from them. Tucker (1963), in measuring summated spike activity from nerve twigs in the gopher, tortoise, and the rabbit, showed that chemoresponsive fibers from the trigeminal nerve responded to many of the same substances that fibers from the olfactory nerve responded to. Another use of group potentials is the monitoring of the condition of the animal. EEG waves may be monitored to determine the depth of anesthesia. The click-evoked potential of the auditory nerve recorded with a gross electrode near the round window of the cochlea is used by some to check on the condition of the animal's ear.

Group potentials may also be utilized for determining where an electrode tip is located within the brain, since many EEG and evoked potentials are of maximum amplitude and of predictable polarities with respect to the location of cell bodies of a particular brain structure. Thus, the slow potentials generated by the cells of the medial superior olivary nucleus in the brain stem have been used by investigators to determine the location of their electrodes (Galambos et al, 1959; Tsuchitani and Boudreau, 1964).

SINGLE-UNIT ACTIVITY

Two types of electrical events can be recorded from a single cell: slow potentials and spike potentials. Single-unit slow potentials are recorded with intracellularly placed microelectrodes, usually within the cell body or large dendritic processes of a neuron or within a receptor. This potential is graded and varies slowly in amplitude when the neuron or receptor is "stimulated." The slow potential is locally generated, is not propagated, and is decremental over space and time. Electrical stimulation of inputs to (a nerve bundle or tract that terminates upon) spinal cord ventral-horn neurons has been demonstrated to result in either a decrease in the amplitude of the neuron intracellular potential (depolarization) or in an increase in the amplitude of the potential(hyperpolarization). Studies involving the electrical stimulation of inputs to spinal cord and cerebellar neurons demonstrated that depolarizing intracellular potentials usually occurred during spike potential generation and that hyperpolarizing intracellular potentials occurred during spike inhibition (Eccles, 1957; 1964). It is believed by some, therefore, that intracellularly recorded slow potentials reflect neural events involved in the generation of nerve impulses; thus, they are often called "generator potentials."

The second electrical event, the single-unit spike or action potential (also called the nerve impulse), can be recorded either intra- or extracellularly from a neuron. It is a rapid voltage shift that appears as a spike or pulse approximately 0.5 to 2.5 msec in duration. The spike potentials generated from a given neuron are uniform in amplitude and shape, provided the neuron has not been injured and the recording situation has not been altered. The spike potential is propagated along the neuron; that is, it travels along the neuron with no decrement in amplitude. It is therefore a response that is transmitted along a neuron, often over great distances.

Although slow and spike potentials are both measures of the electrical output of neurons, studies of slow potentials recorded from receptors or neurons are not reviewed in this book for several reasons. First, it is questionable that the slow potential output of a neuron or receptor is a reliable measure of normal neural activity. Intracellular recording of slow potentials usually involves the injury of the structure by puncturing it with the recording microelectrode. The alteration of the physical state of the structure, which often dies during the experiment, may result in the generation of slow potentials that reflect the abnormal state of the structure. Furthermore, slow potentials are of value to sensory neurophysiology if they are a reflection of the transmission of neural information within a sensory system. If slow potentials are involved in the generation of spike potentials at points of synaptic contact, they would be a measure of neural transmission between components within sensory systems. However, it is not clear that the slow potentials recorded from receptors or neurons are actually related to neural transmission or spike generation.

Slow unit potentials that can be recorded from receptors are called receptor potentials. In those cases where the receptor potential is believed to be involved in the initiation of nerve impulses in the peripheral sensory nerve fibers innervating them, the term "generator potential" is frequently used. Most receptorpotentials that have been studied have been recorded from invertebrates (Loewenstein, 1971). The only mammalian receptor potential that has been studied in any detail is that from the Vater-Pacinian corpuscle (Gray, 1959; Loewenstein, 1971). This potential appears to be produced in the unmyelinated, intracapsular portion of the peripheral nerve fiber, since it can be recorded with most of the lamellar structures of the encapsulated end organ removed from it. The potential is produced by mechanical stresses applied to the nerve terminal in a direction parallel to its long axis. According to Loewenstein (1971), the strain sensitivity is on the order of 10^{-5} cm. or better. The amplitude of this receptor potential grows as the magnitude of the mechanical stimulus increases.

The concept that the receptor potential is a generator potential implies either of two things: (1) that spike production in the peripheral nerve fiber is dependent upon the occurrence of the receptor potential; and (2) that the magnitude of the spike discharge is proportional to the magnitude of the receptor potential. In the case of the Vater-Pacinian corpuscle, it is readily apparent that the second feature does not hold, since spike discharge is not proportional to the amplitude of the receptor potential. Nor is it entirely clear that the first feature holds for the Vater-Pacinian corpuscle, since it is possible to obtain receptor potentials in the absence of spike potentials. Ozeki and Sato (1965) have demonstrated that, in the Pacinian corpuscle with the lamellae removed, the receptor potential elicited by a maintained stimulus is sustained throughout the period of stimulation. The nerve response to such a sustained stimulus, however, is not a sustained discharge but rather a spike or two at the beginning and end of the period of stimulation. They also found that a spike would be produced when the receptor potential was of either sign, i.e., depolarizing or hyperpolarizing. A dissociation of the receptor potential and the nerve spike can also be shown in other stimulus situations. The most effective stimulus for eliciting spike responses from Pacinian corpuscles is rapid vibration. Sato (1961) has demonstrated that both receptor potentials and spikes are produced with vibratory stimuli. It was possible, however, with a high-enough rate of vibration to produce receptor potentials but no spike discharges. It is apparent that the Pacinian corpuscle receptor potential is not directly related to the type of information processed and sent to the central nervous system via the peripheral sensory nerve fiber; and, therefore, measures on this potential are of little value in studying information processing and transmission in the peripheral nervous system.

Most unit slow potentials recorded from CNS neurons have been elicited by electrical stimulation of the inputs to the neuron. Electrical stimulation of an input to a neuron may or may not bear any relationship to the input which would arise when they are naturally activated. When natural stimuli (sound or muscle stretch, for example) are used to stimulate the input to a neuron, the polarity, level, and time course of the intracellularly recorded events are not always correlated with the generation of spike potentials by the neuron. According to Gerstein, Butler, and Erulkar (1968), depolarizing potentials recorded from cat cochlear nucleus cells in response to tonal stimuli applied to the ears were related to the generation of spike potentials in one group of neurons and to the inhibition of spike production in another group of neurons. Also, spikes were generated by a neuron at different slow potential levels that varied from one spike to the next. For some neurons there was a lack of correlation between spike generation and the intracellularly recorded slow potential. Granit, Kellerth, and Williams (1964a) report observing inhibition of spike production that occurred without the expected hyperpolarization of ventral-horn neurons when muscle stretch was used at the natural stimulus. Both Gerstein et al. (1968) and Granit et al. (1964b) argue that this lac k of expected correlation between slow potential shifts and spike generation or inhibition was due to the remoteness of the recording electrode with respect to the spike generator area of the neuron. Thus, under conditions of natural stimulation, the intracellularly recorded slow potentials may be of such a localized nature that they may or may not be related to the generation of spike potentials; and, therefore, may or may not be related to neural transmission within the sensory nervous system.

UNIT SPIKE POTENTIALS

It should be obvious by now that the preferred measure for studying the function of neurons within sensory systems is the spike potential. Spike potentials are rapid electrical transients that are indicative of activity being transmittedfrom one part of a nerve cell to another (Tasaki 1959). Pulses are produced by the transient reversal in cell polarity that travels along the length of the neuron. In sensory ganglion cells the normal mode of transmission is from the periphery to the central nervous system over the dendrites and axons of the nerve cells. Nerve fibers are nondirectional, however, and pulses may be transmitted in either direction. Conduction of nerve impulses in a direction away from the dendrites toward the soma is called "orthodromic" or "dromic" conduction, while the reverse, from axon to cell body, is referred to as "antidromic" conduction. All spikes produced by a single unit are considered to be identical in waveform and amplitude and are transmitted in a nondecremental manner. These observations constitute the "all or nothing" law of neural-pulse transmission of sensory information (Adrian, 1928).

Spike potentials can be recorded from the long dendrites and axons of sensory ganglion cells (Fig. 4-1). They can also be recorded from cell bodies of many neurons, including the sensory ganglion cells. Darien-Smith *et al.* (1965) have estimated that the pulse coming in over a sensory ganglion cell dendrite reaches the central nervous system before it reaches the ganglion cell body; the spike recorded from the soma of the pseudounipolar sensory ganglion cell apparently represents a nonpropagated terminal discharge. Spike potentials apparently cannot be recorded from short dendrites or short axons or from certain cell bodies. It is probable that spikes are produced by neurons only when the activity is to be transmitted over long distances.

For neurons with only one axon, the entire output of a cell must be channeled through that axon. If an electrode records the spike traffic in that axon, an electrical measure is available of the entire output of the cell. Spikes can be recorded both intracellularly and extracellularly from nerve cells or fibers, although in sensory neurophysiology extracellularly placed electrodes are usually preferred to avoid the risk of cell injury with intracellular electrodes. Since all spikes from a single neural unit are considered to be identical in size and shape, the amplitude of spike potentials is unimportant, provided the spikes can be consistently distinguished from either noise or spikes from other units. Measurements consist of counting or otherwise determining the temporal distribution of spike potentials. Whereas there are various uncertainties attending the interpretation of group potentials or unit slowpotentials, no such uncertainties prevail in the consideration of spike trains.

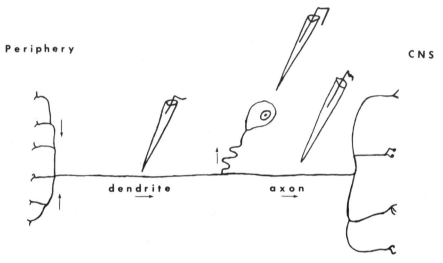

Fig. 4-1. Vertebrate. Spike potentials may be recorded from dendrites, axons, and cell bodies of sensory ganglion cells, as indicated by location of electrodes. The normal direction of pulse transmission is indicated by arrows.

EXPERIMENTAL METHODS IN SENSORY NEUROPHYSIOLOGY

As our earlier chapters indicate, sensory neurophysiology is the study of the function of sensory nervous systems, a function that is broadly defined as the processing of sensory information. Sensory neurophysiology is at a stage of development where the basic activity of experimentation is the observation and quantitative description of sensory neural phenomena. We are presently in the process of collecting data (facts), of developing statements of empirical relationships (mathematical models) between these facts, and classifying these facts and relationships into ordered sets. There are basically two types of data collected in an experiment: measures of stimulus conditions that affect sensory neural activity (stimulus variables or parameters), and measures of spike discharge (response variables) that characterize sensory neural activity. Any stimulus or response variable that can be used to characterize and classify a neuron is a relevant variable to be studied. Thus, studies of spontaneous (nonexperimentor controlled) activity and studies involving measures (stimulus parameters and response variables) of the effects of electrical stimulation of a neuron are relevant to the area of sensory neurophysiology. Quantitative measures of the relevant variables are desirable, for they make possible comparison and use of the results of different investigators. They also form a basis for classification and for describing the stimulus-response relationships in mathematical or graphic form.

EXPERIMENTAL VARIABLES

A sensory system is part of a living or biological system, the organism, and it is affected by numerous internal and environmental variables. In most sensory neurophysiological studies, the variables of interest to the investigator are stimulus parameters and response measures. Experiments are usually designed to minimize the number of extraneous variables affecting the organism, and to control those variables that cannot be omitted so that their effects can be evaluated. Experimental variables such as the health of the animal, the condition of the receptor organ, the anesthetic, the body temperature of the animal, etc., are important influences upon the results of an experiment and should therefore be controlled. They must be controlled with care, to permit replications of experiments that are desired to check results, and to form a basis for estimating the variability of these results.

One important experimental condition that influences the outcome of experiments in sensory neurophysiology is the method of preparation of the animal for experimentation. The method selected determines the general condition or health of the animal and the degree to which such conditions as state of alertness, sleep, and wakefulness can vary during the course of an experiment. A method of preparing the animal that results in a deteriorating condition—e.g., abnormal fluctuations in blood pressure or poor respiration, resulting in gradual death—can only produce results that are typical of dying organisms. Conditions such as state of alertness are known to affect the response of whole organisms to sensory stimuli, and one must assume until it is disproven that they also affect the response of neurons in the sensory nervous system. Although a state of unconsciousness is not the state at which organisms normally use their sensory input, it is a highly stable condition that controls factors such as alertness, fear, and motivation that are difficult, if not impossible, to control and measure in an awake organism placed in a strange environment.

THE PREPARATION

Electrical recordings are usually taken from what is called an "acute preparation." An acute preparation is one in which the animal is sacrificed after the experiment either for histological purposes, or because the surgical exposure is too radical to effect a simple closure. The types of acute preparations most commonly used are heavily anesthetized preparations or decerebrate preparations. Most sensory neurophysiological investigators have elected to utilize deeply anesthetized preparations, usually barbiturate anesthetized, because the animal is unconscious and because use of other pharmacological agents is not required to immobilize the preparation. With proper administration of the anesthetic, the preparation can be held in a deeply anesthetized state for the duration of the experiment. In decerebrate preparations, the brain is usually transected at about the midbrain level, producing an animal with a disconnected forebrain. This condition is a pathological one resulting from destruction of nervous tissue that is often followed by an edemic reaction in the surviving tissue. The brain may swell and occlude blood vessels in the cranial cavity, which results in the slow degeneration of all brain tissues. We have had experience recording from single units in the brain stem of animals made decerebrate anemically; i.e., by ligation of the carotid and vertebral arteries. In our experience, even when anemic decerebration works, the preparation is unstable and pathological.

Because barbiturates sometimes influence the discharge characteristics of neurons, some investigators have chosen to use lightly anesthetized or even unanesthetized acute preparations, in the latter case with all incisions usually infiltrated with a local anesthetic. These lightly anesthetized or unanesthetized preparations can respond to noxious stimuli if they have not been paralyzed. Because these preparations are not fully anesthetized, they must be immobilized with a paralyzing agent often used in combination with a second paralyzing agent. Thus, to avoid one drug, multiple drugs are often used in combination. Paralyzing the preparation may insure a stationary relationship between the stimulus and the receptor organ, but no one is certain of the internal state of the preparation and of its variability. Although precautions can be made to make the experimental animal as comfortable as possible, the animal may be in a highly excited and alarmed state initially in the experiment. It may later "calm down" and vary from a state of wakefulness to sleep during the course of the rest of the experiment. Lightly anesthetized paralyzed preparations appear to be extremely unstable in that single unit responses recorded from such preparations are often non-stationary and highly variable.

Only after we have gained some insight as to the stimulus parameters encoded by a neural structure, and have gained some knowledge of sensory encoding processes under highly stable conditions, will it be feasible to attempt to investigate sensory processing by a preparation in its normal state. The chronic preparation is an unanesthetized, fully conscious, mobile preparation from which single unit activity can be recorded. Recording electrodes are implanted and secured under anesthetic. The animal is allowed to recover from the operation with these electrodes in place. The use of chronic preparations in sensory neurophysiology has been strictly limited to date, although it is expected to increase. One such chronic preparation has been used to record from fibers in the auditory nerve (Simmons and Linehan, 1968).

SPIKE-POTENTIAL RECORDING TECHNIQUES

There are several techniques commonly used by sensory neurophysiologists to measure the spike activity of single units in sensory systems. The

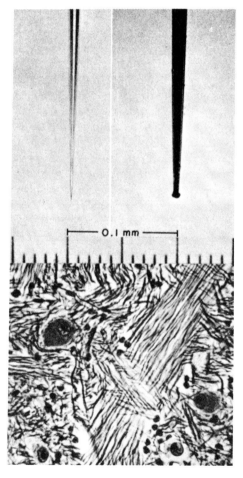

Fig. 4-2. Cat. Two types of electrodes used to record from neural units. Left: Fluid-filled glass micropipette. Right: Metal-filled glass pipette with platinum black tip. Below electrodes is a silver stained (Bodian protargol) section through the cochlear nucleus showing cell bodies and fibers. (Kiang, 1965)

technique depends to a great extent on the type of surgical preparation to be studied. For a study of the spike response in nerve fibers, the technique of dissection is commonly applied. With dissection the nerve bundle is reduced to smaller and smaller filaments until only a single active fiber is left. The small filament is then lifted onto a large wire electrode. Spike activity in fibers can also be studied by inserting a glass (Miller et al., 1962) or metal (Pubols et al., 1965) microelectrode into the nerve bundle. The glass-electrode technique has been utilized for recording from both dendrites or axons of sensory ganglion cells, although it does not work for unmyelinated fibers (Burgess et al., 1968). If the neurophysiologist desires to record from cell bodies, metal electrodes (Hubel, 1957; Marg, 1964) are most often used. There are several different types of metal and glass microelectrodes (Burns, 1961; Gestland et al., 1959; Frank and Becker, 1964). Examples of a micropipette and a metal electrode (Dowben and Rose, 1953) can be seen in Fig. 4-2.

It is desirable to know the anatomical location of a unit from which one has recorded spike potentials when recording in a ganglion or a nucleus in the central nervous system. There are several techniques for marking the site of recording. When tungsten electrodes are used, a small lesion in the tissue can be made by passing current through the electrode. This lesion can subsequently be viewed in a histological section through the brain. Another technique for marking a recording site is to pass current through a stainless steel microelectrode (Green, 1958). The electric current etches off the small metal tip and deposits iron in the neural tissue. By staining this iron deposit with potassium ferrocyanide or ferricyanide (Brown and Tasaki, 1961), one forms a brilliant blue dot by the Prussian blue reaction. A more recent and more exact technique of localizing a unit is to stain the neuron with intracellular injections of dyes through a micropipette (Thomas and Wilson, 1966; Henriques and Sperling, 1966). This procedure stains the neuron and its processes (Fig. 4-3).

Spike potentials may have different shapes and polarities depending upon where one records them. Spikes recorded from fibers with glass pipettes are positive in polarity and monophasic in shape. Spikes recorded extracellularly from ganglion cells apparently may be positive or negative in polarity (Zucker and Welker, 1969; Boudreau et al., 1971) and may have an inflection on the initial rising phase (Bessou et al., 1971). Spikes recorded from cells in the central nervous system are usually negative, but Rosenthal et al. (1966) have described spike potentials from central nervous system neurons of the cortex that vary in polarity from negative to positive, depending upon the extracellular location of the electrode. Spike potentials recorded from cells in the central nervous system are quite frequently biphasic in that they have pronounced positive and negative peaks. In a few cases the shape of the spike can be used to determine the type of cell producing it. In the auditory system, for instance, negative potentials preceded by a small positive potential are seen only in the anterior ventral cochlear nucleus and in the medial trapezoid nucleus (Pfeiffer, 1966).

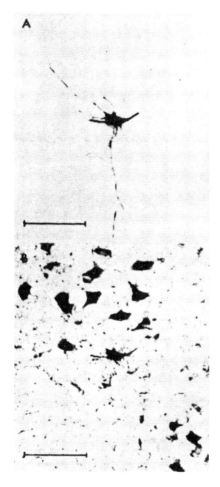

Fig. 4-3. Cat. Intracellular marking with dye from a micropipette of a cell in the central nervous system. Motorneuron marked two hours before the end of the experiment by passing 1.8 μA for one minute through a methyl blue electrode. (A) Cell in unstained section; the staining of the dendrites is extensive. (B) The same after thionin staining, at the same magnification. Some of the dendritic stain has been lost. Scale, 200μ.(Thomas and Wilson, 1966.) Copyright 1966 by the American Association for the Advancement of Science.

SAMPLING

Because there are a large number of sensory neurons in all peripheral sensory systems and because it is impossible to record from all these neurons in any single preparation, an investigator can study only a small portion of the total population of sensory neurons in a peripheral sensory nerve or sensory ganglion. There are many methods for sampling a population of elements.

Most neuroanatomical and neurophysiological studies have relied upon the use of "model" or "judgment" sampling. In judgment sampling, expert choice is used by the investigator to pick "typical" or "representative" results. The difficulty with this method is that experts often hold differing views on the best way to choose representative results or to decide which results are the most representative. Also, judgment sampling depends heavily upon the validity of broad assumptions about the properties and distributions of components within the population. On the other hand, if the population is sampled randomly with unbiased methods, inferences about the population can be made entirely by statistical methods. The ideal method of sampling a population is one in which the probability of selecting any one component in the population is equal. It is difficult to attain this goal because in most cases biased measuring techniques—e.g., the type of microelectrode used—may result in a biased sampling of the neurons making up a population. However, as long as an investigator studies each neuron encountered in the population (subjecting each to the same experimental and stimulus conditions, and obtaining measures from all neurons encountered), the measures obtained from the sample may be considered an unbiased estimate of that segment of the population sampled.

STIMULUS VARIABLES

A sensory stimulus is any physical or chemical agent that when applied to a receptor organ elicits a spike discharge from the sensory neuron under study. Four basic classes of naturally occurring sensory stimuli are electromagnetic (light), ther.nal, chemical, and mechanical; the latter includes acoustic, skin, joint, vestibular, and muscle-system stimuli. In addition, all neurons are responsive to electric current applied to the receptor or neuron itself. In most cases, sensory neurons can be activated by the application of several forms of energy to their receptor organ. Neurons of the visual system can be activated by light, mechanical, and electrical energy applied to the eye, all three eliciting sensations of light. Neurons of the skin system can be activated by mechanical, thermal, and electrical energy applied to the skin. The different types of stimuli capable of activating a sensory neuron are called "effective stimuli"; and the stimulus that requires the least amount of energy to activate a sensory neuron, the "adequate stimulus." Neurons within a given sensory system can be characterized and classified into subsystems on the basis of the form of the adequate stimulus. For example, the skin system can be subdivided into groups of neurons that respond best (with lowest threshold) to thermal stimuli, and those that respond best to mechanical stimuli.

Sensory stimuli can be characterized by stimulus parameters that may be controlled and measured by an investigator. The three parameters that are common to all sensory stimuli are: (1) the energy level, concentration, or intensity of the stimulus; (2) the temporal pattern or duration of the stimulus; and (3) the spatial distribution of the stimulus. A simple visual stimulus is also characterized by its wavelength, a simple auditory stimulus by its frequency. Chemical stimuli can be characterized by many parameters such as the elements contained within the basic compound forming the stimulus—the compound acidity, size, configuration, solubility, etc. When a change in the value of a stimulus parameter results in an alteration in activity of a sensory neuron, that stimulus parameter may be considered an input signal (sensory information) to be encoded by the sensory neuron. All of the stimulus parameters that can be used to characterize a sensory stimulus do not necessarily serve as input signals to a sensory system. The stimulus parameters that do serve as input signals are determined by the capacity of the organism's sensory system to handle those signals. Behavioral studies designed to measure psychophysically the capabilities of a sensory system provide a great deal of information concerning the stimulus parameters that may serve as input signals to that sensory system. However, psychophysical studies of the cat's skin, joint, muscle, vestibular, and chemosensory systems are largely lacking. An investigator must often use his neurophysiological preparation to determine the stimuli and the characteristics of the adequate stimulus that act as input signals to the system under study, as well as to determine the manner in which the input signals are processed.

The more precise the control over the stimulating conditions, the more accurate are the determinable quantitative relationships between stimulus and response measures. Stimulus control is an ever-present problem in sensory neurophysiological investigations. In a proper sensory investigation, stimulus control keeps evolving as the workers discover more and more stimulus parameters that need investigation. In the initial stages of an investigation, stimulus control is often crude since the investigators usually don't know what stimulus parameters are important in eliciting discharge. The study in this book of the skin senses and the chemical senses is largely in this primitive stage of stimulus-control development. The most advanced stimulus control is found in auditory experiments.

RESPONSE VARIABLES

The basic responses recorded from sensory neurons are spike potential discharges. Spike discharges recorded in the absence of an experimenter-controlled stimulus are called "spontaneous discharges" or "spontaneous activity." The spike discharges recorded in the presence of a stimulus assumed constant throughout the duration of an experiment are referred to as "resting" or "background discharges." An "evoked" or "elicited discharge" is activity that is time-locked with the onset of an experimenter-controlled stimulus of relatively brief duration. All three types of spike discharges or spike trains are subject to analysis, as will be described in the section to follow. In addition to the measures derived from spike-train analysis, measures of types of effective and adequate stimuli, stimulus parameters that serve as input signals and threshold and receptive field measures are often routinely obtained in sensory neurophysiological experiments.

To determine the nature of the stimuli and stimulus parameters affecting a sensory neuron, an investigator must examine the response of a neuron to a variety of likely stimuli and stimulus parameters. The threshold of a neuron to a given stimulus is described as that stimulus intensity necessary to elicit a just-noticeable evoked discharge or a predetermined level of discharge. Any stimulus that elicits a discharge is called an "effective stimulus"; that stimulus eliciting a discharge with the lowest threshold is known as the "adequate stimulus." The area of the receptor organ that upon stimulation with an effective stimulus elicits a discharge from a sensory neuron is termed "the receptive field" of that neuron. In most sensory systems the receptive field of a sensory neuron is related to the location of that neuron within the neural structure sampled, i.e., the location of a cell body in a ganglion or nucleus or of a nerve fiber in a nerve, root, or tract. Receptive field measures in combination with histological studies of recording electrode position are often utilized to describe the topological representation of the receptor organ in the neural structure under investigation.

ANALYSIS OF SPIKE TRAINS

A spike train is a temporal sequence of spikes or pulses produced by a neuron. In neural spike processing, all spikes from the same neuron are considered to be identical and to be completely specified by their times of occurrence (Perkel et al., 1967a). Thus, the method of studying spike trains is to precisely describe times of occurrence of the different spikes. Quantitative measures of spike trains can be determined from filmed records of the discharge, by feeding the spike into a counting device, or by processing the spike train with a digital computer. Examples of response measures are latency to first spike of a stimulus-elicited spike train, the total number of spikes in a train, the discharge level or rate in spikes per unit of time, and the average interval between spikes (the reciprocal of discharge rate). By describing quantitatively response variables that characterize the spike trains recorded from a neuron, we quantify the output from that neuron. A comparison of the response variables characterizing the spike train and the stimulus variables eliciting changes in the spike train enables the neurophysiologist to determine quantitatively the means by which information is processed in the nervous system. Inhibition is defined as a decrease in discharge produced by a stimulus.

The different techniques for quantitatively describing spike trains have been described in some detail by Perkel *et al.* (1967a) and Moore *et al.* (1966). In this section we will deal with only a few of the techniques for describing spontaneous activity and elicited discharge patterns so that the reader may understand some of the measures presented in our data chapters (Chapters 6 to 12).

Statistical analyses of spike trains provide quantitative measures of the output of the neuron that may be used for description, comparison, and classification. Most statistical measures of spike activity assume that the activity is stationary, i.e., that its statistical properties do not fluctuate over time, in the case of spontaneous and resting discharge or with repetition of the stimulus in the case of stimulus-elicited discharge. Because specific tests for stationarity of spike trains do not exist, it is difficult to detect and assess the effects of nonstationarity. One method of testing for stationarity of spontaneous or resting activity is to segment the spike train, analyze each segment separately, and test to determine if these sample segments were drawn from the same population. Statistical techniques can be used to detect non-homogeneity in mean rate, mean interspike interval, variance, or other measures of the sampled segments. Trend analysis can also be used for investigating nonstationarities. Individual spikes in most stimulus-elicited spike trains are time dependent. However, if this dependency is the same for each stimulus presentation, all spike trains elicited by the repetitive presentation of the same stimulus are considered to be stationary over all stimulus presentations. If the statistical properties of the stimulus-evoked spike trains do not differ significantly from one stimulus presentation to the next, they are considered to be "stationary." The following analyses of interspike time intervals require that the spike train sampled remain stationary over time.

A measure commonly obtained in sensory neurophysiological studies is the mean rate of discharge, which is calculated by counting the number of spikes occurring in a designated time interval. A higher level of spike-train analysis involves interspike interval time measurements. The interspike interval (ISI) histogram is a frequency histogram of the intervals between successive spikes. Fig. 4-4 illustrates the types of ISI histograms generated by spontaneous-activity spike trains of four types of cochlear nuclear units (Rodieck *et al.*, 1962). The irregularly discharging units 259-2 and 240-1 form ISI histograms that are unimodal and asymmetrical, although they are on different time scales. The ISI histogram of the regularly discharging unit R-4-10 is unimodal and symmetrical. The ISI histogram of unit 261-1 is more complicated because the unit discharged in bursts; thus, there are two peaks in the ISI histogram, one corresponding to the intervals between spikes in a burst, and the other corresponding to the intervals between the bursts. Multiple-peaked ISI histograms do not necessarily indicate recurring

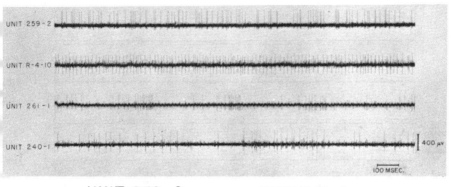

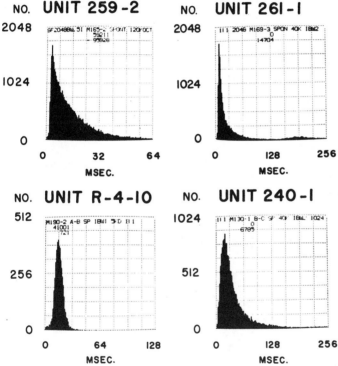

Fig. 4-4. Cat. Upper: Photograph of oscilloscope display of spontaneous activity of four cochlear nucleus units. Lower: Interspike interval histograms of the spontaneous activity of the four units pictured above. (Rodieck *et al.*, 1962.)

bursting in a spike train. A sharp shift in mean discharge rate can also produce a multiple-peaked ISI histogram.

Statistical analysis of interspike interval distributions involves the estimation of the various parameters of the probability distribution of the interspike intervals based upon the sampled spike train. Statistical measures such as mean interval, mode interval, variance, standard deviation, coefficient of variation (standard deviation/mean), measures of skewness and kurtosis can be used to describe the interspike interval distribution. The underlying probability-density function of the interspike interval distribution describes the probability that a neuron will discharge during a time interval elapsed from the occurrence of the immediately preceding spike. The probability-density function and the interspike-interval distribution completely characterize the distribution of a stationary spike train consisting of spikes whose intervals are statistically independent.

Interspike interval measures are not sensitive to the ordering of the intervals sampled and produce order-independent statistical measures. To determine the independence of successive intervals, certain statistical measures have been used to test for, describe, and quantify serial dependence among interspike intervals. The joint-interval histogram, a scatter diagram of pairs of adjacent or successive intervals, was first introduced by Rodieck, Kiang, and Gerstein (1962).

Joint-interval histograms can be plotted for nonadjacent intervals. The kth-order joint-interval histogram is formed by plotting the interval between two adjacent spikes (Si and Si+1) as a function of the interval between two other adjacent spikes (Si+k and Si+k+1), k interspike intervals away. Serial correlation coefficients can be calculated for each order of joint-interval histogram, and plotted as a function of the serial position of the interval to form a serial correlogram (Fig. 4-5). A zero correlogram, within statistical fluctuations, is a necessary condition for independence of intervals (Fig. 4-5,a). Spike trains with serial dependence among intervals produce distinctive serial correlograms, some of which are described by Perkel, Moore, and Segundo (1967). Bursting spike trains produce a dampened oscillation in the serial correlogram (Fig. 4-5, b and c). Regular alterations between long and short interval lengths produce regularly oscillating correlograms (Fig. 4-5, e). Nonstationary, slow oscillations in discharge rate also produce oscillatory serial correlograms. Long-term nonstationary trends, monotonic increases or decreases in discharge rates, contribute a positive component to each serial correlation coefficient (Fig. 4-5, d).

The autocorrelation function involves the time intervals between non-successive spikes. The autocorrelation histogram or autocorrelogram specifies the averaged time sequence of spike potentials following a given spike. The autocorrelogram is formed by accumulating the times following a given spike where other spikes occur, with each spike in a spike train forming the first spike from which the times of occurrence of following spikes are measured. Autocorrelograms differ from serial correlograms in that the former is a function of time; the latter, of the serial position of the interval. The autocorrelation histogram is the sum of the interval distributions of the first-

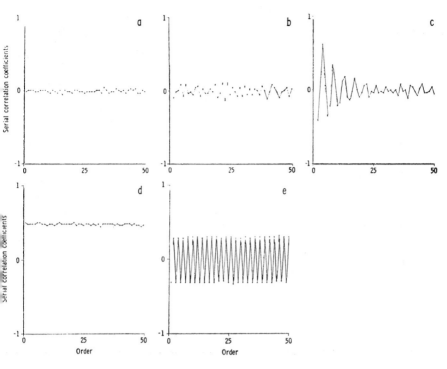

Fig. 4-5. Computer-simulated discharge. Serial correlograms of: a, spike train in which interspike intervals are statistically independent; b, spike train containing irregular bursts of spikes; c, spike train with regular bursting; d, spike train in which mean discharge rate is decreasing monotonically; and e, spike train consisting of alternating long and short interspike intervals. The serial correlogram is a plot of the serial correlation coefficient as a function of the serial position of the interspike interval. Perkel, D.H., Gerstein, G.L. and Moore, G.P. (1967a). Neuronal spike trains and stochastic point processes. I. The single spike train. *Biophys. J.* 7:391-418. Used with the permission of the authors.

order intervals (the interval between successive spikes), the second-order intervals (the interval between a spike and the second spike following), the third-order intervals (the interval between a spike and the third spike following), etc. To test for statistical independence of interspike intervals, the autocorrelation of a spike train is compared with the autocorrelation of the spike train after it has undergone prolonged random shuffling. The shuffling removes any serial dependence in the spike train, but preserves the properties of the original interspike interval distribution. The autocorrelogram produced by the shuffled spike train represents a control case of serial independence. Differences between the autocorrelations of the unshuffled and shuffled spike trains provide a test of serial dependence and indicate the nature of the dependence.

Elicited spike discharges require different types of statistical measures, although time-interval analyses have been used to describe them. Examples of common stimulus-elicited spike trains are illustrated in Fig. 4-6. The stimulus onset is indicated by the ramp curve. Two different types of neural discharge elicited by this stimulus are indicated in the figure. One unit discharges a few spikes only at the onset of the stimulus, whereas the other unit discharges throughout the stimulus duration, although at a somewhat decremental rate. Unit discharge that occurs only at stimulus onset will be known as a "phasic" discharge, while discharge maintained for the duration of the stimulus will be called a "tonic" discharge. In much of sensory literature, the first type is known as a rapidly adapting response, and the second as a slowly adapting discharge. "Adaptation," however, is an interpretive concept and not a descriptive term; as such it has caused endless difficulties and so will not be used in this book.

A customary method of representing stimulus-evoked spike trains is to plot the distribution of spikes in time relative to the onset of the stimulus. The

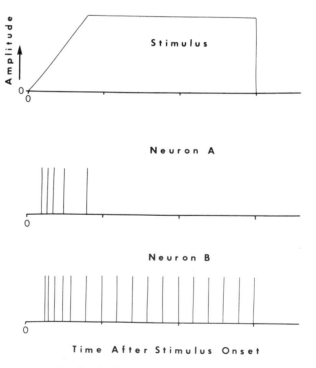

Fig. 4-6. Common types of pulse discharge from two different units to a stimulus applied tonically. Unit A discharges only while the stimulus is changing. This discharge pattern is phasic to this type of stimulus. Unit B discharges tonically to the stimulus.

histogram generated is called the "Post-Stimulus Time histogram" or "PST histogram." The time following stimulus onset is represented on the abscissa in units of time intervals, and the number of spikes that fall into each time interval is represented on the ordinate. Although PST histograms are usually formed by spike trains summed over many repeated stimulus presentations, they may also be formed by the response to a single stimulus presentation. PST histograms of the phasic and tonic discharge illustrated in Fig. 4-6 are presented in Fig. 4-7. A peak in the PST histogram represents a preferred time of spike discharge relative to stimulus onset. The PST histogram illustrates the time relations of the spikes in a train to the stimulus, and emphasizes spike activity that is time-locked to the stimulus. Most spike trains elicited by relatively brief-duration stimuli do not have the characteristic of being stationary over time. It is most often the case that

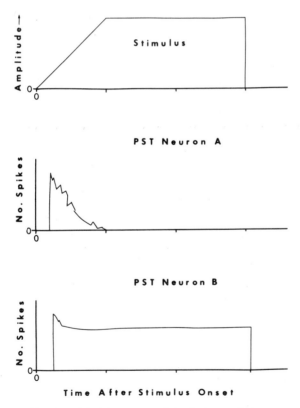

Fig. 4-7. Post-Stimulus-Time (PST) histograms of the discharge of the two units illustrated in Fig. 4-6. In PST histograms the discharge to one or more stimuli is plotted against time. Unit A shows phasic discharge, unit B tonic discharge.

sensory-neuron discharge rate declines from an initial maximum rate following stimulus onset (Fig. 4-7). In some cases, individual spikes in the stimulus-elicited spike train may be time-locked to stimulus onset or to other characteristics of the stimulus.

While PST histograms are useful in studying spike trains that are time-locked to the stimulus, certain aspects of the spike train are lost in calculating PST histograms—for example, the time sequence of spikes contributing to the histogram. Thus, one cannot determine in a multiple-peaked PST histogram whether the spikes occurring in the interval corresponding to the second peak of the histogram were preceded by a spike in the interval corresponding to the first peak. Conditional probability analyses involve the description of the sequence of interspike intervals relative to the onset of the stimulus (Gray, 1966). In this type of analyses, the probability of a spike occurring in a specified time interval relative to stimulus onset, given that the last firing occurred during an earlier time, can be estimated. Thus, the probability that a spike will occur in the interval corresponding to the second peak of the PST histogram, given that the last firing occurred during the interval corresponding to the first peak, can be determined.

RESPONSE TO ELECTRICAL STIMULATION

The response of a neuron to electrical stimulation can also be utilized to characterize and classify sensory neurons. Different nerve fibers conduct at different velocities, with unmyelinated fibers conducting more slowly than myelinated fibers. Instead of conducting impulses continuously along the fiber as do unmyelinated fibers, myelinated fibers conduct in a saltatory fashion in that depolarization proceeds from node to node (Tasaki, 1959). Saltatory conduction is more rapid than continuous conduction. Fibers of the same type (myelinated or unmyelinated) may conduct at different velocities. The conduction velocity of a myelinated neuron is directly proportional to the diameter of the fiber (Fig. 4-8). Conduction velocities of myelinated peripheral nerves can be estimated by multiplying the fiber diameter by a factor of six (Hursh, 1939). This factor seems approximate except for small myelinated fibers (Burgess et al., 1968).

Conduction velocity estimates are made from measures of the latency of a spike following an electrical stimulus, and the distance between the point at which the electrical stimulus was applied and the spike recorded. Velocity estimates made from different parts of a nerve fiber and from the central and peripheral processes of sensory ganglion cells indicate that the conduction velocity of a neuron may differ along its length. According to Iggo (1958), the conduction velocities of the peripheral (dendritic) processes of vagus nodose ganglion neurons are greater near the ganglion than they are peripherally near their terminus. Petit and Burgess (1968) report the conduction velocity estimates of the axonal processes of dorsal-root ganglion cells within the spinal cord were less than those of their dendritic processes in the peripheral nerves. Petit and Burgess (1968) recorded from single fibers in the sural nerve and stimulated these fibers electrically at three points: in the cervical spinal cord, the thoracic spinal cord, and the sciatic nerve. Conduction velocity estimates of the central processes within the spinal cord were calculated from latency differences between spikes elicited with cervical and thoracic spinal

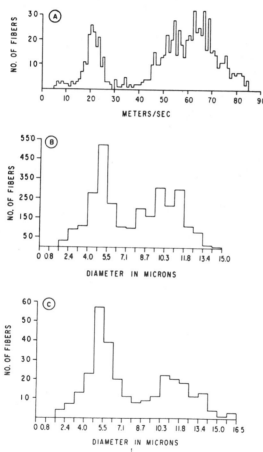

Fig. 4-8. Cat. Comparison of fiber diameter and conduction velocity estimates in a cutaneous peripheral nerve, the sural nerve. A: Sural microelectrode sample (841 fibers). Conduction velocities of all sural fibers studied with microelectrodes. This population is unselected in the sense that every fiber providing a stable potential was included. B: Diameters of the 2,864 fibers found in four sural nerves as determined with the light microscope. An effort was made to measure all the fibers in the four nerves. C: Diameters of 294 randomly selected fibers from two sural nerves as measured from electron micrographs. (Burgess et. al., 1968)

cord stimulation. Conduction velocity estimates of peripheral processes were calculated from the latencies of the spikes with respect to the time of electrical stimulation of the sciatic nerve. Mei (1970) has demonstrated a similar phenomenon for the neural processes of the nodose ganglion of the vagus nerve.

The duration or the width of the spike potential is also related to the size of the nerve fiber (Iggo, 1958; Paintal, 1967). The smaller the fiber, the longer the duration of the spike (Fig. 4-9). Spike width rapidly drops as the fiber diameter becomes larger. In Fig. 4-9, spike width is approximately constant for fibers with conduction velocity above 18 m/sec. The threshold of fibers to electrical stimulation is also related to the fiber diameter (Brown and Hayden, 1971). The smaller the fiber, the higher the threshold to electrical stimulation.

FACTORS AFFECTING VARIABILITY OF SPIKE MEASUREMENTS

There are various factors that may affect the reliability of the measures taken of the spike activity in the nervous system. Any change in spike activity not directly attributable to the stimulus will tend to weaken the quantitative stimulus response relationship sought in sensory neurophysiology. The most common types of variability encountered are those induced by the experimenter. Variability is most often introduced by the experimenter in the form of nonstandardized conditions or by the presence of the measuring instrument itself, the electrode (Stopp and Whitfield, 1963). Nonstandardized conditions can occur when recordings are taken from an animal in which the level of anesthetic fluctuates continuously throughout the experiment. Some investigators have minimized this factor by using long lasting anesthetics.

Injury discharges, a prime source of variability, are defined as changes in the firing pattern (either spontaneous or driven activity) that can be directly attributable to the presence of the electrode. The importance of recognizing injury discharge in a neuron is obvious since sensory neurophysiology involves the quantitative comparison of stimulus and spike-train measurements, and any induced variability in the latter will be reflected in this quantitative comparison and its interpretation.

The types of injury discharges observed depend upon the measuring technique used, whether fibers or cells are being studied and which group of cells one is studying. Fiber discharges studied by the glass-pipette recording technique apparently show few effects of injury since one either maintains contact with them, loses contact suddenly, or loses contact with a short transient burst of spikes. In all cases the change is easily detectable. Recording from fibers with the method of dissection can lead to injury

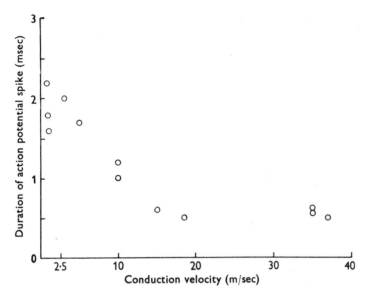

Fig. 4-9. Cat. The duration of the action-potential spike in single fibers dissected from the cervical vagus nerve, each point represents one fiber. (Iggo, 1958)

changes in the spike trains that can affect the measurements. The changes apparently manifest themselves in an erosion in the responsiveness of the fiber. As time goes by, the unit discharges less and less to a constant stimulus.

The type of injury discharge seen with cell-body recordings depends on the type of cell from which one is recording. In the sensory cells of the cat's geniculate ganglion, only the regular discharge units innervating the soft palate and pharynx have been observed to show injury discharges. Injury discharges took the form of a rapid increase in discharge that could often be produced by small advances of the electrode (Fig. 4-10). Geniculate ganglion units innervating the hairs in the inner surface of the ear, and those innervating the tongue, showed no such obvious changes that could be attributable to the presence of the electrode.

In the central nervous system, various types of injury discharge have been seen. Guinan (1969) reports, in recording from the medial trapezoid nucleus, that the complex waveform (positive-negative) of spike potentials generated by the primary type cells can be replaced by a positive-only potential. The most common form of injury discharge shown by neurons in the central nervous system is similar to that shown by the regular discharge units in the geniculate ganglion; i.e., there is an increase in rate of discharge with electrode advancement. This increase in rate may be seen in the spontaneous activity and in the stimulus-elicited discharge. This increase in activity may or may not be followed by loss of contact (frequently with a change in polarity and a "pop"). A more complicated form of injury has been reported for neurons in the cat's superior olive S-segment (Boudreau and Tsuchitani, 1970). S-segment neurons exhibit injury discharges of two types. The first is similar to the increase in discharge shown in Fig. 4-10. The other type is a decrease in spike output evidenced by a lower number of spikes elicited by successive stimuli, and an increase in the variability of intervals that culminate in a previously tonically discharging unit becoming a phasically discharging unit.

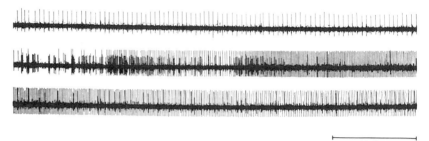

1.0 Sec.

Fig. 4-10. Cat. Injury discharge shown by a sensory ganglion cell in the geniculate ganglion. Top line: Spontaneous activity recorded from the unit before electrode movement. Middle and bottom lines: Increase in discharge occurring during electrode movement. All records continuous in time. (Boudreau et al., 1971.)

Another factor inducing variability in the spike measures is the previous history of stimulation of the cell under study. It has been demonstrated with chemoreceptive cells innervating the tongue that they may change their responsive properties with chemical stimulation (Kruger and Boudreau, 1972). Thus, an unstimulated neuron may respond differently to a stimulus from one that has already been stimulated with chemical substances.

There may also be differences between cats. The neurons recorded from one cat may differ from the neurons studied in another cat. In our own experience, this is a minor source of variability, since, barring pathology, cells from different animals usually differ little more than different cells from the same animal. It is this high degree of similarity among cells from the same sensory system that makes possible the pooling of data from different animals. In most cases, neural responses from different animals are quantitatively similar.

The final source of spike variability encountered is that introduced by differences between functionally distinct neurons. These functional differences may arise because the neurons are members of different sensory systems concerned with different things, or because they are members of the same sensory system but have different roles within that system. These sources of variability are the ones sensory neurophysiology must detect and quantify.

DATA ANALYSIS

The most difficult part of a sensory neurophysiological investigation is the analysis of the data to determine quantitative relationships between stimulus and response variables and between different response variables. With data analysis one uncovers hidden relationships and clarifies those suggested by early experiments. With data analysis cells are grouped into categories and aligned with respect to one another. Sensory neurophysiological data are analyzed by comparing different measures taken under standardized conditions. The quantitative relationships may be presented in either simple histogram form, by plotting one measurement against another, or by other graphic or mathematical manipulations. Examples of graphical presentation of data can be seen in many of the chapters to follow. When properly done, data analysis reveals unknown and frequently unexpected quantitative relationships. In an undeveloped research program, data analysis reveals the weaknesses in stimulus control and the inadequacies in the response measures. Thus, data analysis is frequently followed by a redesign of the experimental conditions.

In data analysis the quantitative description of stimulus and response variables and any mathematical equations relating them should be followed by the classification of data and the empirical rules relating them. Classification has proven to be of the utmost importance to the physical and chemical sciences, where it is possible to define classes precisely enough so that all members of a given class predictably possess properties used to define the class. Furthermore, all scientific laws are based upon classification.

Sensory neurons may be classified on the basis of the stimulus variables affecting them, the response variables characterizing their spike trains, and in terms of the stimulus-response relationships. Variables can be used to define classes when the distribution of their values for the entire sample appears to be heterogeneous. The aim of classification is to form classes or sets of neurons within which the sampled members are relatively homogeneous with respect to the variables used to define the sets. Their variances should be reduced to the extent that the variation among the sampled set is less than their variation in the entire sample. Each set of neurons may be subdivided into smaller sets on the basis of other defining variables. The more precisely the set is specified, the more likely it is that the properties of individual neurons will be shared by the whole set.

Sensory neurons have been differentiated on the basis of response to electrical stimulation. Neurons of the muscle system can be organized into separate sets on the basis of differences in the conduction velocity of their neural processes. The threshold or latency of discharge following electrical stimulation of the sensory receptors may form a basis for classifying neurons into sets, and the adequate stimulus and the stimulus parameters affecting the sensory neuron can be used to classify neurons . The presence or absence of spontaneous activity and the statistical properties of spontaneous activity may form another basis for classifying neurons into separate sets. Similarly, the statistics describing stimulus-evoked discharge trains may also form a basis for classification.

Statistical descriptions of spike trains can be used to characterize and classify neurons. The complexity of the statistical analyses required to describe a spike train differs, depending upon the complexity of the spike train. Stationary spike trains with statistically independent intervals are completely characterized by their interval, probability density, and autocorrelation functions. One of several renewal processes may be used to describe a stationary spike train of independent intervals (Perkel *et al.*, 1967a). The spontaneous activity of cochlear nerve fibers can be described by a Poisson process (Kiang *et al.*, 1965b); like the Poisson process the interspike intervals of cochlear nerve-fiber spontaneous activity are independent. The ISI distribution is a decaying exponential function for intervals longer than the mode interval. The one difference in the statistical properties of cochlear nerve fiber spontaneous activity and the Poisson process is a "dead time" for very short intervals in the ISI histogram of spontaneous activity. However, the Poisson process can describe the discharge of cochlear nerve-fiber spontaneous activity when this dead-time factor is included. Other types of renewal processes can be used to describe spike trains generating nonexponential ISI histograms (Perkel *et al.*, 1967a), provided the interspike intervals are independent. When there is serial dependence between intervals, more complicated statistical analyses are needed to describe the spike train. In special cases of highly patterned spike trains, the degree of complexity of analyses is not too great. In other cases, higher-order interval analyses are required to describe the temporal pattern of discharge. Every attempt should be made to describe the spike train with as few statistical parameters as is necessary to effect a reasonably complete description of the spike train.

5

THEORETICAL SENSORY NEUROPHYSIOLOGY

Strictly speaking, there does not exist any theoretical sensory neurophysiology worthy of the name. Theory in the most advanced sense consists of a mathematical equation or model from which naturally occurring events can be described and predicted. The model is used to represent a naturally occuring system, where a system is defined as a collection of interacting components. In order to develop an adequate model of a system, we must obtain certain basic facts about the system. A fact is a quantitative measure describing some aspect of the structure or function of a system; a theory is a model proposed to describe the order and relationship between an ensemble of facts. The value or utility of a theory is usually based upon its ability — first, to describe known events, and second, to predict events under new conditions. If sufficient facts are incorporated into a theory, the model can predict the response of the system to new conditions. Thus, experiments do not have to be performed on the system, and the model can be used to represent the system under all conditions. Theory in this sense does not exist in sensory neurophysiology because there are very few quantitative measures (facts) describing the structure or function of sensory systems.

Mathematical equations are just the best way to describe a system, not the only way. Prior to the formation of a mathematical model of a complex system, a great many preliminary measures must be taken from the system to determine the number and nature of the system components and some of their properties. Sensory neurophysiology is in this formative stage where the identification of components, and some of the relevant variables, is the major concern. In this stage of development, word or graphic models or other analogies are used to provisionally describe the system under study. In this chapter we will discuss three types of systems: the organism, the nervous system, and the peripheral sensory systems. No attempt is made to specify even a crude model for either the cat or the nervous system, since these systems are too complex. We will use only general word models to provide a proper orientation for the study of sensory systems.

The conceptual model that has been most useful to biology in the past is that an organism is a machine. By virtue of being a machine, different parts of the animal — sometimes even the whole animal — are described as physical systems whose properties can be measured by present techniques or advancements in present techniques. Thus, the circulatory system may be viewed as a hydraulic pumping system and the digestive system as a chemical processing system. The nervous system is that part of the organism that controls all other body parts and directs the organism in day-to-day activities by measuring all aspects of the outside world of concern to the animal, and by controlling and regulating all internal activities.

The types of sensory systems an animal possesses depends to a large extent upon the type of animal it is. Sensory systems are themselves parts of larger neural subsystems that in turn may be parts of even larger neural systems. All of these neural systems are parts of the whole animal, who is in turn a subsystem of a complexly interacting system of other animals, environmental conditions, and so forth. The occurence of some sensory systems are predictable to a certain extent if the animal is known to be a vertebrate or a bird or a mammal or what-have-you. In many cases, however, knowing that the animal is a mammal is insufficient for predicting what type or types of sensory systems will be contained in the organism, since sensory systems may be specifically modified for the particular type of animal. Sensory systems may be modified as well according to the basic design for the particular species.

The basic design of the *Felidae* is obvious. The primary role of the *Felidae* in nature is to kill and eat other animals. The *Felidae* are among the most specialized of the fissiped carnivores: Their front claws are rarely used for support during walking but are kept sheathed and sharp so that they may better grasp other animals. The teeth of the *Felidae* are only suited for eating other animals, and their digestive system is not made for digesting plant substances. The primary difference between most of the *Felidae* is one of size: The larger the species of *Felidae,* the larger the animals it preys upon. Modern *Felidae* evolved just a few million years ago to form one of the major groups of predators feeding on the recently evolved modern mammals. To prey upon these small mammals and other small creatures, small *Felidae* evolved. The basic design of the small *Felidae* is quite similar. As can be seen in Fig. 5-1, the small *Felidae* of Africa are basically similar in shape; similar nervous systems control the different species.

At this point we must digress somewhat and discuss a scientific field of immediate relevance to sensory neurophysiology: systems analysis. At

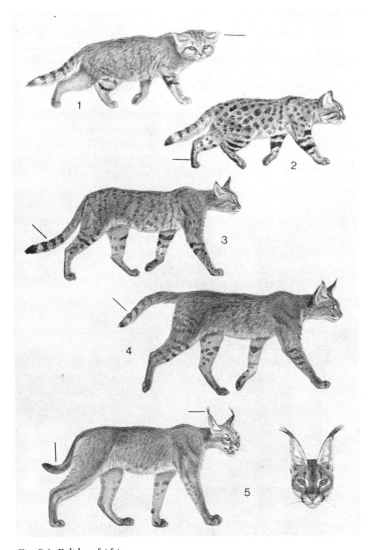

Fig. 5-1. *Felidae* of Africa.
1. Sand Cat, *Felis margarita*
   Small; broadened face; broad ears; almost uniformly sandy buff.
2. Black-footed cat, *Felis nigripes*
   Small; tawny, with large black spots; underparts of feet profusely black.
3. Wild cat, *Felis libyea*
   Larger; indistinct vertical stripes and spots; tail proportionately long.
4. Swamp cat, *Felis chaus*
   Fairly large; rather long legged; no conspicuous markings; ears pointed; tail proportionately
   short.
5. Caracal, *Felis caracal*
   Fairly large; long legged; ears pointed, with long black tassel; uniform reddish fawn.
Illustrated by P. Dandelot. From *A Field Guide to the Larger Mammals of Africa*, Dorst, J. &
Dandelot, P. (1970), Houghton Mifflin Co.

103

present, systems analysis provides much of the theoretical framework within which sensory systems are described and analyzed.

SYSTEMS ANALYSIS

A system can be defined as any single component, or any collection of communicating or interacting components, that performs some function in which an investigator is interested. The components of a system may take any form and may be a structure (a transistor, heart, neuron, or atom) or a force (gravity, magnetism, electricity, etc.). The system is affected by certain variables or input signals and produces an output that the investigator measures. Any aspect of the system may be considered an output, dependent only upon the particular interest of the investigator. All variables that affect the system output may be considered input signals to the system. Thus, a system may receive one or many input signals. An investigator may elect to omit variables from his model of a system, if the variables do not significantly affect the system output, or if the effect of the variable is dependent upon the presence of other input signals, or if the variable cannot be controlled or measured. The input signals and the output measured may take any form — e.g., frequency of a pure tone, amplitude of sound, electrical activity from a neuron. A system can therefore be represented schematically as an input-output device (Fig. 5-2), whose function it is to transform input signals into a system output. In this context, the following are examples of systems: an electrical amplifier, with voltage input and voltage output; the salivary glands, with neural input and saliva output; the heart-lung system, with de-oxygenated blood input and oxygenated blood output; a man, with verbal input and verbal output.

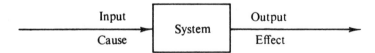

Fig. 5-2. Diagram of a system. In sensory systems the pulse output from single neurons is studied as a function of the stimulus input. The system is described in terms of its input-output properties. From Martens, H. R. and Allen, D. R., 1969 *Introduction to Systems Theory*, C. E. Merrill Publishing Co., Columbus, Ohio. Used with permission of the publisher.

A system may be described experimentally by subjecting it to measurable input signals and observing and measuring the output of the system. The system may be mathematically modeled by an equation that describes in the simplest terms possible the relationship between the input signals and the output measured. The experimental approach to systems is most useful when the system consists of one type of functioning component and the objective is the characterization of this component. However, in most cases a system is composed of an assembly of components that interact or communicate to perform the function in which the investigator is interested. According to the analytical approach to the study of systems, the character and behavior of a multi-component system is determined by the character and behavior of its individual components and by their mode of interaction.

It is a fundamental axiom of systems analysis that each component of a system can be characterized as an input-output device independent of the manner in which that component is interconnected with other components that form the system. Thus, each component of a system can be studied experimentally as a one-component system whose input-output function can be mathematically modeled independent of the system. Furthermore, an investigator can break down his system into any number of components of any level of complexity, provided the components selected can be studied experimentally and are simple enough to be modeled. It is also a basic axiom of systems analysis that a system of interacting components has certain properties that are not obvious properties of the components themselves. The properties of the system as a whole can be described by the rules of interaction between its components. In a system of interconnected components, the input signals of one component are formed by the outputs of other connected components, and the rules of interaction between components can be described by mathematical models describing the relationships between the outputs of the two connected components. Large-scale systems may be analyzed in terms of models of subsystems or sub-assemblies that have been analyzed in terms of their component and interconnection models.

ANALYTICAL APPROACH TO SENSORY SYSTEMS

A sensory system is a complex system of neural and non-neural tissues that serve to provide the non-sensory portion of the nervous system with information concerning the internal state of the body, the position and movement of body parts, or the state of the external environment. In Chapter 3 we classified sensory systems in terms of the body structure forming the receptor organ of the system — e.g., the skin, joint, muscle, visceral, vestibular, auditory, visual, olfactory, and gustatory systems. Each of these sensory systems consists of a non-neural receptor organ, sensory receptors, and sensory neurons. The receptor organ contains the sensory receptors and functions to deliver the stimulus to them. Sensory receptors are specialized nerve endings, neuroepithelial cells, or a complex of nerve endings and non-neural cells that function to measure and encode certain aspects of the internal and external environment (the sensory information). The neural portion of a sensory system consists of all nervous tissue that is involved in processing sensory information received by the sensory receptors. The neurons of a sensory system are usually grouped on the basis of location of their cell bodies into ganglia, nuclei, and cortical areas.

A sensory system is a system of communicating components that together perform the function of processing (encoding and transmitting) sensory information. The components of sensory systems are organized structurally and functionally into subsystems whose outputs serve as input signals to other subsystems of the sensory system. The receptor organ is a structure or system of structural elements that is interposed between the stimulus and the sensory receptors. Receptor organs function to deliver stimulus signals to the sensory receptors with a minimum loss of energy, and often transform the stimulus (input to the receptor organ) into an output that physically resembles but is not identical to the stimulus. For example, light beams reflected or emitted from a viewed object are transformed by the refractive media of the eye into an image that is brighter, smaller, and inverted with respect to the object viewed. The basic form of the stimulus (light) is maintained by the receptor organ and only certain parameters of the stimulus (intensity and spatial characteristics) are transformed. The receptor organ functions as an input-output device whose output serves as the source of input signals to sensory receptors located within it. A model describing the input-output transfer function of the receptor organ provides a means for calculating the receptor organ output without having to measure it directly, and thus provides a measure of the input signals applied to the sensory receptors. The transfer functions of the refractive media of the cat's eye have been described and modeled by Vakkur and Bishop (1963). The sound-pressure-level transfer functions of the outer and middle ear of the cat have also been measured and modeled, the former by Wiener et al, (1965) and the latter by Guinan and Peake (1967). The transfer function of the inner ear has only been grossly described and modeled from data based upon direct observation of the vibration pattern of the cochlear partition of the inner ear of mammals (Bekesy, 1960); and upon behavioral studies of frequency discrimination following destruction of segments of the cochlear partition of the cat's inner ear (Schuknecht, 1960). The transfer functions of the skin, joint, muscle, mouth, nose and vascular and vestibular receptor organs of the cat have not been studied in any great detail and adequate models of these receptor organ systems do not exist.

The output of the receptor-organ system serves as the source of input signals to the sensory receptors located within the receptor organ. The sensory receptors perform a transfer function upon these input signals to produce an output that does not resemble the stimulus or the receptor organ output. It is believed that the sensory receptors transform their input into the release of chemical transmitters or into changes in their electrical state. The released chemicals and/or receptor electrical activity are believed to serve as input signals to the peripheral sensory neurons that contact them. The transfer function of none of the mammalian sensory receptors is known, since no receptor output measure has been demonstrated to be consistently and quantitatively related to receptor-organ output or to the stimulus applied to the receptor organ. Furthermore, no measure of sensory-receptor output has been demonstrated to be consistently related to the spike output of sensory neurons innervating receptors.

The sensory receptors produce an output that provides input to peripheral sensory neurons contacting them (first-order sensory neurons). The peripheral sensory neurons are usually organized into subsystems of sensory ganglia, with neural processes located in nerves, roots, and tracts. The output from most peripheral sensory neurons can usually be measured in spike form. The spike outputs (or some transform of the spike train) of most peripheral sensory neurons serve as input signals to sensory neurons that are organized into spinal-cord or brain-stem nuclei (second-order sensory neurons). These spinal-cord and brain-stem sensory neurons act upon these inputs to produce a spike output that serves as an input to other sensory neurons (third-order sensory neurons), located either within the same nucleus or within other brain-stem nuclei, or that serves as an input to nonsensory neural subsystems. The third-order sensory neurons send their outputs to other sensory neurons (fourth-order sensory neurons) located in the same nucleus, in other brain-stem nuclei, or in a cortical area, or to nonsensory structures.

If the outputs of any neural structure (nucleus, nuclear complex, or cortical areas) of a sensory system could represent the "final" output of the entire sensory system, the stimulus information-processing function of the system could be described in terms of the stimulus applied to the receptor organ and the response recorded from neurons in that neural structure. However, there is no such neural structure in any of the sensory systems. All sensory information must first be processed by the peripheral sensory nervous system, but all sensory information processed by a given sensory system does not appear to be processed by each of the spinal-cord or brain-stem nuclei, thalamic nuclei, or cortical areas constituting a sensory system; that is, a single nucleus or cortical area appears to receive only part of the sensory information processed by the system as a whole. Also, it is highly probable that some sensory information may leave a sensory system at the level of the spinal cord or brain stem and may not reach "higher" sensory neural structures. Thus, sensory information processing by sensory nervous systems can only be studied by investigating the processing of sensory information by each of the neural structures making up the sensory nervous system.

To utilize the systems-analysis approach in the study of sensory systems, we must first identify the system component to study, characterize it independently of the system, and determine the variables that act as input signals to this component. Next, we must study quantitatively the relationship between system-component outputs and develop mathematical models of the functional structure of system-component communication in terms of input and output signals. We can then formulate a mathematical model for the entire system on the basis of these preliminaries.

In Chapter 3 we identified the single neuron as the basic functioning unit of the nervous system, and in Chapter 4 designated the single-unit spike potential as the most unambiguous measure of single-neuron functioning. We will now identify a neuron as a sensory neuron if the majority of the input signals entering the soma and/or dendrites of the neuron arise directly or indirectly, by way of interconnections with a chain of neurons, from the sensory receptor system. Thus, the input signals to a sensory neuron are represented primarily by the outputs of sensory receptors or of other sensory neurons to which it is connected. Although we can study some of the characteristics of a sensory neuron with electrical stimulation of the neuron as an input, we are unable to specify or measure naturally occurring input signals that can be functionally related to spike output of a sensory neuron. Investigators have not demonstrated any consistent functional relationships between any measure of receptor activity and the spike output of peripheral sensory neurons connected to a receptor, or any relationships between the spike outputs of interconnected sensory neurons. Because we cannot identify or measure the input signals to a sensory neuron, we will not at this time identify the sensory neuron as the sensory component of sensory nervous systems. Rather, we will identify as a sensory component any combinations of sensory neurons, sensory receptors, and sensory receptor organs for which a naturally occurring input signal can be specified.

The original source of naturally occurring input signals to sensory structures is the physical or chemical stimulus that when applied to a receptor organ is capable of exciting neurons within the sensory system. For sensory systems whose receptor organ input-output transfer functions are known, the simplest spike-producing component we can identify consists of a peripheral sensory neuron and the receptors with which it is in direct contact. This peripheral or "first-order" sensory component can be treated experimentally as a one-component device, with input signals applied to its input terminals (receptors) and with output measured from the sensory neuron. The peripheral sensory component may be described to be a simple communications system (Fig. 5-3) that consists of an encoder and a

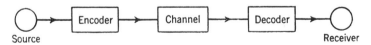

Source   Receiver

Fig. 5-3. Diagram of a communication system. A sensory component may be considered a communication system. A signal (stimulus) is delivered to the system. This signal is encoded into a series of pulses and sent out over the nerve fiber to other parts of the nervous system. The goal in sensory neurophysiology is to determine the nature of the input signals and the manner in which they are neurally encoded. From *An Introduction to Information Theory* by F.M. Reza, Copyright © 1961 by McGraw-Hill, Inc. Used with permission of McGraw-Hill Book Company.

communications channel. The source of the input signals to the encoder is the receptor-organ output. The encoder, which consists of the receptors and the synaptic terminals of the peripheral sensory neuron, transforms the input signals into a spike train that is generated and transmitted by the communications channel. The communications channel consists of the nerve-impulse conducting portion of the peripheral sensory neuron. The encoding process of the peripheral sensory component involves the transformation of the input signal applied to the sensory receptor into the spike output measured from the peripheral sensory neuron. When the sensory neuron whose output is measured is one or more neurons removed from the sensory receptor, those sensory neurons interposed between the receptors and the sensory neuron recorded from form part of the transform or encoder device. The model of the encoding process of an "Nth-order" sensory component would describe the relationship between the input signal applied to the receptors and the output measured from the Nth-order neuron. As the number of intervening neurons increases, the number of unknown transfer functions that combine to form the observed input-output relationship increases.

Although we can treat all orders of sensory components as simple input-output communication devices, we have elected to review in most of the following chapters of this book only studies of peripheral sensory components for several reasons. The number of sensory structures interposed between the measurable input signals and the sensory neuron whose output is measured is minimized, thus minimizing the number of neurons and unknown transfer functions that are represented by the modeled component. This minimizes the number of facts that must be discovered to describe the input-output function of the neuron studied. For example, the input signals representing the sensory information received by a peripheral sensory neuron could be specified after its receptor-organ and sensory-receptor transfer functions have been described. Once the input signals to the peripheral sensory neuron have been specified, the input-output function of this neuron can be described. However, the input signals representing the sensory information to be encoded by a higher-order sensory neuron cannot be described until the transfer functions of the receptor organ, sensory receptors, and all inter-connecting, lower-order sensory neurons are first described. Furthermore, more is known about the anatomical interconnections of peripheral sensory neurons than is known about centrally located sensory neurons.

THE PERIPHERAL SENSORY COMPONENT

The basic unit of a sensory system to be considered in most of the following chapters is the peripheral sensory component, consisting of a single peripheral sensory neuron from which spike potentials are recorded and the sensory receptors with which the neuron is connected. The locations and types of receptors that a peripheral sensory neuron innervates are important characteristics that determine the input signals affecting the output of the peripheral sensory component. Most sensory receptors are distributed within a receptor organ to form two-dimensional receptor surfaces. In the cochlea of the ear the receptor surface forms a spiral, in the eye it forms the posterior two thirds of the inner wall of a sphere, in the ampulla of the ear it forms the surface of a dome, and in the vestibule of the ear it forms two slightly curved surfaces. Other receptors are distributed in three dimensions to form receptor bodies such as skin receptors that are distributed along the width, length, and depth of the cutaneous and subcutaneous covering of the body, and the tendon organs and muscle spindle end organs that are distributed three dimensionally within tendons and striated muscles. The location of a receptor within the receptor organ is an important factor in determining which input signals reach it, since the distribution of receptor-organ output varies along the receptor surface or body. A stimulus applied to a localized area of the visual, skin, joint, muscle, and chemosensory receptor organs is transmitted by the organ to receptors in a localized area of the receptor surface or body. Application of a specific stimulus parameter to the auditory and vestibular receptor organs — e.g., frequency of tone or movement of the head in one direction — is transformed by the receptor organ into a spatially distributed output that is also localized along the receptor surface. There may be morphological differences between receptors of a sensory system that determine the input signals affecting the output of a peripheral sensory component. For example, the rod and cone receptors of the eye differ structurally and chemically, and also appear to differ with respect to spectral sensitivity. A peripheral visual component that contains only cone receptors would be affected by different wavelengths of light than one containing only rod receptors.

The peripheral process of a peripheral sensory neuron usually branches repeatedly near its terminus and sends its terminal processes to several receptors. The terminal processes may fan out to innervate receptors scattered over a large area of the receptor surface, or may remain concentrated and innervate a few receptors in a localized area of the receptor organ. The area of the receptor organ containing the receptors innervated by a peripheral sensory neuron is called the receptive field of a sensory component. The receptive field of a skin component can be described by the dimensions and location of the skin area that when touched, heated, or cooled will result in spike output from that component. The receptive field of a visual component can be specified in terms of the size, shape, and location of the retinal area that when lighted will result in spike output from that component. In those cases where the spatial distribution of the receptor organ output represents a transform of a stimulus parameter — e.g., frequency transformed to place of maximal vibration along the cochlear partition — the receptive field may be described in terms of the stimulus parameter represented. For example, the receptive field of an auditory component is usually given in terms of the frequencies and intensities of pure tones that elicit spikes from the component (response area or tuning curve) because it is more convenient and more accurate at this time to represent it in this manner.

EXPERIMENTAL APPROACH TO SENSORY SYSTEMS

The object of endeavors in sensory neurophysiology is to find out what sensory information each sensory system is processing, and what general language is employed in transmitting the information to the central nervous system. The general plan of attack is to break each sensory system down into its basic components and determine what each of the components is doing. In sensory systems, some aspect of the internal or external body environment is precisely measured, and the information obtained is encoded into a series of pulses and transmitted to other neural structures. Sensory neurophysiology provides a means for measuring and interpreting the pulse-coded messages transmitted in the nervous system.

In sensory neurophysiology the output of a component is described as a function of its input. The more exact measurements are for describing both the input and output of a component, the more precise can be the functional description of that component. If one is dealing with inputs that can be calibrated in terms of physical or chemical quantities, as can be done with most sensory systems, the inputs to a sensory component can be precisely quantified (provided, of course, a relevant variable is being measured). Since spike trains from a single sensory component consist of identical discrete pulses, and since these spike trains are often highly stable from one identical input presentation to another, equally exact measures can be obtained for the spike train. The establishment of a functional relationship between these two measures is the goal in sensory neurophysiology. As will be observed, this goal is not easily obtained because the nature of the input is usually imperfectly understood, the output is often the function of more than one distinct input, the output language (pulse code) may be inadequately understood, and messages may be encoded within a population of similar sensory components; thus the output from a single component may be intrepretable only with respect to the population discharge.

A peripheral sensory component and its central (output) connections are illustrated schematically in Fig. 5-4. The input signals to the component have been spatially distributed upon the receptor surface by the receptor organ and are represented as arrows labeled S1 and S2. The receptive portion of the sensory component is indicated in this diagram as distinct structures to emphasize that different types of receptors may act upon different input

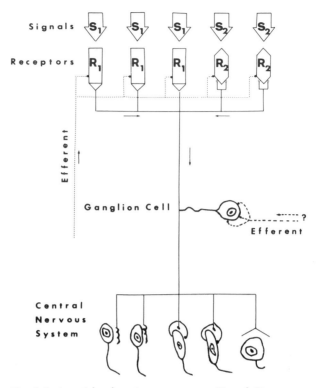

Fig. 5-4. A peripheral sensory component. S1 and S2 are two different sensory input signals that are distributed over the receptor surface by the receptor organ. These signals are measures of internal or external events. R1 and R2 are two different types of receptors that form the input terminals of the peripheral sensory component. The ganglion cell is the nerve-impulse conducting portion of the peripheral sensory component. Efferent fibers conduct impulses from the CNS toward the receptor or ganglion cells. The central process of the ganglion cell branches and terminates upon a number of cells in the central nervous system.

signals, and that the terminal processes of a peripheral sensory neuron may contact one or more receptors of the same type or may contact one or more types of receptors. However, we will not be treating the receptive portion of a peripheral sensory component as distinct structures but rather as the input terminals of the peripheral sensory component. As illustrated in Fig. 5-4, a peripheral sensory component is a multi-input or multiport input-output device that accepts multichannel information. Since the input signals applied to the peripheral sensory component are spatially distributed over its input terminals, the output of the component is related to the distribution of the receptor-organ output across the input terminals of that component. The implications of this structural relationship are tremendous when it comes to determining the nature of the input signals processed by a peripheral sensory component. For example, a peripheral sensory neuron innervating hair follicles of the skin innervates more than one hair follicle: If any one of these hairs is moved, the neuron will produce a spike output; but the more hairs that are moved simultaneously, the greater is the number of spikes produced by the neuron. That more complicated interactions than this additive effect can occur has been demonstrated by Miller (1971) in the chemosensory system of the rat tongue. According to Miller, the discharge elicited in a chorda tympani fiber by applying one chemical to a fungiform papilla could be inhibited by simultaneous application of a different chemical onto another fungiform papilla to which the nerve fiber was connected.

Also indicated in Fig. 5-4 is an efferent input (a nerve fiber conducting nerve impulses from the central nervous system toward the periphery) to the receptive portion of the peripheral sensory component. Efferent fibers terminating upon sensory receptors and upon sensory neuron terminal processes abound in sensory systems. Muscle spindle end organs appear to be innervated by three types of efferent fibers that differ in their origin and effect. Auditory receptors and their sensory terminal nerve fibers appear to receive efferent terminals of at least two types, the crossed and uncrossed olivocochlear fibers. Efferent inputs to the cell bodies of peripheral sensory neurons have been observed less frequently (Ramón y Cajal, 1909) and are also indicated in Fig. 5-4. Efferent inputs can profoundly affect the output of peripheral sensory components. Both the spontaneous and stimulus-evoked activity of muscle-spindle sensory neurons are affected by the presence or absence of the efferent inputs to the muscle-spindle receptors. The spike output of spiral ganglion cells of the cochlea can be depressed by the electrical stimulation of efferent fibers in the olivocochlear bundle. In most neurophysiological studies, the peripheral sensory component is treated as if it is independent of its efferent connections, which is in keeping with the principals of systems analysis. However, in order to develop an adequate and complete model of the peripheral sensory component as it functions within the sensory system of which it is a part, the effects of efferent inputs upon component output must also be described.

Having identified the sensory system component to be studied, the function of this component may be examined experimentally. The components are usually studied independently of their efferent and central connections, but in contact with their receptor organ, since it is most convenient to manipulate the stimulus parameters (input signals) applied to the receptor organ. The input signals to the peripheral sensory component may be described in terms of receptor-organ output, where the receptor-organ transfer function is known; or in terms of the stimulus parameters applied to the receptor organ. While in some cases the stimulus parameters that serve as input signals to sensory systems are known, in many cases they are not. For example, the stimulus parameters that serve as input signals to the auditory and visual systems are fairly well understood; while those of the vestibular, skin, and joint systems are partially known and those of the olfactory, gustatory, visceral, vascular, and muscular systems are poorly understood. The less that is known about the stimulus parameters affecting a sensory system, the more difficult it becomes to determine the manner in which sensory systems process sensory information. An investigator must determine what stimulus parameters serve as input signals and the manner in which they are encoded.

The peripheral sensory component output is measured or recorded from the neural processes or cell body of the peripheral sensory neuron. Thus, the number of peripheral sensory components existing in a sensory system are determined by the number of peripheral sensory neurons connecting the system sensory receptors to the central nervous system. For example, each spiral ganglion of the auditory system contains approximately fifty thousand neurons; therefore there are bilaterally approximately one-hundred thousand peripheral sensory components in the auditory system. Because of the large number of peripheral sensory components in all sensory systems, and because of the difficulties involved in recording from a large number of neurons in any single preparation, an investigator can measure the output of only a small portion of the total population of peripheral sensory components in a given animal.

There is evidence, both anatomical and neurophysiological, that the peripheral sensory components of sensory systems form heterogeneous populations. For example, the location of the input terminals of a peripheral sensory component within the receptor organ is not identical for all peripheral sensory components of a sensory system. The components may also differ with respect to the types of receptors forming their input terminals and thus would differ in the input signals that affect component output. The neural portion of peripheral sensory components also may differ with respect to degree of myelination and fiber-diameter size and thus would differ with respect to response to electrical stimulation. Peripheral sensory components have also been demonstrated to differ with respect to temporal pattern of spontaneous activity and of stimulus-evoked activity. For example, peripheral sensory components of the skin system that differ with respect to the receptor type forming their input terminals — e.g., body hair, vibrissae, tactile pads, Vater-Pacinian corpuscles, etc. — also differ with respect to the type of stimuli they are affected by, the temporal pattern of spontaneous and stimulus elicited discharge, and conduction velocity measures (see Chapter 9). The skin system is, in fact, a complex system consisting of many subsystems of similarly functioning sensory components that process the different types of sensory information elicited by contacting the skin with mechanical and thermal stimuli.

It is most probable that the population of peripheral sensory components of each sensory system consists of a variety of groups or sets of components, each of which are affected by different input signals and/or have different response characteristics. We will call these groups of components "common function sensory sets," and define a set as a group of components affected by similar input signals that are encoded into a common code. Components belonging to the same set must have properties similar to one another and certain properties that are distinct from components of other sets. In the following chapters, each common function set of a sensory system is treated as a subsystem and is often called a "sensory system."

Common function sensory sets may be defined operationally on the basis of measurements taken on the responses of all elements of the component population. However, at present it is not entirely clear just what response measures can be utilized to determine the characteristics or properties of components forming a common function set. Anatomical distinctions can be made on the basis of cellular geometry and chemistry, and on the basis of anatomical locations and connections. The receptors and neurons of components in different sets may be different in shape or in size, have larger fibers, or stain differently because they have different chemical processes occurring within them. The neurons of components in different sets may connect with anatomically distinct receptors and probably with different nuclei in the central nervous system. Neurophysiological measures can be used to distinguish between different sets. Various measures that have been utilized are: (1) types of stimuli and stimulus parameters that affect peripheral sensory components, (2) responses to electrical stimulation, (3) spontaneous activity patterns, and (4) stimulus-elicited discharge patterns.

Peripheral sensory components can also be classified into sets on the basis of the types of "neural codes" utilized in processing sensory information. The most commonly occurring code in sensory systems is that of labeled communication channels (Perkel and Bullock, 1968). Each peripheral sensory component consists of a channel that is labeled by the location of its input terminals (receptors) and by its types of input terminals. When a component produces an output, it signals that a certain region of the receptor organ has been stimulated and that a certain input signal has been applied to the receptor organ. Because the labeled channels are the carriers of the codes embodied in the component spike output, they can affect the requirements for such coding. For example, if there are a large number of similarly labeled channels, accuracy of coding within a given channel is not necessary because similar information can be represented by separate channels.

The number of other possible coding schemes available for encoding sensory information corresponds to the number of distinctive features of the output measured. In most cases, when a receptor organ is stimulated with a "natural" (in contrast to an electrical) stimulus, peripheral sensory components respond by producing an output that consists of a discharge of one or more pulses. Because of the all-or-none character of the spike potential, the amplitudes of the spikes are not available for encoding sensory information. The duration and shape of spikes forming a spike train are also unavailable as coding devices because they are relatively uniform for all spikes forming the train. Thus, the spike potentials forming a spike or pulse train differ only with respect to their times of occurrence or interspike intervals.

Communication and information theory have described models of different types of pulse codes, some of which may be utilized by components of the sensory nervous system (Harmon, 1963; Schwartz, 1970). An example of a simple pulse code is one in which there is no systematic change in the intervals between spikes, the information being represented by the number of spikes or the duration of the spike train. For example, an input signal of *value one* may elicit five spikes forming a spike burst of 100 msec. duration, and an input signal of *value two* may elicit 10 spikes forming a spike burst of two-hundred msec duration. The rate or frequency code illustrated in Fig. 5-5, is a class of codes in which the intervals between spikes form the basis of the code. The value of the input signal may be encoded by the value of the instantaneous rate (the reciprocal of the current interval between successive pulses), or by the rate averaged over some period of time. The information in a spike train may also be described by the statistics describing the interspike interval distribution formed from a spike train. Thus, it may be the case that the mean rate and mean interspike interval of a spike train remain constant

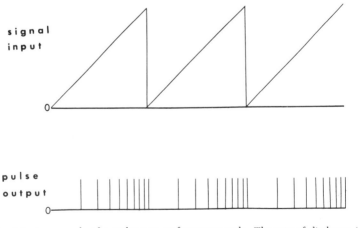

Fig. 5-5. An example of a pulse rate or frequency code. The rate of discharge is proportional to the amplitude of the input signal. The signal rises from zero to some positive values. No pulses are emitted at zero-input levels in this illustration.

for all values of the input signal, while the value of the variance or the mode of the interspike interval distribution varies systematically with changes in the input signal. The temporal pattern of a spike train may encode information in terms of the sequence of ordering of interspike intervals. Such spike trains would show some degree of serial correlation or tendency toward nonrandom ordering of interspike intervals. In the example illustrated in Fig. 5-6, the spike intervals are ordered in structured sequences that are grouped to form a "word." Another possible neural pulse code is a pulse position code. This coding process would require highly regular spontaneous activity acting as a carrier train that is modulated to form the coded message. A change in the value of the input signal would cause a change in the position of the

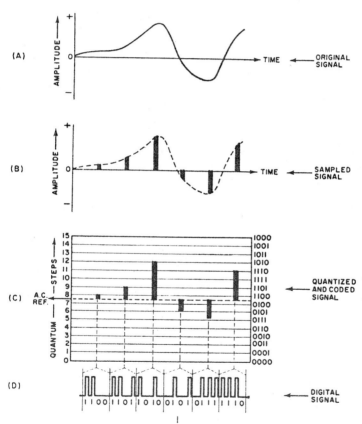

Fig. 5-6. A temporal pattern pulse code in which groups of pulses are used to encode the signal. The original signal (A) is sampled at fixed intervals (B) and the signal amplitude is quantitized (C) into incremental levels and (D) encoded into equivalent digital signals (Silver, 1970).

pulses of the carrier train, depending upon the direction of change of the input signal. The preceding are but a few examples of the many types of pulse codes that may be utilized by components of the sensory nervous system.

There is evidence from several sensory systems that the spikes from components in the same common function set are time-locked with respect to one another. Thus, simple auditory stimuli evoke discharges across the ordered set of cochlear nerve fibers wherein the time of firing of each activated unit is probabilistically related to the nature of the stimulus and its position within the ordered set (Kiang *et al.*, 1965). Hunt (1961) has shown that vibratory stimuli applied to the hind limb will elicit phase-locked discharge from a group of fibers connected to Vater-Pacini corpuscles. In the geniculate ganglion of the cat, there is a group of cells that are responsive to movements of the tissues of the soft palate and nasopharynx (Boudreau *et al.*, 1971). These neurons are often found to discharge spontaneously at high regular rates. We have often recorded from two or more units simultaneously where the spontaneous discharges were of the same frequency and often in phase with one another. These facts suggest that information may be carried by the phase relationship of interneuronal discharge. If interfiber-discharge phase relationships are important in encoding information, information may be transmitted with no change in frequency or interspike intervals.

If each of the common function sensory sets contains a homogeneous population of peripheral sensory components, models can be derived from the data of all component members of a set. The larger the number in a sample of a set, the greater the probability that the model derived from the sample is representative of the population from which the set was sampled. However, if the classification of components into sets is incomplete, or if a sample consists of components from two or more differing sets, large numbers of components within a sample will not assure a representative model. Because the input-output functions of different common function sensory sets differ, the grouping together of measurements from components of different sets may confuse or obliterate the functional relationships existing between the stimulus and measured response. Therefore, care must be taken to determine the properties of different sets and to classify each component into its proper set. The aim of a sensory neurophysiological study is to characterize common function sensory sets within which the sample components are relatively homogeneous in the response measures used to characterize them.

MODELING

There are two approaches that can be taken in mathematical modeling; one is a purely descriptive one, the other is a theoretical one. A purely descriptive model describes the input-output relationship without giving any physiological meaning to the parameters that occur in the model. For example, in descriptive modeling the parameters a and b (intercept and slope) of a straight-line function describing the relationship between mean discharge rate (output) and stimulus intensity (input) are only considered to be characteristics of the model describing the function. The model becomes a theoretical one when these parameters are treated as hypothetical constructs and are given physiological meaning, e.g., when the intercept is interpreted to represent component threshold and the slope, to represent component time constant of excitation and decay. In theoretical models, restrictions are placed upon the values that the parameters can take on the basis of indirect measures of values the physiological process or hypothetical construct that they represent have taken. Because the science of sensory neurophysiology is in its infancy, it would seem most profitable at this time to accumulate as many facts (descriptive models) as possible before entering into the area of constructing and testing hypothetical constructs and theoretical models.

It is often the case that several models are capable of describing the input-output relationship of a peripheral sensory component. For example, it may be that the relationship between stimulus intensity and spike discharge can be described in terms of the mean rate of discharge, the mode and variance of the interspike interval distribution and the temporal pattern of discharge. The selection of one model over another as the encoding scheme utilized by a peripheral sensory component can only be based upon whether the code affects the sensory neuron with which the component synapses — i.e., upon whether the code is readable and used by the receiving neurons. At present we are unable to determine whether a code is read and used by the sensory neurons making contact with the central process of a peripheral sensory neuron. The selection of a single model to describe the input-output function of a component on the basis of a calculated a priori "best guess" of the input-output function of the component should be avoided. It seems most profitable at this time to create a descriptive model of peripheral sensory components based upon the collection of mathematical functions that describe all of the input-output relationships of the stimulus-evoked spike train. In the ideal case, all aspects of a stimulus-evoked spike train would be described in the model, assuming that any one or perhaps several of the aspects may be utilized as the encoding process. The resulting descriptive model may be overspecified, but it could be simplified when it becomes possible to determine which aspect of the spike train is read and used by the second-order sensory neurons.

In the chapters to follow we will examine in detail the structure and function of the cat's peripheral sensory systems as revealed by anatomical and neurophysiological studies. In no case has the type of neural code employed by a sensory system nor the exact nature of the input signals been determined. The data from sensory neurophysiological experiments are presented with little or no interpretive comment. In most cases the illustrations are derived from published journal articles. In presenting data, we have concentrated on measures that might separate different neural groups — e.g., common function sets or sensory subsystems. We have tried to utilize the same measures (e.g., spontaneous activity, fiber diameter, conduction velocity, etc.) for comparing different neural systems, but in many cases these were not available for different sensory systems. In the different sensory systems to be presented, many of the factors discussed in this chapter come into play, but the study of sensory systems is still in its infancy and techniques of analysis of spike trains and their interpretations are tentative at best. Hence this chapter can be no more than a crude guideline for a rapidly evolving science.

6
SENSORY SYSTEMS OF THE JOINTS

The basic shape of vertebrates is determined by the internal bony frame known as the skeleton (Romer, 1970). The skeleton of the cat is composed of approximately 287 bones (Fig. 6-1). These bones form a dense protective covering for the central nervous system, and perform certain vital functions relating to the internal ionic environment. In addition, the bones supply a rigid framework for supporting the organism in different positions. The bones of the skeleton are segmented and joined together at specialized regions known as joints, which allow movements of the bones relative to one another. It is by positioning and repositioning the bones at joints that the cat moves his body and limbs. When an animal shifts to a new position or engages in a movement, many bones must be repositioned in order to achieve this movement and to maintain balance during the movement.

The skeleton may be considered to be a collection of struts (bones) held together by various ties (muscles and tendons). These struts and ties form triangles for the disposition of forces similar to the principles used in bridge building (Gray, 1968; Roberts, 1967). In the limbs, the triangles are formed by two struts and a tie. During movements the disposition of the struts and ties change to compensate for the redistribution of forces. Thus, in Fig. 6-2, we see the disposition of the struts and ties of the pectoral girdle when the cat is standing in a position in which his weight is symmetrically distributed on the two forelimbs. When one foreleg is lifted, the bones must be repositioned to support the new weight distributions of the forequarters (Fig. 6-2).

The bones are more than a series of struts and ties, however. They are also a series of levers and bearings and are used to move the cat around and to grasp prey. The running ability of an animal is a function of the articulations of bones (Hildebrand, 1959); thus, the cheetah achieves its rapid speed by virtue of its swiveling shoulder blades and its flexible spine (Fig. 6-3).

The movement of bones is made possible by specialized structures known as joints. The most common joint connecting movable bones is the synovial

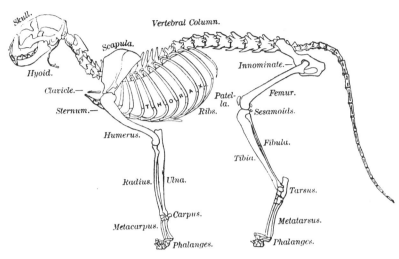

Fig. 6-1. Cat. The skeleton of the cat (Jayne, 1898).

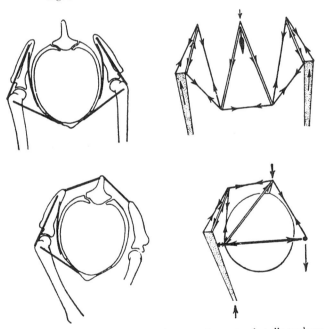

Fig. 6-2. Cat. Top: Position of the bones in the pectoral girdle to show the disposition of struts and ties when the weight is symmetrically supported on the two forelimbs. Bottom: Position of the pectoral girdle to show the disposition of struts and ties when one forelimb is lifted from the ground (Roberts, 1967).

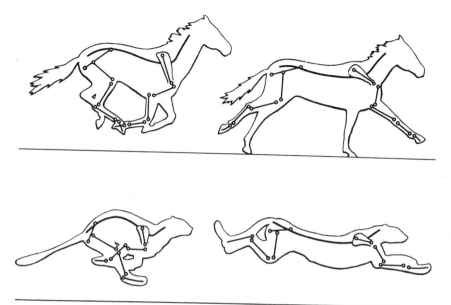

Fig. 6-3. Mammal. The position of some of the bones of the skeleton of the galloping horse and cheetah. The animals are shown in positions of maximum flexion and extension of the spine and maximum rotation of the scapula on the spine. From "How Animals Run" by M. Hildebrand. Copyright © 1960 by Scientific American, Inc. All rights reserved.

joint, shown in schematic form in Fig. 6-4. Basically, this joint consists of the ends of two separate bones enclosed within a fibrous capsule and supported by various ligaments and tendons. The ends of the bones that meet are covered with special articular cartilage, and lubricated with a special fluid known as synovial fluid. Within the capsule, there may be fat pads and menisci that may function during bone movements (Barnett *et al.*, 1961). The position of the bones within the joints is determined by the geometry of the bony surfaces and the constraints on bone movement imposed by the fibrous capsule, the ligaments, and the muscle-tendon connections.

Various types of synovial joints may be distinguished (Barnett *et al.*, 1961). A simple joint is one consisting of a single pair of articulating boney surfaces enclosed within a fibrous capsule. In a compound joint, such as the elbow, more than two articulating surfaces may be found within the same capsule. In a complex joint, such as the knee joint, an intra-articular fibrocartilage subdivides the intra-capsular cavity of a compound joint. In the knee joint, there are actually four bones (the femur, the tibia, the fibula, and the patella), held together by a complex of supporting structures. The knee joint of the cat is the only cat joint that has been studied to any degree by both anatomists and neurophysiologists. A view of the cat's knee joint can be seen in Fig. 6-5.

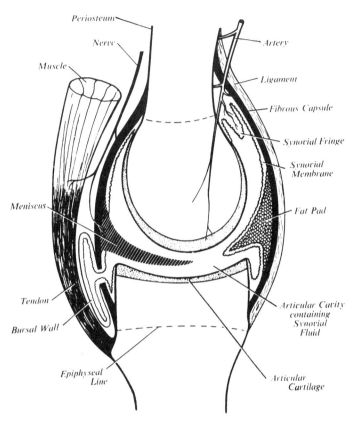

Fig. 6-4. Mammal. Schematic representation of a synovial joint. From Barnett, C. H. Davies, D. V., and MacConaill, M. A.: *Synovial Joints. Their Structure and Mechanics* (1961). By permission of Longman Group, Ltd.

The bone movements made possible by joints are of two basic types: spin and slide (MacConaill, 1966). A spin movement involves a partial or complete rotation of a bone about its long axis. In a slide movement, one bone slides along the surface of the other bone. During any one of these movements, a number of forces are set up in a joint (Frost, 1960). Many joints are also active in the support of the weight of the animal. Thus, the movements of bones within joints must be accomplished while the joints perform simultaneously the function of support. Presumably, it is some aspect of the forces occurring during movement and support that the sensory systems of joints must measure; the bones can then be accurately positioned relative to one another so that movement and support can be accomplished.

In neurophysiological studies on joint systems, the usual stimulus situation is one in which the bones of an anesthetized animal are passively moved. The

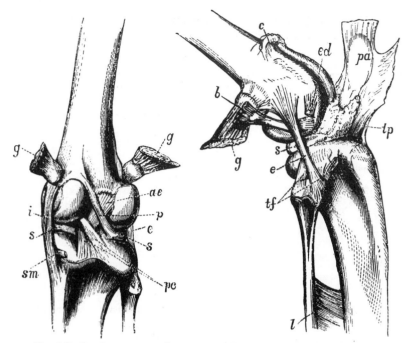

Fig. 6-5. Cat. Ligaments with some muscular insertions of the knee joint.
Reproduced with permission from Mivart, G. (1881): The Cat. John Murray,
London.

Left: Seen posteriorly
ac. Anterior crucial
   ligament
b. Biceps muscle
c. Upper attachment of
   capsular ligament
e. External lateral ligament
ed. Extensor longus
   digitorum
g. Gastrocnemius
i. Internal lateral
   ligament

Right: Seen externally
l. Inter-osseous
   ligament
p. Posterior ligament
pa. Patella
pc. Posterior crucial
   ligament
s. Inter-articular
   cartilage
sm. Semi-membranosus
tf. Tibio-fibular
   ligament
tp. Ligament of the
   patella toward
   its insertion

stimulus measured is therefore considered to be the joint angle or rate of
movement of the bones. This type of stimulation does not provide for all
possible bone movements within joints, nor does it approximate the normal
situation in which the weight of the animal is being supported by the bones
and joints. When a cat is walking, for instance, there are constant changes in
the weight supported by the different legs as a function of the leg position
(Manter, 1938). As we shall see later, many of the fibers innervating receptors
in the knee joint are activated only when the leg is fully extended or fully

Table 6-1. Composition of Primary Articular Nerves to the Knee Joint (Freeman and Wyke, 1967)

(Figures in parentheses are Percentages of the total nerve-fiber counts)

	Posterior articular nerve			Medial articular nerve		
	Total number of fibers (mean)	Myelinated fibers (mean)	Un-myelinated fibers (mean)	Total number of fibers (mean)	Myelinated fibers (mean)	Un-myelinated fibers (mean)
Sasaoka (1939 a,b)	225	159 (70.5)	66 (29.5)	-	-	-
Gardner (1944)	286	171 (59.8)	115 (40.2)	266	144 (54.1)	122 (45.9)
Skoglund (1956		176	-	-	145	-
Fidel-Osipova et al. (1961)	-	150	-	-	120	-
Freeman & Wyke (1967)	387	224 (58)	162 (42)	291	157 (54)	131 (46)

flexed, or when the leg is rotated with a twist. These results suggest that some of the sensory systems would only function in stimulus situations more closely approximating those occurring during normal cat locomotion.

NEUROANATOMY OF JOINTS

The nerves innervating the knee joint have been described by Poláček (1963; 1966) and Freeman and Wyke (1967). The nerves supplying the sensory innervation to the knee joint arise from a number of dorsal-root ganglia and spinal nerves that may also supply sensory fibers for the muscles, skin, and bone (Poláček, 1963; 1966). These nerves are somewhat inconstant in their appearance. The fibers innervating the knee-joint branch off from a number of major nerve trunks, frequently from more-than one point of origin (Freeman and Wyke, 1967).

In the cat, three main articular nerves have been distinguished as well as some accessory nerves that are highly variable and may or may not be present. The three primary articular nerves innervating the knee joint of the cat (Freeman and Wyke, 1967) are the posterior articular nerve, the medial articular nerve, and the lateral articular nerve (Fig. 3-9). These nerves are distributed to different parts of the knee joint. They contain both myelinated and unmyelinated fibers (Table 6-1), with the myelinated fibers constituting about 58 percent of the 387 fibers in the posterior articular nerve and 54 percent of the 291 fibers of the medial articular nerve. A distribution of the fiber diameter reveals a great heterogeneity with diameters as large as 16 microns present (Fig. 6-6). Skoglund (1956) demonstrated with electrical

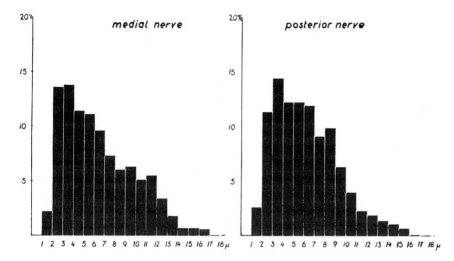

Fig. 6-6. Cat. Diagrams showing the distribution of different fiber sizes in the medial and posterior nerve to the knee joint in the cat, plotted against percentage of total number of fibers in ten nerves of each (Skoglund, 1956).

stimulation that the fibers of the medial articular nerve enter the spinal cord via the fifth and sometimes sixth lumbar dorsal roots, and the posterior articular nerve via the seventh lumbar and sometimes first sacral root.

Fibers of joint receptor systems are generally believed to enter the spinal cord and project without interruption to the dorsal-column nuclei of the brain stem via the large ascending dorsal-column fiber tracts. However, Burgess and Clark (1969b) recorded from individual joint fibers while they electrically stimulated the cervical dorsal columns, and they found that only a small percentage of the joint fibers could be activated. It is likely that each of the different joint sensory systems that have been identified has a different central projection. Since classification of peripheral joint fibers has only recently been attempted (Burgess and Clark 1969a), central projections of the different fiber groups have not been worked out in any detail.

The heterogeneity of fiber size displayed by the histogram of articular nerve fibers shown in Fig. 6-6 bespeaks a complexity of sensory systems supplying the joint tissues. The variety of nerve endings found in the joint tissues fulfills this expectation. The receptors in the joints have been described by several workers, most of whom seem to be in fair agreement as to the classifications of these receptor end organs. The end organs commonly found in the joint tissues of the cat are (1) free nerve endings; (2) encapsulated corpuscles; and (3) spraylike endings. These different types of receptors can be seen schematically in Fig. 6-7. Some indication of the distribution of these different types of receptors and the relative caliber of

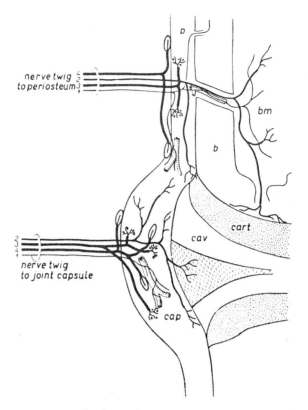

Fig. 6-7. Mammal. Scheme of joint innervation: p - periosteum, b - bone, bm - bone marrow, cart - joint cartilage, cap - joint capsule, cav - joint cavity; 1 - vasomotor nerve fiber, 2 - free endings bearing nerve fiber, 3 - spraylike endings bearing nerve fiber, 4 - encapsulated corpuscles bearing nerve fiber (Poláček, 1966).

fibers supplying them can also be gained from this diagram. In addition to these receptors in the capsule or joint proper, distinct receptors similar to Golgi tendon organs can be found on the ligaments (Boyd, 1954; Freeman and Wyke, 1967). These ligament receptors are formed by terminals of large (12 microns or greater) myelinated fibers. The fibers supplying these receptors run with the sensory fibers of the joint capsule.

Free nerve endings are the receptors most entensively distributed around the joint tissues. Besides being found in the capsule, free nerve endings are abundant in the menisci or discs, the edges of the articular cartilage, the periosteum of the bone, bone marrow, adipose tissue, and blood vessels (Poláček, 1966). The fibers supplying free nerve endings are both myelinated and unmyelinated. Poláček (1966) separates the free nerve endings of myelinated fibers into two types: simple and those with arborizations. Freeman and Wyke (1967) divide free nerve endings into three types on the basis of the location, types (plexes or simple terminals), and kind of parent fiber (myelinated or unmyelinated).

The spraylike endings and the encapsulated corpuscles are formed by myelinated fibers only. These two types of receptors have been studied extensively by Poláček and his associates. These investigators have utilized a variety of species in their studies (Frankova, 1968; Sklenská, 1965; 1968; 1969), and have also examined the endings and encapsulated corpuscles found in other parts of the cat's body, such as the vagina, skin of the nose, foot pads, and tongue. The end organs found in these other tissues resemble in morphology those found in the joint tissues; Chapter 9 discusses some of the findings in more detail.

The spraylike endings and the encapsulated corpuscles take a variety of shapes and Poláček could not establish any hard-and-fast categories. Examples of different spraylike endings can be seen in Fig. 6-8. In the cat, the spraylike endings outnumber the encapsulated corpuscles about three to one. Spraylike endings (also known as Ruffini endings) are characterized by (1) a ramifying terminal fiber; (2) an inner core of special cells interdigitated between the ramifying terminal fibers; and (3) a thin, inconstant capsule that surrounds the nerve endings and inner core (Poláček, 1965; 1966). Examples of the different types of spraylike endings found in the cat and other animals and their frequency of occurrence can be seen in Fig. 6-8. As can be observed, different animals have different types of spraylike endings. Those of the cat tend to be primarily of one type (simple ramifying fiber with a capsule), but examples of other morphologically distinct types are also present. These end organs tend to occur in clusters (up to eight) derived from the same parent nerve fiber. The diameter of the fiber near the end organ averages about 3.7 microns (Poláček et al., 1969). Spraylike endings are widely distributed in joint tissues; they occur in the joint capsule predominantly but may also be found in the bone marrow, fibrous cartilage, periosteum, and adipose tissue (Poláček, 1966).

The encapsulated corpuscles are found in the joint capsule and in the periosteum of the bone (Fig. 6-7). These end organs are characterized by a nerve terminal and inner core material that are surrounded by a distinct capsule consisting of several layers or lamellae. As was true of the spraylike endings, morphologically distinct varieties of encapsulated corpuscles may be distinguished (Hromada and Poláček, 1958; Poláček, 1961). As can be observed in Fig. 6-9, the terminal fiber and its capsule may take a variety of shapes. The types of end organs found differ within different species. The cat's encapsulated corpuscles are thinner and longer than those in other animals and are primarily of the paciniform type; i.e., containing an unbranched terminal fiber (74.5 percent in Fig. 6-9). Corpuscles containing

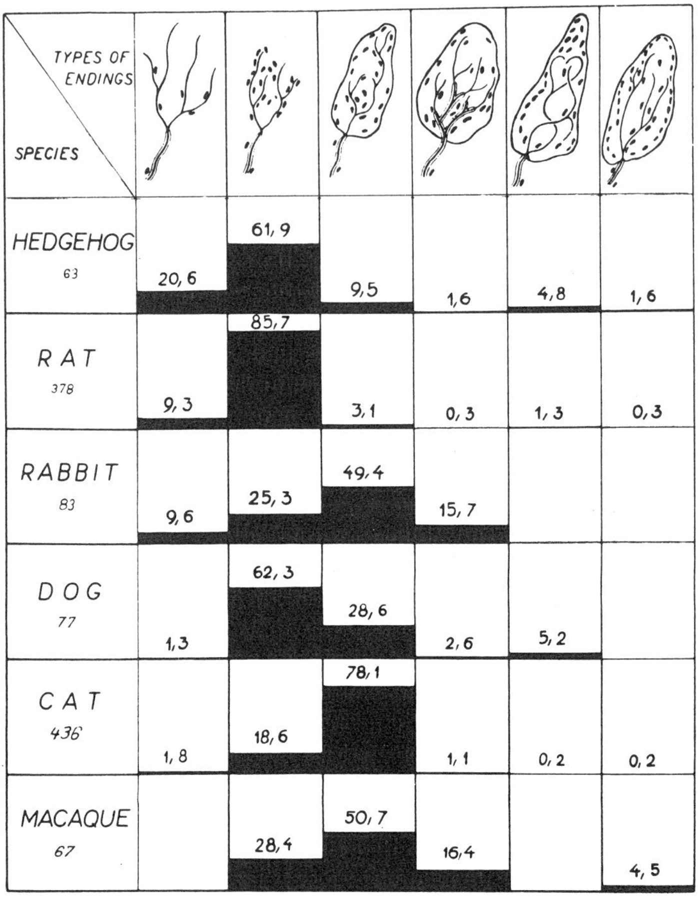

Fig. 6-8. Mammal. Species differences of occurrences of varieties of spraylike endings in the joint capsule. Numbers give the percentage of occurrences (Poláček, 1966).

an inner core and branched terminal fiber, the Golgi-Mazzoni type of corpuscle, occur less frequently (3.2 percent in Fig. 6-9). More complicated types with divided capsules, the branched corpuscles, may also be found. As with spraylike endings, a single parent nerve fiber can form more than one encapsulated corpuscle (Fig. 6-10). Encapsulated corpuscles are usually arranged side by side, but may be found strung out on the nerve fiber in a rosarylike arrangement. The diameters of the last myelinated segment of fibers forming encapsulated end organs are slightly greater (4.77 microns on

Species	Hedgehog	Rat	Rabbit	Cat	Dog	Macaque	Man newborn after Hromada
Number of corpuscles	20	433	13	94	30	62	100
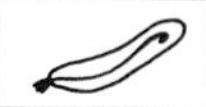	60,0 %	77,8 %	92,3 %	74,5 %	46,7 %	56,5 %	89,0 %
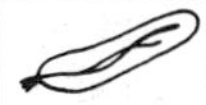	10,0 %	10,9 %	7,7 %	3,2 %	13,3 %	8,1 %	5,0 %
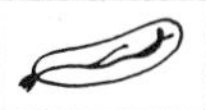		3,7 %			23,4 %	4,8 %	3,0 %
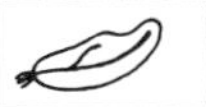		0,15 %		1,1 %		1,6 %	2,0 %
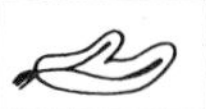	5,0 %	3,7 %		9,6 %		4,8 %	
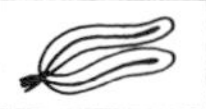		2,5 %		7,5 %		1,6 %	
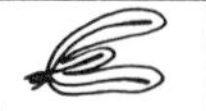		0,25 %		2,1 %			
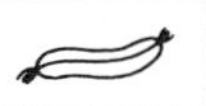	25,0 %	0,7 %		2,1 %	3,3 %	1,6 %	
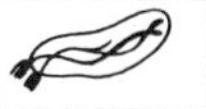		0,25 %			3,3 %		
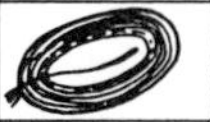						21,0 %	1,0 %
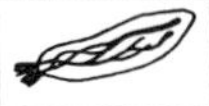					10,0 %		

Fig. 6-9. Mammal. Species differences in occurrence of varieties of encapsulated joint corpuscles (Poláček, 1961).

the average) than those forming spraylike endings (Poláček *et al.*, 1969). The parent fiber of the terminal fibers supplying spraylike endings are five to eight microns and eight to twelve microns for encapsulated corpuscles (Freeman and Wyke, 1967).

Poláček (1966) believes that the different types of receptors found in the joints are evolutionarily related to one another but asserts together with Boyd (1954) and Freeman and Wyke (1967), that all receptors formed by a single parent fiber are of the same type; i.e., only spraylike or only encapsulated corpuscles. The same fiber may form morphologically distinct spraylike or encapsulated endings, however. Freeman and Wyke (1967) describe small unmyelinated fibers that innervate spraylike endings and encapsulated corpuscles (their type I and type II endings) formed by the myelinated fibers. Hromada and Poláček (1958) also describe unmyelinated fibers innervating corpuscles and tissues surrounding them.

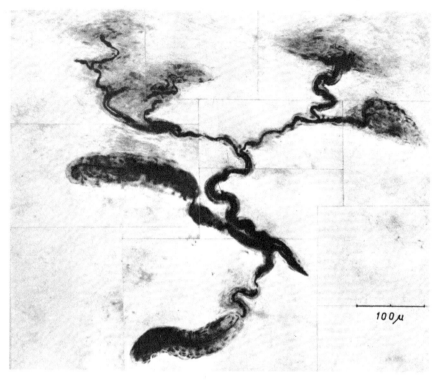

Fig. 6-10. Cat. Two encapsulated corpuscles and four spraylike endings in the joint capsule. The corpuscles are borne by the one and the sprays by the other nerve fiber. Mounting of 11 photos (Poláček, 1966).

NEUROPHYSIOLOGY OF JOINTS

There have been several investigations in which the responses of single fibers in articular nerves have been measured. Andrew and Dodt (1958) and Andrew (1954) have recorded from fibers innervating the medial ligament of the cat's knee joint. Boyd (1954) and Cohen (1955) have recorded from fibers in the posterior articular nerve; and Skoglund (1956) has recorded from fibers in the medial and posterior articular nerves. We shall report in some detail upon the study of Burgess and Clark (1969a), because it is the only neurophysiological study of a joint system nerve that has attempted to systematically characterize and classify all units encountered in the nerve.

These investigators recorded from fibers in the dorsal roots, L6 and L7, of anesthetized cats. Fibers were determined to be of posterior articular nerve origin by electrical stimulation of this nerve peripherally. This technique of electrical stimulation also provided estimates of single fiber conduction velocity. The experimental stimulus setup is illustrated in Fig. 6-11. The lower leg was moved in a variety of manners while the thigh was held rigid. With this apparatus, they were able to move the lower leg from flexion to extension and twist the tibia, or perform a combination of the two movements. Other stimulus conditions included were pressure on the knee and intravenous injections of succinylcholine, which is known to activate fibers innervating muscle spindles (Smith, 1963).

Altogether, 278 myelinated nerve fibers were studied; and on the basis of unit responses to their stimulus conditions, the population was divided into eight fiber types (14 units could not be activated by any form of stimulation). The primary criterion for classification was whether the unit responded tonically or phasically to leg movements. Three tonically responding types of fibers and two phasically responding types were identified. The tonic units were classified into three categories, depending upon whether they responded at leg flexion, extension, or both. The flexion-extension fibers, the extension, and most of the flexion fibers could also be activated by pressure on the back of the knee. None of them responded to succinylcholine injections. The tonically responding fibers constituted the majority (209) of

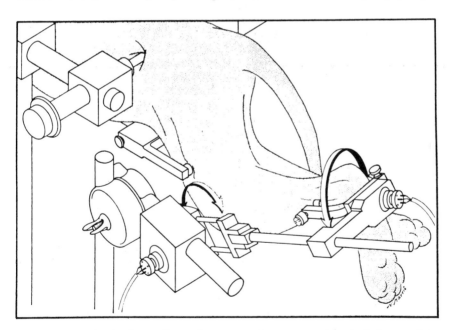

Fig. 6-11. Cat. Sketch of assembly used to measure knee-joint angle and tibial twist. Slide bearings were used at knee pivot to accommodate slight misalignments and a shift in the center of rotation as joint was moved. Joint position was monitored with potentiometers (Burgess and Clark, 1969a).

the fibers in the posterior articular nerve, although 197 of these fibers responded only during marked flexion or marked extension or both. Only four fibers were activated specifically at intermediate joint positions. Twisting the tibia enhanced the discharge of most fibers.

The conduction velocities of the three tonic fiber classifications can be seen in the upper three histograms of Fig. 6-12. The flexion fibers seem to exhibit a bimodality in their conduction-velocity distribution, indicating that units from separate neural groups may be classified together.

Also shown in Fig. 6-12 are the conduction-velocity measurements for the two types of phasically responding fibers identified by Burgess and Clark. These two fiber types were called "phasic fibers" and "corpusclelike fibers." No distinction between the two is evident with respect to conduction velocity. Phasic fibers responded to joint movement with a transient response, although a low-level sustained discharge could be produced in about 25 percent of the cases with a strong twist and maximum extension. All but three phasic fibers could be activated by pressing on the lateral, medial,

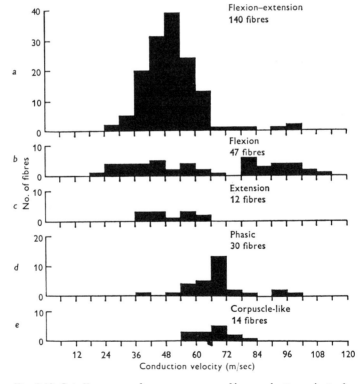

Fig. 6-12. Cat. Frequency of occurrence versus fiber conduction velocity for the various fiber types studied. Posterior articular nerve (Burgess and Clark, 1969a).

Table 6-2. Summary of Fiber Types (Burgess and Clark, 1969) Cat Posterior Articular Nerve (278 fibers)

Receptor type	Number observed	Conduction velocity m/sec (95% or more fall into range shown)	Discharge	Type of response
Flexion-extension	140 (50.4%)	30-70	Tonic	Discharge only at or near the extremes of flexion and extension
Flexion	47 (16.9%)	20-70, 80-110	Tonic	Discharge only at flexion with tibia not twisted, but 60% respond at most joint angles with outward tibial twist (see text)
Extension	12 (4.3%)	38-65	Tonic	Discharge only at or near full extension
Phasic joint	30 (10.8%)	50-100	Intermediate	Predominantly phasic but capable of low-rate sustained discharge, respond to movement over part or all of range
Corpusclelike	14 (5.0%)	55-83	Phasic	Respond with variable sensitivity only during joint movement
Other receptors	4 (1.4%)	-	Tonic	Some response at intermediate joint angles (see text)
	11 (4.0%)	12-33	Variable	Possible nociceptors, respond only to bending and twisting procedures considered noxious
	6 (2.2%)	34-107	Tonic	Muscle-spindlelike, discharge increases in response to succinylcholine (0.1-0.2 mg I.V.)
	14 (5.0%)	5-125	-	Not activated, six had conduction velocities below 30 m/sec.

or patellar aspects of the knee, a form of manipulation that could also produce steady discharge. According to Burgess and Clark the discharge patterns of corpusclelike fibers were apparently similar to those seen with fibers innervating Vater-Pacini corpuscles (see Chapter 9). They were activated by light taps and joint movements in any direction; their responses to joint movements were phasic.

Additional fiber types identified by Burgess and Clark were muscle-spindlelike fibers that responded to injections of succinylcholine (Smith, 1963), intermediate joint angle responders, and very high threshold units responding only to vigorous bending or twisting procedures. Some of the characteristics of these and other fiber types identified in the posterior articular nerve can be seen in Table 6-2, modified slightly from Burgess and Clark (1969a).

Electrical stimulation of fibers in the cervical dorsal columns of the spinal cord excited only a small percentage of the posterior articular nerve fibers. Nerve fibers projecting into the cervical dorsal columns were of the phasic responding types, with all the corpusclelike fibers projecting and half of those classified as phasic joint fibers projecting. Their conduction velocities ranged from 48 to 84 m/sec.

The occurrence of two peaks on the flexion fiber histogram in Fig. 6-12 is most likely due to the inadequacy of the stimuli utilized for classifying cells. The complexity of the knee joint (Fig. 6-5) suggests that a joint movement may have different effects at the three different joint surfaces, and will differentially stimulate the receptors in the various articular tissues. Since the different types of receptors are distributed about three different articular surfaces, the same movement could differentially stimulate the receptors of the same type, depending upon the surface in which they are located. The fact that most fibers are not activated unless the tibia is twisted suggests that most neurons are not activated unless a "load" is placed on the tissues. More natural stimulation techniques, perhaps ones simulating various leg movements, are suggested. The influence of the contraction and relaxation of the various muscle groups used to regulate joint position is unknown.

The classification of cells according to whether their discharge is tonic or phasic has had some applicability in the analysis of the skin senses. In an absence of knowledge about relevant stimulus parameters, this response measure must always be used with caution. In the auditory system, for instance, it is possible to activate a cell phasically only at the onset of tone (using a fast stimulus-rise time) of one frequency and to activate the cell tonically by using another frequency. The fact that tonic-phasic is not an adequate criterion for many joint fibers is indicated by the fact that Burgess and Clark could tonically activate some phasic units by certain tibial motions.

7
THE VESTIBULAR SYSTEM

The peripheral vestibular system comprises a number of small oriented sensory surfaces equipped with specialized hair-cell receptors. These sensory surfaces are contained in fluid-filled chambers buried deep in the hardest bone in the body. Apparently the primary functions of these organs are to measure head movements and to establish the position of the head relative to the pull of gravity. The information obtained from these organs is utilized in the performance not only of head movements but also in the positioning of other parts of the body (Fig. 7-1).

The sensory surfaces of the vestibular system, and the chambers in which they are located, are oriented at different angles with respect to one another so that they are differentially affected by head movements in different directions. One end of the receptor cells is anchored in tissue that is firmly fixed to the bone while the hairs at the other end project into a gelatinous covering that overlies each sensory surface. The coverings of two of the sensory surfaces contain dense crystals of calcite. When head displacements (either static or dynamic) occur, the sensory surface and the covering may be differentially affected. The hair cells interposed between the two surfaces apparently measure the stresses and strains set up between them.

ANATOMY OF THE VESTIBULAR ORGANS

Within the petrous portion of the temporal bone are several interconnected cavities and chambers known as the bony labyrinth (Fig. 7-2). The structures of the bony labyrinth form the inner ear and may be separated into three parts: the cochlea, the vestibule, and the semicircular canals. The latter two structures contain the receptor surfaces of the vestibular system; the former, the receptor surface of the auditory system. The membranous labyrinth is located within these hollow structures, but does not completely fill them. The fluid perilymph almost surrounds the membranous labyrinth completely.

Connective tissue trabeculae support and attach the membranous labyrinth to the wall of the osseous labyrinth (Fig. 7-3). The membranous labyrinth consists of the cochlear duct, the semicircular ducts and the utricle and saccule that occupy the lumen of the vestibule. The membranous labyrinth contains the fluid endolymph and the receptor surfaces of the auditory and vestibular systems. The following paragraphs will describe only the vestibular portion of the inner ear. The auditory portion of the ear will be dealt with in Chapter 10.

The osseous vestibule is a pyramidal-shaped cavity that communicates with the cochlea rostrally and with the semicircular canals caudally. The medial wall of the vestibule contains two depressions, the elliptical and spherical recesses. The elliptical recess is located caudodorsally and contains the membranous utricle. The spherical recess is located anteroventral to the elliptical recess and contains the membranous saccule. The vestibular crus separates the two recesses. A number of small openings through which nerves enter the vestibule occur near the recesses. The oval window is an opening in

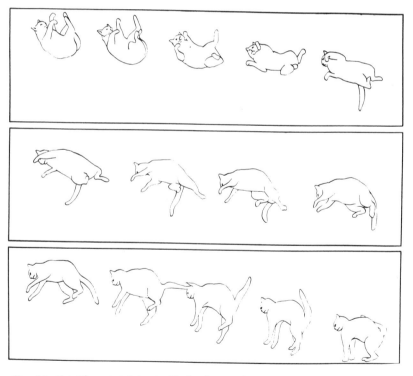

Fig. 7-1. Cat. The cat righting itself after being released upside down in midair. The vestibular system is one of the sensory systems utilized in this behavior. (Artwork by M. Berman redrawn from Marey, 1894.)

the lateral wall of the vestibule that is normally closed off from the cavity of the middle ear by the footplate of the stapes (Fig. 7-3).

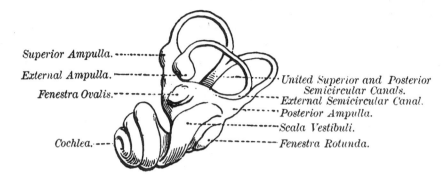

Superior Ampulla.

External Ampulla.

Fenestra Ovalis.

United Superior and Posterior Semicircular Canals.
External Semicircular Canal.
Posterior Ampulla.
Scala Vestibuli.

Cochlea.

Fenestra Rotunda.

Fig. 7-2. Cat. A cast of the bony labyrinth of the cat. Within these bony chambers is enclosed the membranous labyrinth that contains the receptors of the vestibular and auditory sensory systems. (Jayne, 1898.)

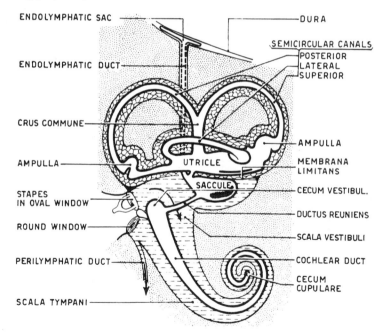

ENDOLYMPHATIC SAC

DURA

SEMICIRCULAR CANALS
POSTERIOR
LATERAL
SUPERIOR

ENDOLYMPHATIC DUCT

CRUS COMMUNE

AMPULLA

AMPULLA

UTRICLE

MEMBRANA LIMITANS

SACCULE

CECUM VESTIBUL.

STAPES IN OVAL WINDOW

DUCTUS REUNIENS

ROUND WINDOW

SCALA VESTIBULI

PERILYMPHATIC DUCT

COCHLEAR DUCT

CECUM CUPULARE

SCALA TYMPANI

Fig. 7-3. Mammal. Schematic showing some of the gross features of the membranous labyrinth. The receptor surfaces (maculae) of the saccule and utricle appear as dark bands within their cavity. The macula of the utricle is located anteriorly, near the ampulla of the superior canal and the macula of the saccule is located below. Reprinted with permission from Iurato, S., *Submicroscopic Structure of the Inner Ear,* © 1967 Pergamon Press, Ltd.

There are three semicircular canals located caudal and slightly superior to the vestibule. These bony canals are curved tubes, each of which is continuous at two ends with the space of the vestibule. From their position in man, the canals have been named the horizontal, lateral, or external canal, the superior or anterior (vertical) canal, and the posterior (vertical) canal. Each canal forms about two thirds of a circle and lies at approximately right angles to the other two canals (Fig. 7-2). The bony canals measure about 0.28 mm in diameter, but at one end become enlarged into an osseous ampulla about 0.9 mm in diameter (Fernández and Valentinuzzi, 1968). The ampulla of the horizontal canal is located at its anterior end, as is the ampulla of the anterior canal. Both open into the anterior end of the utricle, close to one another. The ampulla of the posterior canal is directed away from the other two and opens into the opposite end of the vestibule. The narrow end or crus of the horizontal canal opens into the vestibule near the ampulla of the posterior canal. The nonampullated ends of the two vertical (anterior and posterior) canals unite to form the common crus, through which they communicate with the vestibule.

The horizontal canals of the two ears lie in the same plane. Fernández and Valentinuzzi (1968) have measured the orientation of the semicircular canals of the cat with respect to the three planes of the skull. The horizontal canal is parallel with the horizontal plane of the skull and forms 90-degree angles with the sagittal and frontal planes of the skull. The anterior and posterior canals lie in nearly vertical planes, each forming a 90-degree angle with the horizontal plane of the skull and with the horizontal canal. The anterior canal forms a 36.5-degree angle with the sagittal plane and a 53-degree angle with the frontal plane. The posterior canal forms a 53-degree angle with the sagittal plane and a 36.5-degree angle with the frontal plane. The anterior and posterior canals form a right angle between them that opens laterally. The anterior canal of one ear is therefore nearly in the same plane as the posterior canal of the other ear, whereas the posterior, or anterior, canal of one ear is at right angles to its fellow of the opposite ear, as well as to the other two canals of the same ear.

The membranous labyrinth is a system of epithelial ducts and sacs filled with a clear fluid, the endolymph. Located within the membranous labyrinths are the sensory receptor surfaces of the ear; the organ of Corti, the macula sacculi, the macula utriculi, and the cristae ampullaris. The membranous labyrinth lies enclosed within the bony labyrinth. Within the vestibular portion of the ear, thin connective-tissue membranes forming a spider's-weblike network connect the periosteum that lines the bony labyrinth to the membranous labyrinth. The membranous and bony labyrinths are generally separated by a perilymphatic space. The outer aspect of the membranous labyrinth is in contact with the periosteum of the bony labyrinth only in certain places. Detailed measurements on the physical dimensions of the osseous and membranous portions of the cat labyrinth have been made by Fernández and Valentinuzzi (1968) and are summarized in Table 7-1. The following description of the membranous labyrinths is based primarily upon the observations of Lindeman (1969) on guinea-pig, rabbit, monkey, cat, and human ears.

In the vestibule are the membranous utricle and saccule (Fig. 7-3). The utricle and saccule lie just medial to the oval window on the medial wall of the vestibule. Their medial aspects are attached to the wall of the bony labyrinth by periotic connective tissue and by fibers of the vestibular nerve that enter their maculae. The lateral aspect of each is a free surface. Thus the utricle and saccule are partially supported by the perilymph in which they float. The utricle is an irregularly shaped tube with an oval cross-section. The utricle lies in an oblong groove in the medial wall of the vestibule, the elliptical recess, above the saccule. The sensory epithelium of the utricle is situated in a dilatation of the anterior part of the utricle, the utricular recess, and is called the macula utriculi (Fig. 7-3). With the head in the erect position, the macula utriculi lies with its main plane parallel to the horizontal plane of the head. The sensory epithelium of the macula utriculi rests upon a cushion of connective tissue, blood vessels, and nerve fibers that is fixed to bone anteriorly. The saccule is a flattened, irregular-shaped sac that lies in a groove in the medial wall of the vestibule, the spherical recess. The upper portion of the saccule projects up to the utricle and has a broad attachment to the utricular recess, but does not communicate with the utricle along this site of contact. A subepithelial layer of connective tissue, blood vessels, and nerve fibers attach the sensory epithelium of the saccule, the macula sacculi, to the bone forming the medial wall of the vestibule. With the head in an erect position, the macula sacculi is approximately vertical and at right angles with the main plane of the macula utriculi.

The surface of the macula utriculi faces toward the top of the head, whereas that of the macula sacculi faces outward toward the ear. The macula sacculi is hook shaped with an anterior part that bulges outward in a superior direction. The macula of the utricle is kidney shaped with the anterior part curving upward, much like the front end of a sled. The maculae of the utricle and saccule are covered with gelatinous mantles within which are embedded crystals of calcite (Fig. 7-4). These coverings are known as "statoconial membranes," and the calcite crystals as "statoconia" or "otoliths." The oblong statoconia are of different sizes and are arranged in layers. The sizes of statoconia and the density of the layers vary depending upon which region of the macula they overlie (Fig. 7-11). The saccule and utricle together are frequently termed the "otolith organs." The overlying statoconial membranes of the maculae have the same shape as the receptor surfaces. The sensory epithelia of the two maculae are not uniform in appearance; rather, stripes can be seen in the central portion of the two maculae. These stripes

Table 7-1. Intrinsic Metric Characteristics of Cat Labyrinth (Fernandez & Valentinuzzi, 1968)

	HC Canal			AVC Canal			PVC Canal			Sacculus	Utriculus
	Osseous	Memb.	Ampulla	Osseous	Memb.	Ampulla	Osseous	Memb.	Ampulla		
r (cm)	0.014	0.011	0.064	0.014	0.013	0.058	0.013	0.012	0.069	0.053	0.07
R (cm)	0.17	0.17		0.20	0.20		0.15	0.15			
L (cm)	1.06	1.06		1.13	1.13		1.00	1.00			
Circle area (πR^2) cm²	0.09	0.09		0.13	0.13		0.07	0.07			
Cross-section area (πr^2) x 10^{-4}cm²	6.1	3.8	128.7	6.3	5.3	106.8	5.3	4.4	148.6	88.0	154.0
Volume (10^{-6}cm³)	493	403	546	580	533	400	437	373	696	616	1.36

HC, HHORIZONTAL CANAL; AVC, anterior canal; PVC, posterior canal; r, radius of cross-section area; R, radius of curvature of canal; L, length of the canal as a circle.

correspond to distinctions in the overlying statoconial membranes and in the organization of the receptor cells in the sensory epithelium. The region of the stripes has been termed the "striola" (Werner, 1940). The striola can be used to divide the receptor surface of the maculae into a pars interna (the medial portion of the macula sacculi and the superior portion of the macula utriculi) and a pars externa (Fig. 7-4). The position of the statoconial membrane has been shown to be affected by the pull of gravity and centrifugal forces (De Vries, 1950).

The saccule is connected to the utricle by way of the saccular and utricular duct, and to the cochlear duct by way of the ductus reuniens (Fig. 7-3). The endolymphatic duct arises at the meeting of the saccular duct and utricular duct. The endolymphatic duct leaves the cavity of the vestibule and ends in the cavity of the skull in the endolymphatic sac. The utricle is continuous with the semicircular ducts at five openings: one at each of the ampullae; one at the crus of the horizontal canal; and one at the common crus.

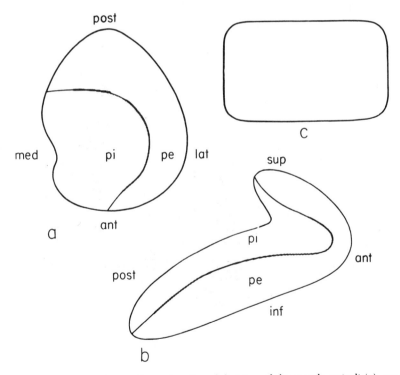

Fig. 7-4. Guinea pig. Diagram illustrating the subdivisions of the macula utriculi (a), macula sacculi (b), and the sensory epithelium of the crista ampullaris (c). Each of the maculae is divided into two areas, the pars interna (pi) and the pars externa (pe), generally with opposite morphological polarization of the sensory cells. (Lindeman, 1969.)

The three membranous semicircular ducts lie in the bony semicircular canals. The ducts are eccentrically placed in the canals, with their convex sides close to the periosteum. In general, there is a perylymphatic space between the canals and ducts that is crossed by a fine network of fibrous tissue and blood vessels. The perilymphatic space between the roof of a membranous ampulla and the periosteum is also crossed by a fine network of fibrous tissue and blood vessels. The basal part of the membranous ampulla is in contact with bone. A septum of connective tissue, blood vessels, and nerve fibers projects into the cavity of the ampulla at its base to form a transverse ridge called the crista ampullaris (Fig. 7-5). The crista ampullaris is covered by sensory epithelium over which a gelatinous substance, the cupula, extends to the roof of the ampulla and out to its lateral walls. The sensory epithelium of each cristae is formed by a rectangular-shaped sheet of epithelium (Fig. 7-4). Lindeman (1969) divides the sensory epithelium of the cristae into a central and a peripheral zone. The crista extends across the ampulla and has been described to be oriented with the long axis vertical to the plane of the semicircular duct. However, according to Lindeman (1969), the cristae of the guinea pig are not found at right angles to the plane of the semicircular ducts.

In addition to the five major receptor surfaces described above, in the cat, the lion, and some other animals (Gacek, 1961; Igarashi, 1965) the vestibular labyrinth contains a small sensory organ that Benjamins (1913)

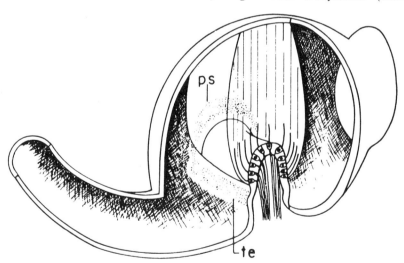

Fig. 7-5. Mammal. Schematic drawing illustrating the architecture of the ampulla. The crista, traversing the ampulla, is covered by sensory epithelium. The hairs of the sensory cells protrude into the cupula, which is assumed to extend from the surface of the epithelium to the roof of the ampulla and outward to the plana semilunata (ps) on the side walls of the ampulla. The transitional epithelium (te) is located at the base of the crista. (Lindeman, 1969.)

has termed the "crista neglecta." In the cat, this structure is located on the floor of the utricle, 800 to 900 microns from the crista ampullaris of the posterior canal and about 1.0 mm from the entrance of the common crus into the utricle (Fig. 7-6). It is circular or ovoid in shape with a diameter of 200 to 300 microns. The sensory area consists of a mound containing both receptor and supporting cells surrounded by a ridge of transitional epithelium (Montandon et al., 1970). No statoconia are contained in the covering membrane. The receptor cells are of the same types as those found in other vestibular end organs and have both afferent and efferent nerve terminals.

MECHANICS OF THE VESTIBULAR ORGANS

The vestibular end organs can be stimulated in several ways (Dusser de Barenne, 1934). Either natural stimulation can be used or electrical or thermal (caloric) stimulation. Natural stimuli include static displacements of the head and linear and angular movements. When head movements are in a straight line, e.g., progressing in any dimension of space, the movement is termed "linear." Head movements in other directions, e.g., rotational

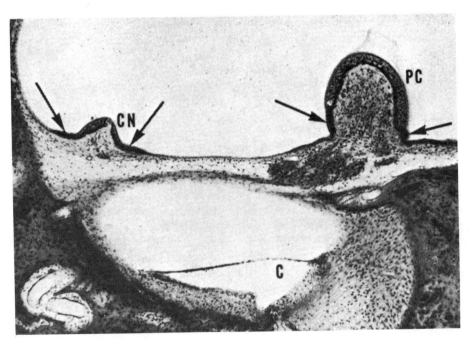

Fig. 7-6. Cat. Photomicrograph of the posterior canal crista (PC) and crista neglecta (CN). Arrows indicate the location of transitional epithelium. C: cochlear duct of basal turn of the cochlea. (Montandon et al., 1970.) Reproduced with the permission of Dr. Montandon & The Annals of Otology, Rhinology & Laryngology.

movements around any axis in space, are referred to as "angular." To produce these movements, the animal can be moved back and forth as in an automobile, or up and down as in an elevator (linear movements), or the head can be rotated about a fixed point as on a swing or spinning barber's chair (angular movements). It is also possible to produce static displacements of the statoconial membranes by centrifugal forces set up when the animal is rotated off center.

The stimulus affecting the vestibular receptors is believed to arise from a mechanical displacement of either the statoconial membranes in the saccule and utricle or of the cupulae in the ampullae of the semicircular canals. This displacement is thought to occur during head movements because of gravity effects or from forces set up by the head movements themselves. There have been no experimental studies on the mechanical movements of the cupulae or the statoconial membranes in any mammal. The displacements of statoconial membranes of the fish have been studied by de Vries (1950). Using x-ray photography, he measured the displacements of the statoconial membranes to static forces developed by placing the decapitated fish heads at different angles to the force of gravity and by centrifugal forces set up by rotation of the head. Displacements by gravitational forces were about 0.1 mm for the statoconial membrane of the saccule and about 0.005 mm for the statoconial membrane of the utricle. The saccular statoconial membrane tended to rotate about the center of its spherical surface when its displacements occurred in the plane of the sacculus. The statoconial membrane of the sacculus could also be displaced with low-frequency vibration of the head.

The mechanism for stimulating the vestibular receptors of the semicircular canals is believed to be displacements of the cupula induced by angular movements of the head with respect to inertial space. When angular accelerations of the head in any canal plane occur, the endolymph fluid within the canal tends to lag behind the canal structure owing to the inertia of the fluid. This lag is equivalent to a movement or flow of endolymph in the canal and results in the displacement of the cupula. Cupular displacements have not been measured in mammals. Steinhausen (1931) has measured cupular displacements in fish to angular accelerations and to caloric stimulation. With a turning motion in the plane of the canal, the force of the endolymph moves the cupula. By direct manometric measurement, Dohlman (1941) found cupular movement in living fish form pressure changes equal to 0.05 mm of water. With cessation of an angular movement, the cupula will regain its normal position although several seconds may elapse before it does so.

FINE STRUCTURE OF THE VESTIBULAR ORGANS

The basic features of the sensory epithelium are the same in the maculae and cristae (Lindeman, 1969). A basement membrane separates the sensory epithelium from the subepithelial tissue. The sensory epithelium consists of sensory receptor cells and supporting cells (Fig. 7-7). The supporting cells extend from the basement membrane up to the surface of the sensory epithelium. The sensory cells extend from the surface of the sensory epithelium down to a varying depth, but never as far as the surface of the basement membrane. Numerous nerve fibers and nerve endings are located between the sensory and supporting cells. The free surface of the sensory cell gives rise to a number of sensory hairs, consisting of one kinocilium and a number of stereocilia. The stereocilia are attached to a cuticular plate at the free surface of the receptor cell. The kilnocilium originates from a basal body located in a cuticular free area of the cell surface. The supporting cells surround the sensory cells and enclose nerve fibers in the basal region of the epithelium. On their free surface the supporting cells are covered by microvilli. Receptor and supporting cells can be distinguished when viewed in a surface preparation. The sensory cells have a round or oval shape and are surrounded by supporting cells which are more polygonal. Lindeman (1969) reports that in the cat a sensory cell is surrounded symmetrically by a rosette of supporting cells.

There are two basic types of sensory receptor cells; Type I and Type II hair cells (Wersäll, 1956; Smith, 1956). The Type I hair cells are goblet shaped and are enveloped almost entirely by a single nerve ending known as a "chalice" or "calyx" (Fig. 7-7). According to Lindeman (1969), one or more highly granulated bud-shaped nerve endings contact the chalice ending. Type II hair cells are more uniformly cylindrical and receive primarily bud-shaped nerve endings of two types in the guinea pig, richly and sparsely vesiculated. An intermediate type of hair cell has also been observed, innervated by parts of a chalice ending and also by bud-shaped endings making direct contact with the hair cell. Lindeman (1969) counted 11,250 hair cells in the macula sacculi of the cat and 26,350 in the macula utriculi. In their studies on the cat's vestibular nerve, Gacek and Rasmussen (1961) found that the macula saculi was innervated with 2,089 myelinated fibers and the macula utriculi by 2,694 myelinated fibers.

Type I and Type II hair cells are intermixed in all the vestibular sensory surfaces. Lindeman (1969) has measured their distribution in the cristae and maculae in the guinea pig. In the striola of the maculae, about two thirds of the cells are of Type I, whereas the two cell types are about equally distributed in the periphery. The density of cells is also less in the striola; cells in the striola have larger surface areas (as seen from above) than cells in the periphery. The sensory epithelia of the cristae could be divided structurally into a central region and a peripheral region. There are fewer cells in the central region than in the periphery. Type I cells constitute about 60 percent of the hair cells found in both the central regions and the periphery of the sensory epithelium of the cristae.

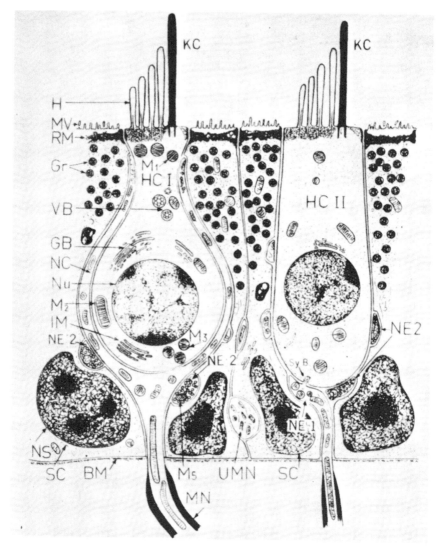

Fig. 7-7. Mammal. Schematic drawing of two vestibular sensory cells with surrounding supporting cells. HCI = hair cell Type I, HC II = hair cell Type II, H = sterocilia, KC = kinocilia, MV = microvilli, RM = reticular membrane, Gr = granules in supporting cells, VB = vesiculated bodies, GB = Golgi complex, NC = nerve calyx Nu = nucleus, IM = intracellular membranes with ribosomes NE1 = sparsely granulated nerve endings, NE2 = richly granulated nerve endings presumably with efferent functions, Sy B = synaptic bar, NS = nucleus of a supporting cell, BM = basement membrane, M1 - M5 = mitochondria, SC = supporting cell, UMN = unmyelinated nerve, MN = nerve with myelin sheath. (Engström et al., 1965.)

It is possible to distinguish two types of hairs projecting from Type I and Type II sensory cells: a long hair known as the "kinocilium," and shorter hairs called the "stereocilia" (Fig. 7-7). In the guinea pig, there are between fifty and one-hundred stereocilia on each sensory cell. The kinocilium is located eccentrically on the sensory-cell free surface (Fig. 7-8). It is the longest of the hairs and appears to be more flexible than the stereocilia. The stereocilia are arranged in parallel rows in a regular pattern. Their lengths vary considerably but regularly, with the stereocilia nearest the kinocilium longest and the length gradually diminishing away from the kinocilium (Fig. 7-8). A cell can be considered oriented or polarized with respect to the location of the kinocilium. When the orientation of cells is considered with respect to the different sensory surfaces, it is found that the cells of the crista lateralis are arranged with the kinocilia directed toward the utricle (Fig. 7-8). The cells of the other two cristae are polarized away from the utricle. The orientation of hairs of macula receptor cells is not uniform; rather, the location of the kinocilium depends upon the location of the sensory cell with respect to the striola. Sensory cells on either side of the striolae are polarized in opposite directions. In the cat and in the rabbit, the periphery of the macula sacculi is scalloped with the cells reversing polarity again (Fig. 7-9).

INNERVATION OF THE VESTIBULAR ORGANS

The innervation of the vestibular organs is quite complex. Both myelinated and nonmyelinated fibers travel in the vestibular nerve, although in all cases the myelinated fibers lose their myelin before entering the basement membrane of the sensory epithelium. The fibers innervating the vestibular end organs differ markedly in diameter. The fibers are loosely described as thin, medium, and thick by most investigators, although Wersäll (1956) provides diameter measurements of one to two microns, three to six microns and six to nine microns for these groups in the posterior ampullary nerve of the guinea pig. The summits of the cristae are innervated by the thick fibers and some medium fibers (Lindeman, 1969). The slopes of the cristae are innervated by medium fibers and thin fibers. The thick fibers to the central summit region of the cristae branch to innervate a small number (usually three or four) Type I cells with the large calyx endings, which almost completely envelop the cell. (Fig. 7-10) More than one Type I cell may be contained in the same calyx. The medium-sized fibers may innervate many Type I cells with calyces or Type II cells with bud-shaped endings. The smallest fibers innervate Type II cells and the calyces on Type I cells. Fibers innervating Type II cells exhibit much branching and innervate many cells. There are two types of endings on Type II cells, sparsely and richly vesiculated. The richly vesiculated endings are believed to be of efferent origin. The richly vesiculated endings are also present on the calyx endings of

MORPHOLOGICAL POLARIZATION

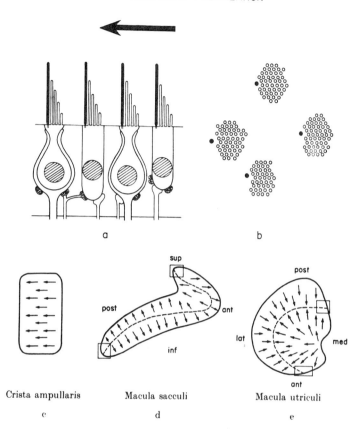

Crista ampullaris   Macula sacculi   Macula utriculi

c   d   e

Fig. 7-8. Guinea pig. Diagram illustrating the morphological polarization of the sensory cells and the polarization pattern of the vestibular sensory epithelia. The morphological polarization (arrow) of a sensory cell is determined by the position of the kinocilium in relation to the stereocilia: a—section perpendicular to the epithelium, (note increasing length of stereocilia toward the kinocilium); b—section parallel to the epithelial surface; c—the sensory cells on the crista ampullaris are polarized in the same direction; d—macula sacculi; e—macula utriculi are divided by an arbitrary curved line into two areas, the pars interna and the pars externa, with opposite morphological polarization. On the macula sacculi the sensory cells are polarized away from the dividing line; on the macula utriculi toward the line. Constant irregularities in the polarization pattern are found in areas corresponding to the continuation of the strioia peripherally (rectangles in d and e). (Lindeman, 1969.)

POLARIZATION PATTERN

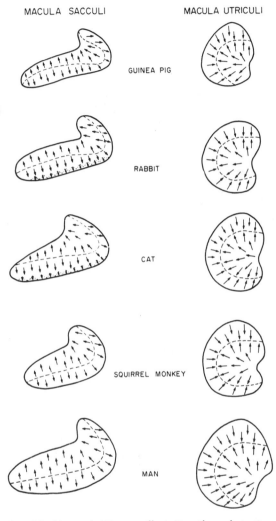

Fig. 7-9. Mammal. Diagram illustrating the polarization pattern in different species of mammals. In the macula saculi of the rabbit and cat, a marginal, antero-inferiorly located zone contains sensory cells, morphologically polarized in a direction opposite to that of the sensory cells in the remaining part of the pars externa. (Lindeman, 1969.)

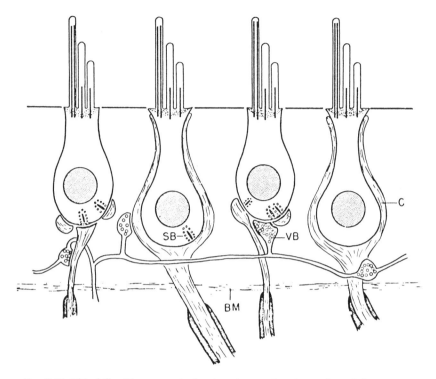

Fig. 7-10. Chinchilla. Diagrammatic drawing showing four hair cells and their nerve endings and the relationships of vesiculated boutons (VB) to hair cells, chalice terminals (C), other boutons and nerve fibers in the chinchilla maculae. BM, basement membrane; SB, synaptic bar. It is believed the efferent nerves form a sort of horizontal plexus as drawn. (Smith and Rasmussen, 1965.)

Type I cells. The innervation of the maculae is similar to that found in the cristae. The large fibers preferentially innervate Type I cells in the striola with calyx-type endings.

Lindeman (1969) has summarized his anatomical studies on the macula utriculi and macula sacculi of the guinea pig in diagrammatic form. His figures are reproduced here as Figs. 7-11 and 7-12. These figures illustrate the regional differences in the statoconial membranes. Some of the differences in the distribution of the hair cells, their polarization, and their innervation patterns can also be seen in these diagrams.

The innervation of the vestibular end organs is of both afferent and efferent origin. The fibers innervating the sensory epithelium of the vestibular system are contained in the vestibular portion of the eighth cranial nerve, the other portion being the acoustic nerve. Peripherally, the vestibular nerve forms several branches as it divides to innervate the different vestibular

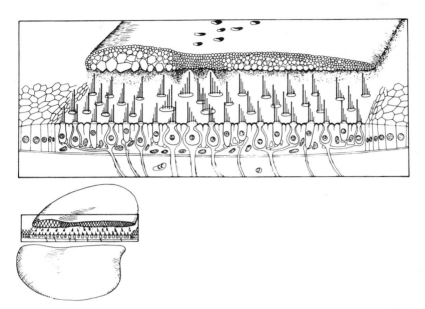

Fig. 7-11. Guinea pig. Diagram illustrating the regional differences in the structure of the macula utriculi and the statoconial membrane. Regional differences can be shown concerning the thickness of the statoconial layer; size of the statoconia; structure of the gelatinous substance; structure of the sensory hairs; size and density of the sensory cells and size of the nerve fibers. Note the change in the morphological polarization of the sensory cells in the middle of the striola. (Lindeman, 1969.)

end organs of the membranous labyrinth. Branching initially just inside the internal auditory meatus, the vestibular nerve divides into a superior and inferior division (Fig. 7-13). The superior division innervates the ampullae of the anterior and horizontal canals, the macula of the utricle and, via Voit's nerve, the anterosuperior portion of the macula of the sacculi. The inferior division of the vestibular nerve divides and innervates the macula of the sacculi and, via the posterior ampullary nerve, the ampulla of the posterior canal. The crista neglecta is innervated by a small branch of the posterior ampullary nerve (Montandon *et al.*, 1970), which contains about thirty-five fibers with sheath diameters ranging from 1.0 to 3.6 microns (Gacek, 1961).

There are approximately twelve thousand myelinated nerve fibers in the vestibular nerve of the cat (Gacek and Rasmussen, 1961). The fiber-diameter composition varies in the peripheral and central portions of the vestibular nerve and in the different parts of the superior and inferior divisions of the nerve (Gacek, 1969). Gacek and Rasmussen (1961) studied the diameters of the fibers in the peripheral portions of the vestibular nerve in the cat and other animals. A histogram of fiber diameters (Fig. 7-14) revealed a unimodel distribution with a mode value between two and three microns and a maximum diameter of ten microns.

THE VESTIBULAR GANGLION

The majority of the fibers of the vestibular nerve arise from cell bodies located in the vestibular ganglion or Scarpa's ganglion. The cell bodies of Scarpa's ganglion form a band of cells stretching obliquely across the vestibular nerve just inside the internal auditory meatus. The approximately 12,000 cells (Gacek, 1969) of Scarpa's ganglion are almost exclusively of the bipolar type, with the peripheral fiber issuing from one end of the cell body and the central process from the other (Fig. 7-15). According to Alexander (1901), the cells in the cat's Scarpa's ganglion vary from 16 to 24 microns in diameter and can be grouped into large and small cells, with large fibers issuing from the former and small fibers from the latter. Ballantyne and Engström (1969), utilizing electron microscopy, found that there were two cell-size groups in the guinea pig's vestibular ganglion, one between 15 and 27 microns and the other between 27 and 37 microns. Most of the vestibular ganglion cells are covered with myelin, although the myelin covering is not uniform from cell to cell nor on different parts of the same cell. According to Ramón y Cajal (1909), some multipolar cells can be seen in Scarpa's ganglion (Fig. 7-15). Fibers terminating within the vestibular ganglion can also be seen in Fig. 7-15. These fibers enter the ganglion via an anastomosis with the

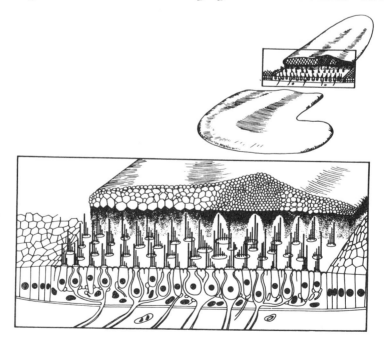

Fig. 7-12. Guinea pig. Diagram illustrating the regional differences in the structure of the macula sacculi and the statoconial membrane. (Lindeman, 1969.)

nervous intermedius portion of the facial nerve. These fibers make synaptic contacts with unmyelinated cells within the ganglion in the mouse (Ehrenbrand and Wittemann, 1970).

The cells of Scarpa's ganglion form two distinct groupings: a rostral one associated with the superior division of the vestibular nerve, and a caudal grouping associated with the inferior division. Gacek (1969) traced the connections of Scarpa's ganglion to the vestibular end organs in the cat by

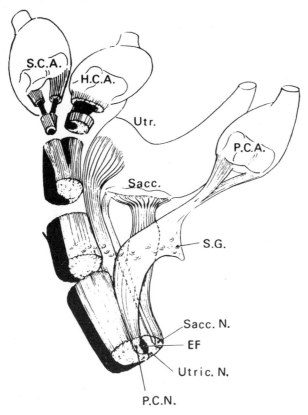

Fig. 7-13. Cat. Drawing from a dorsal view of the right vestibular nerve and end organs summarizing the peripheral location of first order neurons. The dark and light areas in the superior division represent the location of large and small caliber neurons respectively to the superior and horizontal canal cristae as explained in text; this nerve is segmented in the drawing in order to demonstrate the change in position of the large and small fibers in the nerve trunks. EF, efferent fibers; H.C.A., horizontal canal ampulla; P.C.A. and P.C.N., posterior canal ampulla and nerve; S.C.A., superior canal ampulla; S.G., Scarpa's ganglion; Sacc. and Sacc. N., sacculus and sacculan nerve; Utric and Utric N., utriculus and utricular nerve. (Gacek, 1969.)

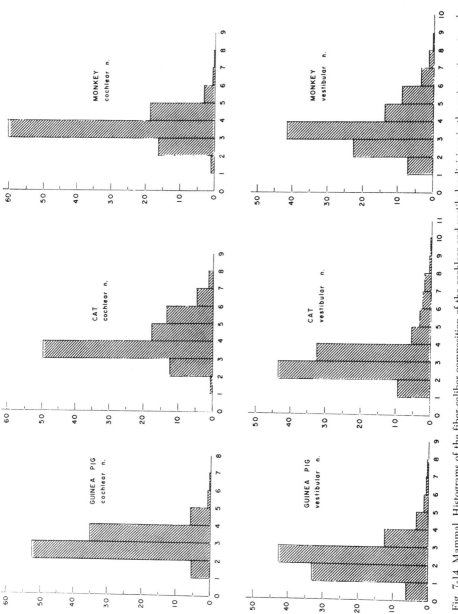

Fig. 7-14. Mammal. Histograms of the fiber-caliber composition of the cochlear and vestibular divisions in the guinea pig, cat, and monkey. Each graph represents the mean values of the data from at least two specimens. Ordinates, percentage composition;

dissecting the peripheral fibers. He found that the fibers to the macular end organs arise from the ventral portions of Scarpa's ganglion, with the fibers to the utricular macula originating from the most ventral and caudal region of the superior-division ganglion and the fibers to the saccular macula originating from a mass of cells in the main saccular nerve of the inferior-division ganglion. The fibers to the cristae originated from dorsal portions of Scarpa's ganglion (Fig. 7-13). The superior and horizontal canal cristae were innervated by a mass of cells in the most rostral portion of the superior-

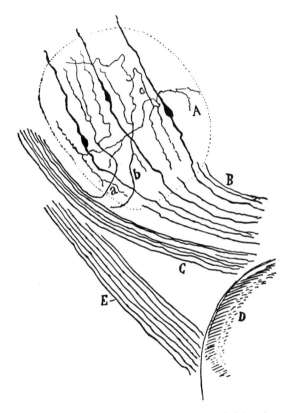

Fig. 7-15. Mouse, Scarpa's ganglion as revealed by the
Golgi technique.
A. Scarpa's ganglion.
B. Internal branches of the vestibular nerve.
C. Nervus intermedius.
D. Brain stem.
E. Facial nerve.
a, b. Fibers coming from the nervous in-
termedius.
c. Intra-ganglionic terminal branches.
(Ramón y Cajal, 1909.)

division ganglion and another cell group in the dorsal caudal region of the superior-division ganglion. The ganglion cells innervating the posterior canal crista were located in the dorsal portion of the inferior division ganglion. This description of the location of ganglion cell bodies projecting to the vestibular end organs is in most respects similar to that given by Lorente de Nó (1926) and Voit (1907). According to Gacek (1969), the two cell groups innervating the superior and horizontal canals give rise to fibers of different diameters. Fibers of large diameter originate from the rostral portion of the superior-division ganglion and small-size fibers originate from the dorsal caudal region of the superior-division ganglion. As the fibers traveled toward the periphery, the large fibers tended to form the core of each ampullary nerve and the small fibers surrounded them. The large fibers were destined for the crest of the cristae, and the smaller fibers for the slopes of the cristae. Even smaller fibers innervated more peripheral regions of the cristae. Fibers in the inferior division of the vestibular nerve were mainly of small diameter with large fibers scattered among them.

PROJECTION TO THE CENTRAL NERVOUS SYSTEM

The central projections of the cells of Scarpa's ganglion have been described by Gacek (1969) in the cat. By making small lesions in the different cell groups in the vestibular ganglion, he traced their peripheral and central connections with fiber-degeneration techniques. A line drawing summarizing the central course and termination of the different cell groups innervating the canal cristae is presented in Fig. 7-16. The cell groups of origin of the large and small fibers of the vestibular nerve innervating the superior and horizontal canal cristae project in part to distinct locations within the brain stem. The large and small fibers innervating the superior canals are illustrated with a thick line and a thin line respectively (Fig. 7-16). The small fibers from the superior semicircular canals project to the interstitial nucleus of the vestibular nerve (N.I.V.), the cerebellum, to ventral and dorsal parts of the superior vestibular nucleus (S.V.N.), to parts of the medial vestibular nucleus (M.V.N.), and to cells in the dorsal vestibular nucleus (D.V.N.). The large fibers project to these nuclei also, but as can be seen they project to different locations in the superior and medial vestibular nuclei. The fibers from cells that innervate the posterior canal are indicated with a dark medium-width line, which indicates the termination of both large and small posterior canal fibers since these could not be studied independently.

The central terminals of the fibers from cells innervating the maculae of the saccule and utricle are also shown by Gacek in line drawings in Fig. 7-17. As can be seen, the central terminations of the cells innervating the otolith organs are quite dissimilar from the terminations of the cells innervating the

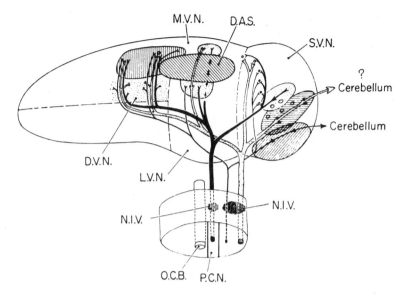

Fig. 7-16. Cat. Line drawing summarizing the central course and termination of semicircular canal neurons in the vestibular nuclei. The large and small fibers innervating the superior canals are illustrated with a large line and a thin line respectively. Large and small fibers innervating posterior canals are indicated with a medium-sized line. DVN—dorsal vestibular nucleus; MVN—medial vestibular nucleus; S.V.N.—superior vestibular nucleus; L.V.N.—lateral vestibular nucleus; N.I.V.—interstitial nucleus of vestibular nerve; O.C.B.—olivo-cochlear bundle; D.A.S.—dorsal acoustic stria; P.C.N.—posterior canal nerve. (Gacek, 1969.)

cristae of the canals. Neurons innervating the otolith organs do not synapse in the interstitial nucleus of the vestibular nerve, nor do they apparently send axons to the cerebellum. The fibers from neurons innervating the utricle terminate on a few neurons of the lateral vestibular nucleus (L.V.N.), but the main projection of the ascending limb is to a rostral part of the medial vestibular nucleus. Fibers of utricular origin also terminate in the dorsal vestibular nucleus. The central destination of fibers from cells innervating the macula of the saccule is quite distinct from that of fibers from any other vestibular end organ. As can be seen in Fig. 7-17, these fibers terminate on a small part of the lateral vestibular nucleus, the dorsal vestibular nucleus, and a small brain stem group called "Group Y" by Brodal and Ponpeiano (1957).

Comparison of the diagrams in Figs. 7-16 and 7-17 reveals that neurons innervating different vestibular end organs project to dissimilar parts of the brain stem. The dorsal nucleus receives inputs from all vestibular end organs.

EFFERENT INNERVATION

In addition to receiving fibers from Scarpa's ganglion, the vestibular end

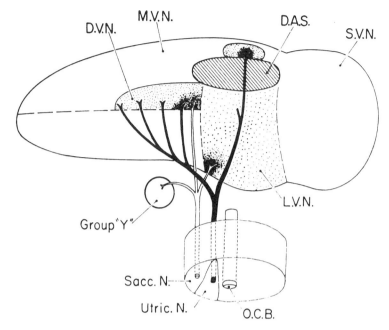

Fig. 7-17. Cat. Line drawing summarizing the central course and termination of neurons supplying the otolith endorgans. (Gacek, 1969.)

organs receive fibers originating from various regions within the brain stem. Rossi and Cortesina (1963), using acetylcholinesterase staining, demonstrated in the rabbit that the efferent fibers in the eighth nerve arise from five locations. Two of these fiber bundles corresponded to the crossed and uncrossed olivocochlear bundles of Rasmussen (1946; 1960). One of the other three efferent tracts (the uncrossed efferent reticular bundle) arose from cells in the reticular substance of the medulla. The "direct ventral vestibular efferent bundle" arose from a small nucleus near the lateral vestibular nucleus. The "direct dorsal efferent vestibular bundle" originated from the anterior caudal part of the lateral vestibular nucleus. These five bundles fuse as they emerge from the brain stem. The resulting single bundle courses with the vestibular nerve and then distributes to the cochlear and vestibular end organs.

According to Rasmussen and Gacek (1958) and Gacek (1960), the efferent fibers of the eighth nerve travel in a single bundle in the central portion of the vestibular nerve. At a point near Scarpa's ganglion, the efferents to the cochlea diverge via the vestibulocochlear anastomosis. The efferent vestibular fibers, numbering about four hundred (Gacek et al., 1965), continue peripherally in both the superior and inferior divisions of the vestibular nerve to innervate all of the vestibular end organs. Pratt (1969), utilizing histochemical stains, studied the efferent fiber input to the maculae of the saccule and utricle. He found that the fibers were not distributed to the central portions of the maculae. The efferent fibers innervated only the peripheral portions of the maculae. Prior to penetrating the basement membrane of a maculae, each efferent fiber divided into several branches. The branches formed neural plexes that surrounded the sensory cells at their bases. The efferent fibers are believed to be the small fibers forming the richly vesiculated endings on the Type II cells and on the calyx endings of the Type I cells.

NEUROPHYSIOLOGY OF THE VESTIBULAR NERVE

The classic studies on the vestibular system have been performed on the isolated labyrinth of the thornback ray (Lowenstein and Sand, 1940; Groen *et al.*, 1952). The anatomy of the vestibular end organ in this organism is different from that of the mammalian vestibular end organ (no Type I cells have been identified, for instance). The most complete study of unit activity in the vestibular nerve of a mammal has been performed by Goldberg and Fernández (1971a; 1971b) on the squirrel monkey. We will report extensively on the findings of Goldberg and Fernández, since anatomical studies of the mammalian inner-ear structures, including the cochlea, demonstrate that they are highly similar across species. It must be realized, however, that one of the major utilizations of vestibular end-organ information is undoubtedly for the control of posture and locomotion; and in these respects, there are marked differences in the arboreal squirrel monkey and terrestrial cat.

Goldberg and Fernández recorded unit activity with fine tipped glass pipettes from units in and near Scarpa's ganglion, which in the squirrel monkey is not buried in the internal auditory meatus as it is in the cat. It is probable that they recorded from both cells and fibers, since injury discharges were reported (Goldberg and Fernández, 1971a). The apparatus used for inducing precision movements of the head of the squirrel monkey is depicted in Fig. 7-18. With this device they studied the response of units to constant angular accelerations (Goldberg and Fernández, 1971a) and to sinusoidal oscillations of the head (Fernández and Goldberg, 1971). We shall only report on those aspects of their work relating to unit classification.

The vestibular units were divided into two groups, canal units and otolith units, on the basis of how they responded to manual movements of the device shown in Fig. 7-18. An "otolith unit" was "unresponsive to angular accelerations but was sensitive to changes in head position relative to the vertical meridan" (Goldberg and Fernández, 1971a). A "canal unit" responded to angular accelerations. Only reports on the activity of canal units were available at the time of this writing. Canal units were further subdivided into three groups, depending upon the plane of effective angular acceleration. These three groups were labeled horizontal-canal, superior-canal, and posterior-canal units in accordance with the assumed crista innervation. All the units that were studied exhibited some degree of spontaneous activity. This spike activity could be increased or decreased, depending upon the type of unit and the direction of head movement. Horizontal-canal units were excited by rotations that would deflect the cupula toward the utricle (i.e., toward the kinocilium) and inhibited by

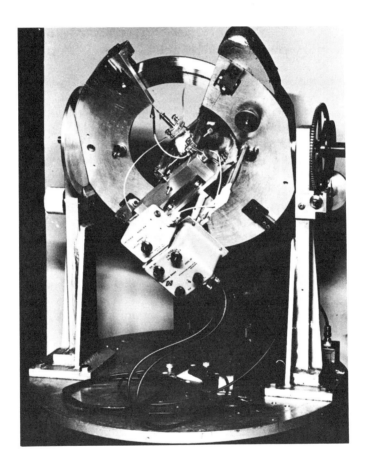

Fig. 7-18. Monkey. Photograph of animal in stimulating apparatus. Microelectrode is mounted in Davies' chamber. Rotating device below, superstructure above. Animal pivoted out of standard position for illustrative purposes. Negative-capacitance cathode follower mounted on front of animal platform. Output of cathode follower led to AC amplifier (black box) with a gain of 1000. Leads pass through center of device to slip rings. (Goldberg and Fernández, 1971a.)

rotations in the opposite direction. Posterior-canal units and anterior-canal units were excited by rotations in their respective planes from the utricle and inhibited by rotations toward the utricle.

The spontaneous and evoked discharge patterns of canal units were studied in some detail. Examples of spontaneous activity, termed "resting discharge" by Goldberg and Fernández (1971a), can be seen in Fig. 7-19. Spikes tended to be emitted continuously at fairly high rates. Rates varied from near zero to about 180 spikes/sec. with an average for the population of

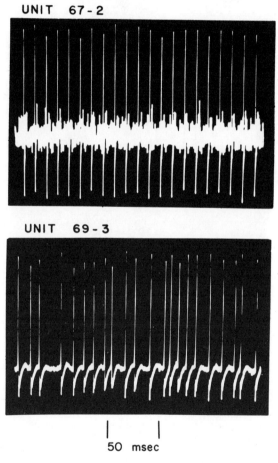

Fig. 7-19. Monkey. Action potentials recorded during resting activity. Photographs from tape-recorded data. Recording bandwidth: 100-1000 Hz. Resting discharge: unit 67-2 (superior canal, above), 97 spikes/sec.; unit 69-3 (horizontal canal, below), 98 spikes/sec. Positive is upward. (Goldberg and Fernández, 1971a.)

91.3 spikes/sec. As can be seen in Fig. 7-19, some fibers emit spikes separated by regular intervals whereas others emit spikes separated by irregular intervals. Interspike-interval (ISI) histograms of spontaneous and evoked discharge were unimodal for any unit, but varied from highly symmetrical distributions to highly skewed distributions, depending on the unit (Fig. 7-20). Rotating an animal at a constant angular acceleration changed the rate of firing but did not change the basic shape of the ISI distribution (Fig. 7-20).

Since the mean and standard deviations of the interval histograms of a unit driven at different rates tended to be related, Goldberg and Fernández

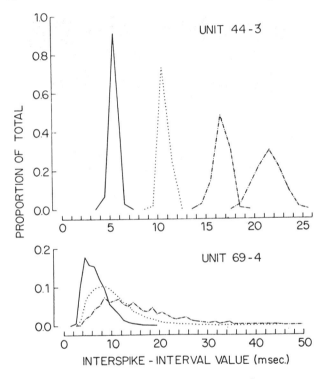

Fig. 7-20. Monkey. Interspike-interval histograms for two units. SOLID LINES, histograms during excitatory response; DOTTED LINES, during resting activity; BROKEN LINES, during inhibitory response. A: unit 44-3 (posterior canal). Stimulus conditions, each based on single presentation, for histograms (from left to right): 3.4-5.0 sec. after start of 60-deg/sec.[2] excitatory acceleration; resting activity; 8.0-10.0 sec. after start of 30-deg/sec.[2] inhibitory acceleration; 3.4-5.0 sec, 60-deg/sec[2] inhibitory acceleration. B: unit 69-4 (superior canal). Stimulus conditions, each based on 5 presentations, from left to right: 15.0-20.0 sec. after start of 15-deg/sec.[2] excitatory acceleration; resting activity; 10.0-15.0 sec. after start of 15-deg/sec.[2] inhibitory acceleration. (Fernández & Goldberg, 1971.)

(1971b) measured the coefficients of variation (standard deviation divided by mean interval) at a mean interval of 12.5 msec for a large number of units. The resulting distribution of the values of the coefficients of variation is clearly bimodal (Fig. 7-21), and suggests that two separate groups of units can be partially distinguished on the basis of their discharge patterns. The two modal values of this distribution are at coefficient of variations of 0.0579 and about 0.42. As can be seen in Fig. 7-21, there are more regularly discharging units in this sample of 142 than irregularly discharging units.

With the apparatus pictured in Fig. 7-18, it was possible to place the animal's head in a plane corresponding to the plane of the canal assumed to be innervated by the unit and to sinusoidally oscillate the animal's head about this plane. The response of a unit to sinusoidal head movements is seen in Fig. 7-22. The responses of regular and irregular units were studied to sinusoidal stimulation at a number of stimulus frequencies. From graphs

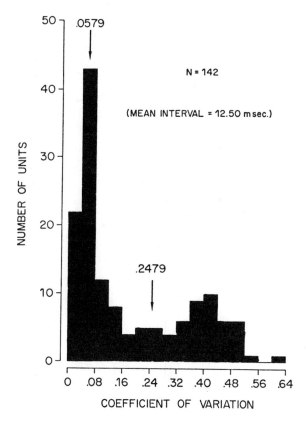

Fig. 7-21. Coefficient of variation at mean ISI interval of 12.5 msec, 142 units. (Goldberg and Fernández, 1971.)

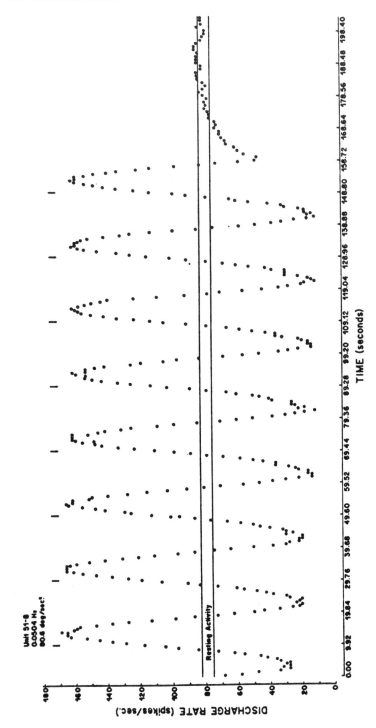

Fig. 7-22. Monkey. Response of unit 51-8 (superior canal) to 8 cycles of a sinusoidal stimulus, 0.0504 Hz, 80.6 deg/sec.[2]. Stimulus ends at 158.72 sec. Each point, average discharge rate for 1/40th of sine-wave cycle (0.496 sec.). Vertical marks, instants of peak excitatory acceleration. Lower and upper horizontal lines, respectively, resting discharge before and after stimulation. (Fernández and Goldberg, 1971.)

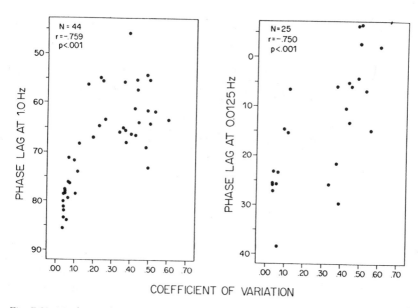

COEFFICIENT OF VARIATION

Fig. 7-23. Monkey. Relations between coefficient of variation at mean ISI rate of 12.5 msec. and phase lags at 0.0125 Hz (left) and 1.0 Hz (right). N, number of units; r, rank-order correlation coefficient; p, significance of correlation (t-test). (Goldberg and Fernández, 1971b)

such as those presented in Fig. 7-22, Goldberg and Fernández derived a measure relating the phase of pulse discharge to the phase of sinusoidal oscillations. It was found that the phase of discharge tended to lag the phase of stimulation. When the phase lag measured for each unit was plotted against the coefficient of variation for each unit, the population seemed to fall into two clearly separated groups, especially for sinusoidal stimuli of 0.0125 Hz (Fig. 7-23). Thus, there seem to be two major unit groups in the monkey's vestibular nerve, regular and irregularly discharging units. Kiang (1971) has reported that these two unit groups can also be detected in the vestibular nerve of the cat.

8
SENSORY SYSTEMS OF MUSCLE

Muscle is the means by which the body converts chemical energy into mechanical energy. With muscles the cat howls, breathes, defecates, pumps blood, expels the contents of the bladder, erects hairs, and otherwise performs the mechanical functions required to attain mobility and sustain life. Three major types of muscle have been distinguished: heart muscle, smooth muscle, and skeletal muscle. These three kinds of muscle have quite different structures, perform different kinds of tasks and are influenced by different kinds of sensory systems. We will discuss in this book only skeletal muscle. The elucidation of some of the complexities of skeletal muscle innervation is one of the best examples in sensory neurophysiology of the interplay between neuroanatomy and neurophysiology and their interdependence.

The different muscles classified as striated or skeletal on the basis of structure have quite different tasks: Some control the anal sphincter, some move the eyes or the tongue, others move bones. The sensory innervation of these different types of muscles is different (Cooper, 1960). In fact, some of the muscle sensory systems discussed in this chapter are found only in the somatic muscles of the trunk and limbs. The sensory systems of the somatic muscles of the cat's tongue, facial muscles, and eye muscles are different, at least in part.

This chapter then is concerned with the sensory systems of the muscles of the trunk and limbs. These muscles also have different tasks. Some are concerned primarily with moving bones, others in stabilizing them. In addition to moving bones, the muscles must hold the skeletal frame rigid, counteract the pull of gravity, and maintain a stable body position. To perform these tasks, the skeletal muscles work in coordinated groups. Different muscles contract and others relax in the performance of complicated movements. How well these muscles perform is as well seen in the cat as any other animal. The cat is capable of greater acrobatic feats than any other ground animal. He can leap over six feet straight up in the air from a sitting position. He can climb trees with a squirrel-like agility. He can hold himself motionless in almost any position for an indefinite period. In the wild, a cat's survival is to a great extent dependent upon his athletic abilities.

Skeletal muscle consists of bundles of long cylindrical fibers known as extrafusal muscle fibers. Individual fibers are bound together by connective tissue into fasciculi. These fasciculi in turn are bound together into longer bundles known as muscles. Each fiber, each fasciculus, and each muscle is encased in connective tissue. Muscles are attached to bones by tendons formed from connective tissue, or to one another by large bands of connective tissue known as aponeuroses. Muscles accomplish their mechanical functions by contracting. Muscle fibers shorten or contract in response to nerve impulses brought to them by efferent motor fibers that leave the spinal cord via the ventral roots. Each motor fiber innervates more than one muscle fiber. The skeletal muscles are attached to the bones in several layers. Some of the muscles of the legs of the cat are illustrated in Fig. 8-1. These muscles have been the most frequent subject of study by both neurophysiologists and neuroanatomists. The muscles receive both afferent and efferent nerve fibers (Fig. 8-2). Some of the features of the sensory systems of muscles are reviewed in detail in the following pages. An additional treatment of various aspects of muscle neurophysiology can be found in the recent book by Granit (1970).

NEUROANATOMY OF MUSCLE

The complex neural innervation of muscles has occupied the attention of neuroanatomists from Ramón y Cajal and Ruffini to many present-day investigators. The description of the innervation of the muscle presented in this book is largely that which has been worked out by Barker and his associates. It has only been after many years of work by Barker and his associates, and others, that some of the measurement variables have been enumerated and some of the details worked out. As we shall see, their task has been a formidable one, and even now our understanding of muscle innervation is incomplete.

AFFERENT INNERVATION OF MUSCLE

The complexity of the sensory systems of the muscle is mirrored in the heterogeneity of the nerve fibers innervating a muscle. The sensory nerve fibers are both myelinated and nonmyelinated; and nonmyelinated fibers may outnumber the myelinated fibers (Stacey, 1969). Distributions of nerve-fiber-diameter measurements disclose multiple peaks for both the myelinated and nonmyelinated sensory fibers (Fig. 8-3). It has been the unfortunate custom in muscle work to designate certain nerve-fiber-diameter

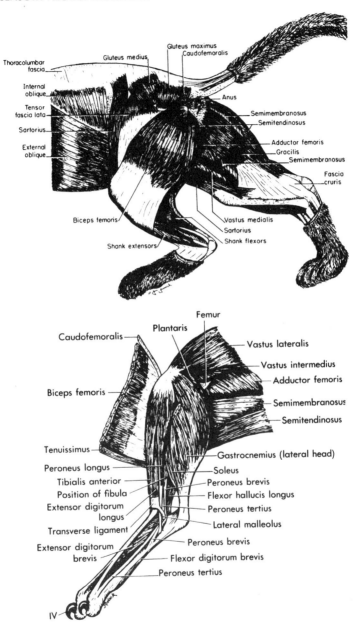

Fig. 8-1. Cat. Top: Superficial pelvic and thigh muscles. Lateral muscles can be seen on the left leg and medial muscles on the right leg. Bottom: Lateral view of the shank muscles of the cat after reflection of the biceps femoris and removal of the crural fascia. From Walker, W.F. (1972), A *Study of the Cat*, Second Edition, W.B. Saunders Co., Philadelphia.

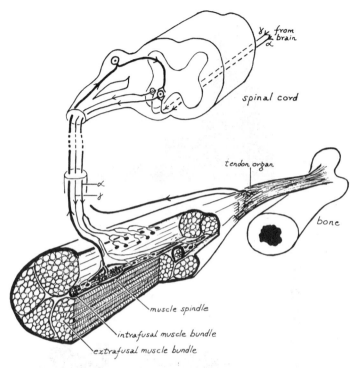

Fig. 8-2. Cat. Schematic diagram of the structure and innervation of muscles, tendon organs, and muscle spindles of skeletal muscle (simplified). (Barker, 1963.)

sizes with numerals. Thus, Group I fibers are 12 microns in diameter or larger, those in II are 4-12 microns, in III, 1.0-4.0 microns; and non-myelinated fibers are designated group IV. In some cases, these numerals correspond to definite peaks in the fiber-diameter distribution, but these peaks are not all present in the tibialis posterior muscle nerve examined in Fig. 8-3. The diameter of a nerve fiber does not remain constant; rather, it may change as it approaches its peripheral destination (Adal and Barker, 1962). In general, sensory fibers get smaller as they approach their final termination. Thus, a distribution of fiber diameters taken near the nerve origin may be quite different from a distribution of diameters of the nerve near its insertion. Stacy (1969) traced sensory fibers that formed free endings in muscle and found that the different terminal twigs were of different diameters.

Parent fibers branch to form terminal fibers that form sensory nerve endings of various types. These endings and their associated structures are sensory end organs. The different types of sensory end organs found in

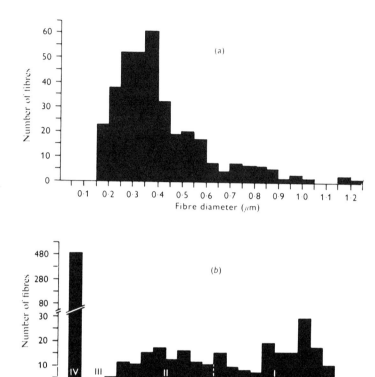

Fig. 8-3. Cat. The diameter of sensory nerve fibers in the de-efferentated and sympathectomized tibialis posterior muscle nerve of the cat. The top figure (a) was constructed from diameter measurements, made from electron micrographs, of 357 nonmyelinated fibers from two tibials posterior muscle nerves. The bottom figure (b) is a composite histogram of the total sensory-nerve-fiber component compiled from both electron microscopic and light miscroscopic observations of two tibials posterior muscle nerves. Reproduced with permission from Stacy, M. J., (1969) *Journal of Anatomy, 150:* 231-254.

muscle have been enumerated by Barker (1962, 1967) and by Stacey (1969). The schema for sensory innervation devised by Stacey on the basis of his observations and those of Barker on traced silver-stained material is presented in Fig. 8-4. The different types of sensory end organs recognized by Stacey are (1) free nerve endings, (2) paciniform or encapsulated corpuscles, (3) tendon organs, and (4) muscle spindles. As indicated in Fig. 8-4, parent fibers of different diameters innervate these sensory end organs.

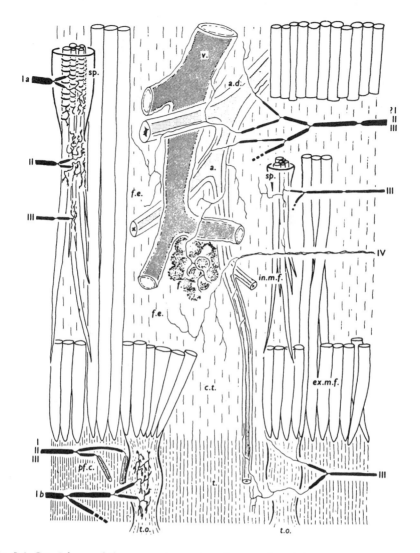

Fig. 8-4. Cat. Schema of the sensory innervation of mammalian skeletal muscle, based on observations of de-efferentated and sympathectomized cat sketetal muscle impregnated by the modified de Castro method, and on previous observations of Barker (1962).

The muscle spindle (sp.) on the left possesses a primary and two secondary endings, one of which is supplied by a group III stem fiber. The tendon organ (t.o.) on the left is innervated by a Group Ib fiber, but a much wider range of innervation is possible (see Barker, 1962). Paciniform (encapsulated) corpuscles (pf.c.) receive their innervation from stem fibers of all three myelinated fiber groups. The nerve fibers on the right of the figure are those that supply free endings (f.e.). They fall within the Group II, III, and IV diameter ranges and possibly also Group I. The axon terminals of the endings lie in association with intrafusal (in.m.f.) and extrafusal (ex.m.f.) muscle fibers, the capsules of spindles (sp.) and tendon organs (t.o.), tendon tissue (t.) at musculo-tendinous junctions, the adventitia (a.d.) of arterioles (a.) and venules (v.), fat cells (f.) and connective tissue (c.t.). Reproduced with permission from Stacy, M.J., (1969) *Journal of Anatomy, 150:* 231-254.

The free nerve endings are formed by the branched unmyelinated portion of the parent fiber. Free nerve endings constitute the bulk of the sensory end organs found in muscle. They occur in the most diverse type of tissue (fat, blood vessels, between extrafusal and intrafusal muscle fibers, in the capsules of tendon organs, etc.), and their parent fibers include all the unmyelinated sensory fibers. Two examples of free nerve endings can be seen in Fig. 8-5. Encapsulated corpuscles are formed by the terminal unmyelinated portion of myelinated fibers. Around these terminal fibers are several lamellae. A single parent fiber usually forms more than one encapsulated corpuscle. They are found near tendon organs and at musculo-tendinous junctions. They are apparently similar to the encapsulated corpuscles found in the joints and the skin (Poláček, 1966). True Vater-Pacinian corpuscles are found under the fascia of some cat muscles (Barker, 1967).

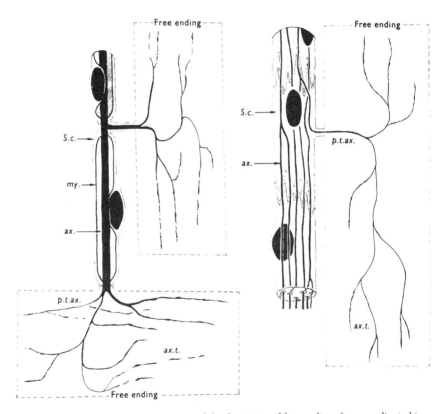

Fig. 8-5. A diagrammatic representation of the derivation of free endings from myelinated (on the left) and nonmyelinated (on the right) nerve fibers. S.c., Schwann cytoplasm; my., myelin; ax., axon; p.t.ax., preterminal axon; ax.t., axon terminal. Reproduced with permission from Stacy, M.J., (1969) *Journal of Anatomy, 150:* 231-254.

Although the free nerve endings and the encapsulated corpuscles of the muscles seem similar to sensory end organs found in other tissues, skeletal muscle contains two unique sensory structures: the Golgi tendon organ and the muscle spindle. The tendon organ consists of collagen tendon bundles forming dense fascicles into which extrafusal muscle fibers insert (about 10 muscle fibers for each tendon organ in the cat). The parent nerve fibers usually innervate only one tendon organ or at most two. Terminal branches of large-diameter sensory-nerve fibers form a complex interlacing network around the collagen fibers, and the whole tendon organ is surrounded by a capsule (Fig. 8-6). Tendon organs are found at either end of a muscle where it connects with the bone and at tendonous aponeuroses connecting muscle to muscle.

The structure that has captured the fancy of neuroanatomists from the time of Ramón y Cajal to the present is the unique muscle spindle (Fig. 8-7). Muscle spindles consist of modified muscle fibers (intrafusal muscle fibers) and their complex afferent and efferent nerve terminals. The central part of the muscle spindle is enclosed in a connective tissue capsule, and the whole spindle is embedded in the body of muscle. The number of spindles and their distribution vary widely from muscle to muscle. In the cat, no muscle spindles are found in the extraocular eye muscles, the tongue, the facial musculature (Cooper, 1960; Matthews, 1964) or in the tympanic muscles

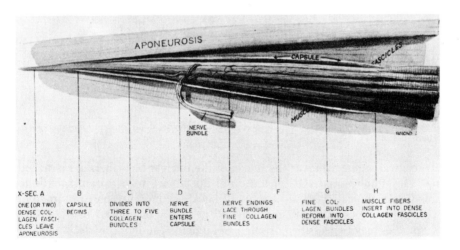

X-SEC. A	B	C	D	E	F	G	H
ONE (OR TWO) DENSE COL- LAGEN FASCI- CLES LEAVE APONEUROSIS	CAPSULE BEGINS	DIVIDES INTO THREE TO FIVE COLLAGEN BUNDLES	NERVE BUNDLE ENTERS CAPSULE	NERVE ENDINGS LACE THROUGH FINE COLLAGEN BUNDLES		FINE COL- LAGEN BUNDLES REFORM INTO DENSE FASCICLES	MUSCLE FIBERS INSERT INTO DENSE COLLAGEN FASCICLES

Fig. 8-6. Cat. This longitudinal view illustrates the way in which a tendon organ typically originates at the musculotendinous junction. The tendon organ begins to appear as a spur of dense collagen fascicles (G) projecting inward among extrafusal muscle fascicles (H). As the fascicles become isolated from the aponeurosis, they acquire a capsule (B) in which several lamellae are distinguishable. (Bridgman, 1968)

(Blevins, 1963; 1964). Fernand (1970) has shown that in the large infrahyoid muscle, the number of spindles varied from zero to 20. The arrangement of the muscle spindles in some muscles of the cat is shown in Fig. 8-8. Barker and Chin (1960) have shown that although the number of spindles may vary from cat to cat, identical pairs of muscles on different sides of the body tend to have the same number of spindles.

The intrafusal muscle fibers within a cat muscle spindle are of two types: nuclear bag fibers and nuclear chain fibers (Boyd, 1956; 1962). These intrafusal muscle fibers can be distinguished by their length, diameter, internal structure, and histochemistry. Nuclear bag fibers are large and long and extend outside the capsule. Nuclear chain fibers are smaller and usually terminate within the capsule (Bridgman *et al.*, 1969). Both types of intrafusal muscle fibers have many nuclei in the central region of the fiber where the capsule bulges. The nuclei of the nuclear chain fibers are arranged in a line in

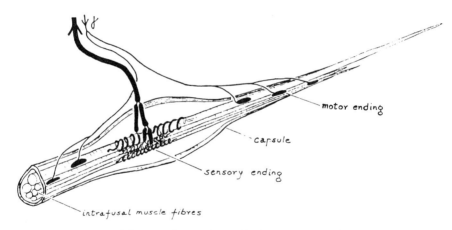

Fig. 8-7. Cat. Simplified diagram of a muscle spindle showing motor and sensory innervation. (Barker 1963)

the central region whereas the nuclei of the nuclear bag fibers are bunched up. The number and type of intrafusal fibers vary widely from spindle to spindle. In the cat there are two to 12 intrafusal muscle fibers per spindle, with the low fibered spindles composed primarily of nuclear bag fibers.

Spindles may be classified as single or tandem. Tandem spindles share one or more intrafusal muscle fibers with the same intrafusal muscle fiber entering two separate capsules. Tandem spindles occur in groups of two, three, or five spindles (Barker and Ip, 1961). Barker (1963) has observed that a single continuous intrafusal fiber may form a nuclear bag in one spindle capsule and a nuclear chain in another capsule in a tandem spindle. Barker

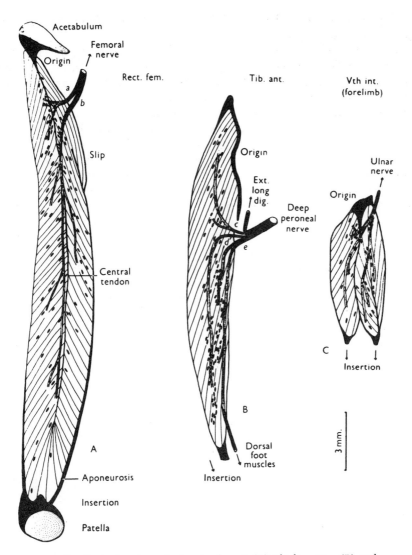

Fig. 8-8. Cat. Projection plans of cat rectus femoris (A), tibialis anticus (B), and Vth interosseus of forelimb (C) showing distribution of spindle and nerve supply. Spindles shown as black oval symbols; nerve branches a-e shown black up to point of entry into muscle. Reproduced by permission from Barker, D. & Chin, N. K., (1960) *Journal of Anatomy 94:* 473-486.

and Ip (1961) estimate that about 20 percent of the spindles in a muscle may be of the tandem type.

Both the afferent and efferent neural innervation of the intrafusal muscle spindle fibers take a complex form. Two types of afferent endings have been distinguished on the basis of fiber size and location. These two types of endings have been designated primary and secondary endings (Barker and Ip, 1960). Primary endings are formed by large fibers (Fig. 8-9) and are located on the central parts of the intrafusal muscle fibers. Secondary endings are formed by smaller diameter nerve fibers and are located on either side of the central area of the spindle. Primary endings form regular spirals around the intrafusal muscle fibers. Secondary endings may form spirals or irregular "flowerspray" endings, depending upon their location. Primary endings are located on both nuclear-bag and nuclear-chain intrafusal muscle fibers, whereas secondary endings are concentrated on nuclear-chain intrafusal muscle fibers (Barker, 1967). The sensory nerve fibers lie in troughs on the surface of the intrafusal fibers about which they entwine. The sensory endings of the central region of nuclear-bag fibers may take an anulospiral form or have a cagelike configuration (Scalzi and Price, 1971). The number of primary and secondary endings in a muscle spindle depends on the type of spindle and on the type of muscle in which it is located. Table 8-1 was prepared by Barker (1962) and demonstrates that the ratio of primary to secondary endings varies from 0.7 to 1.7, depending on the muscle. Similar variations in primary endings to tendon organ ratios occur in different muscles.

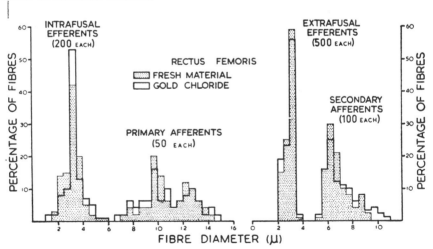

Fig. 8-9. Cat. Quantitative comparison of the external, internodal diameters of equivalent samples of sensory and motor nerve fibers from rectus femoris as measured in the fresh state, teased in mammalian Ringer's solution, and in teased gold chloride preparations. (Adal and Barker, 1962)

Table 8-1. Proportional Distribution of Afferent Endings in Various Cat Muscles (Barker, 1962)

MUSCLE	NO. STUDIED	TOTAL NO. ENDINGS				RATIOS			
		P	S	TO	PC	P:S		P:TO	
						range	av.	range	av.
rect. fem	9	920	899	705	114	0.9-1.5:1	1.0:1	0.7-2.4:1	1.3:1
soleus	3	164	130	92	6	1.0-1.4:1	1.3:1	1.7-1.9:1	1.8:1
ST	3	411	489	257	10	0.7-1.0:1	0.85:1	1.2-1.85:1	1.6:1
mesial FDL	1	51	47	17	2	-	1.1:1	-	3.0:1
V pes int.	4	108	64	99	34	1.3-2.3:1	1.7:1	0.9-1.6:1	1.1:1
IV intercostal (int. & ext.)	1	49	67	17	10	-	0.7:1	-	2.9:1

P: primary   TO: tendon organ   S: secondary   PC: paciniform corpuscle

Muscle spindles are also classified as simple, intermediate, or complex on the basis of the number and types of afferent endings found on their intrafusal muscle fibers (Fig. 8-10). Simple spindles are those that are innervated by one primary nerve fiber. Intermediate spindles have a secondary nerve fiber in addition to the primary nerve fiber. Complex spindles are characterized by one or more primary endings and two or more secondary endings. The nerve fibers supplying the primary ending of the simple spindles are of smaller diameter than the primary nerve fibers of intermediate and complex spindles (Fig. 8-11).

EFFERENT INNERVATION OF MUSCLE SPINDLES

Intrafusal muscle fibers are innervated by nerve fibers other than the afferent primary and secondary nerve fibers. These other nerve fibers are efferent nerve fibers that are carrying information to the spindle. The description of the efferent innervation of intrafusal muscle fibers has been laboriously compiled by Barker and others over the last 10 years (Barker, Stacey, and Adal, 1970). These workers relied primarily on a special type of silver stain to reveal the finer complexities of the nerve endings, although gold chloride stains, enzyme stains, and electron microscopy were also used. According to these workers, there are three different types of efferent endings on intrafusal muscle fibers: trail endings, p1 plate endings, and p2 plate endings. The trail endings are the most common and are usually intracapsule on either side of the afferent primary ending. These trail endings consist of a number of diffuse ramifications that sometimes extend over the entire pole of the intrafusal muscle fiber. Trail endings are formed by myelinated and non-myelinated nerve fibers and are found on both nuclear-bag and nuclear-chain intrafusal muscle fibers. The efferent p1 plate terminals are located near the poles of the intrafusal muscle fibers and may lie outside the central capsule. The p1 plates resemble the efferent plates on extrafusal muscle fibers in both light and electron microscopy; and p1 plates degenerate at the same rate as extrafusal plates following sectioning of the ventral roots. The majority of p1 fibers end in only one plate, and this one usually in the pole of a nuclear bag fiber (75 percent of p1 plates). The p2 plate endings are found in the same location as p1 plates but they can be distinguished by their appearance in silver and electron microscopy. About 90 percent of p2 plates are located on nuclear bag fibers and 10 percent on nuclear chain fibers. Examples of efferent endings as revealed by silver staining can be seen in Fig. 8-12.

The different types of efferent endings were not uniformly distributed along the intrafusal muscle fibers. Nerve fibers forming each of the three types of endings could branch and supply both nuclear-bag and nuclear-

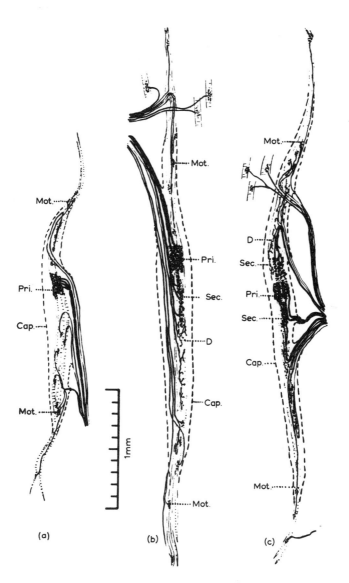

(a)

(b)

(c)

Fig. 8-10. Cat. Drawings of muscle spindles in teased gold chloride preparations. Structures projected and outlined, further details filled in from microscope studies. a. Extensor digitorum longus. Simple spindle with primary ending, Pri; and motor end-plates, Mot. b. Tibialis anticus. Intermediate spindle with primary ending, Pri; and one secondary ending, Sec. Both poles have motor end-plates, Mot; but between the end-plates of the lower pole and the secondary ending, there is a diffuse mass of endings, D, supplied by small nerve fibers. c. Soleus. Complex spindle with primary ending, Pri; and two secondary endings, Sec. There are motor end-plates, Mot. at the poles; but between these and the secondary endings, especially in the upper half of the spindle, there are regions with diffuse endings, D, supplied by small nerve fibers. The scale applies to a, b, and c. Note the greater length of the capsule, Cap., when there is a secondary ending, All the spindles have some of their intrafusal muscle fibers running beyond the capsules, and they sometimes have small end-plates on them here. (Cooper, 1960)

181

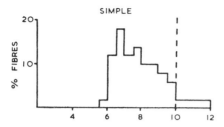

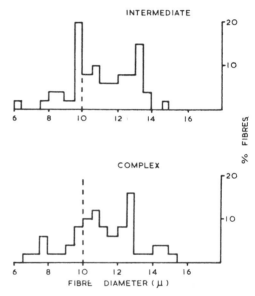

Fig. 8-11. Cat. Site measurements of the external, internodal diameters of primary nerve fibers supplying different types of muscle spindles. Fifty fibers in each sample; rectus femoris, teased gold chloride preparations. (Adal and Barker, 1962)

chain intrafusal muscle fibers. Bag fibers received both trail endings and both kinds of plate endings. Chain fibers received primarily trail endings, but also 25 percent of p1 and 10 percent of the p2 endings. The different endings arise from nerve fibers of somewhat different diameters. The nerve fibers forming p1 plates were similar in diameter to nerve fibers forming similar endings on extrafusal muscles (Fig. 8-13). Nerve fibers forming p2 plate endings were slightly larger in diameter on the average than nerve fibers forming p2 plates; the nerve fibers forming trail endings showed a wide range of diameters. Some of the nerve fibers forming trail endings were even unmyelinated (Fig. 8-13).

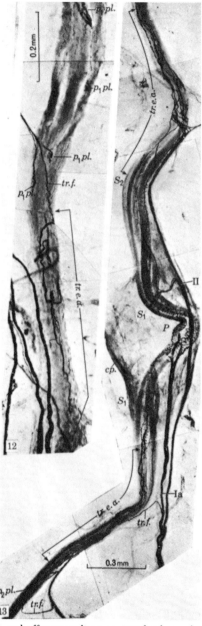

Fig. 8-12. Cat. Afferent and efferent endings on intrafusal muscle fibers. Primary (P) and secondary (S) afferent endings. Efferent endings: p1 plates, p2 plates, and trail endings (tr.e.a.). Fibers supplying trail endings, tr.f. (Barker *et al.*, 1970) Reproduced with the permission of The Royal Society.

Barker, Stacey, and Adal (1970) have summarized the efferent innervation of the muscle spindle with the diagram shown in Fig. 8-14. This figure illustrates the different types of nerve endings and where they are found. As can be seen, some p1 plates are formed by nerve fibers that also supply p1 plate endings on extrafusal muscle fibers.

NEUROPHYSIOLOGY OF MUSCLE SENSORY SYSTEMS

Muscle receptors are studied by moving or activating the muscles within which they are situated. The most common method of stimulating receptors is to move a bone to which one end of a muscle is attached or to attach a

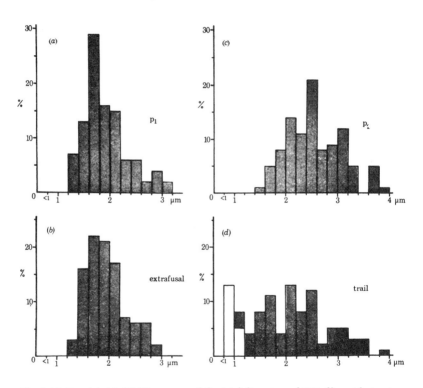

Fig. 8-13. Cat. (a), (c), (d) Histograms of the total diameters of 100 efferent fusimotor fibers, or fiber branches, supplying each type of motor ending in peroneal spindles as measured in teased silver preparations up to 0.5 mm from spindle entry: (b), similar histogram of 100 terminal branches of extrafusal nerve fibers. Unstippled columns in (d) indicate nonmyelinated trail fibers. (Barker *et al.*, 1970) Reproduced with the permission of The Royal Society.

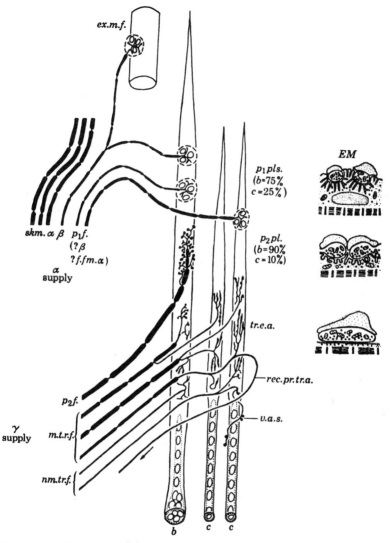

Fig. 8-14. Cat. Schematic diagram of the motor innervation of nuclear-bag (b) and nuclear-chain (c) muscle fibers in the cat, based on observations made on spindles from the peroneal and soleus muscles. Nonmyelinated trail fibers (nm.tr.f.) in just over one third of the spindles. Less than 5 percent of spindles have recurrent preterminal trail axons (rec.pr.tr.a.) leaving them. Some pl fibers (plf.) can be identified as collaterals of fibers (β) that also innervate extrafusal muscle fibers (ex.m.f.); this is not possible for the majority, which may either be connected to beta fibers or to fast fusimotor alpha fibers (f.fm.a). Sketches of the ultrastructure of the myoneural junctions of the three types of fusimotor ending are shown on right under EM. Other lettering: pl pls, pl plates; p2pl., p2 plate; p2f., p2 fiber; skm. α, skeletomotor alpha fibers; tr.e.a., trail-ending area; v.a.s, vesicular axonic swelling. (Barker *et al.*, 1970) Reproduced with the permission of The Royal Society.

muscle to a servocontrol device while the other end of the muscle is secured to a bone that is fixed in place. Moving the bones apart stretches or lengthens the muscle while moving them together shortens the muscle. Muscle receptors can also be stimulated by contracting (shortening) the muscle by electrical stimulation of the motor fibers in the ventral root. Other stimuli used are pressure on the muscle or vibrating stimuli applied directly to the muscle or to the tendon longitudinally.

The complexity of the muscle sensory system is presaged by the heterogeneity of sensory nerve fiber diameters (Fig. 8-3) and the diversity of sensory end organs as described in the previous section. The attack on this complexity by neurophysiologists has followed the form of differentiation and grouping of peripheral nerve-fiber types on the basis of conduction velocity and response to various stimulus parameters, since in the main these two characteristics seem to go together. Nerve fibers with diameters below 1.0 micron (as indicated by conduction velocity measurements) are considered to be unmyelinated fibers. Although unmyelinated fibers outnumber myelinated fibers in muscle sensory nerves, they have been little studied, since the techniques for isolating single muscle afferents (dissection of dorsal roots) prejudice against isolation of unmyelinated fibers. The general procedure followed to study muscle afferents is illustrated in Fig. 8-15: Nerve fibers are isolated by dissection of the dorsal roots, and the muscle is moved by anchoring the bone to which it is attached at one end while the other end of the muscle is attached to a servocontrol that can move the muscle in various ways.

The myelinated fibers (i.e., those with diameters greater than 1.0 micron as indicated by conduction velocity estimates) are separated into stretch afferents and nonstretch afferents, depending upon whether or not they are responsive to stretching of the muscle. This classification of fibers tends to break down along fiber diameter estimates with stretch afferents being greater than four microns in diameter and nonstretch afferents being less than four microns in diameter. Since stretch afferents are larger in diameter than nonstretch afferents and therefore much easier to isolate than nonstretch afferents, special efforts must be taken to isolate nonstretch afferents. These efforts have been taken by Besson and Laporte (1961a, 1961b) and by Paintal (1960).

Out of thirty-one nerve fibers with estimated fiber diameters between 1 and 4 microns, Paintal (1960) found that only two could be stimulated by stretching the muscle. Six of the thirty-one nerve fibers could not be discharged to any type of mechanical stimulation, whereas twenty-three could be discharged by local pressure directly applied to the muscle but not stretching. Some pressure-responsive nerve fibers were of large diameter similar to stretch afferents; also, some nerve fibers could not be activated by any form of mechanical stimulation.

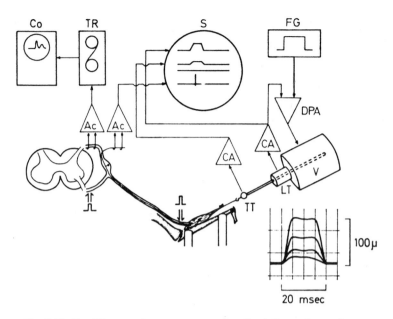

Fig. 8-15. Cat. Diagram of an arrangement for stimulating and recording
from muscle sensory neurons. AC, a-c coupled amplifier; CA, carrier
amplifier; Co, averaging computers; DPA, differential power amplifier; FG,
function generator; LT, co-axial capacitive length transducer; S, recording
oscilloscope; TR, tape recorder; TT, strain ring tension transducer. Superimposed photographs of rhomboid stretch profiles employed in experiments
shown in lower righthand corner. (Stuart *et al.*, 1970)

Muscle afferents with diameters greater than four microns are usually
classified as stretch afferents. Hunt (1954), in a systematic study of the
sensory fibers to the soleus and medial gastrocnemius muscles, only found
three nerve fibers out of 628 nerve fibers with diameters greater than four
microns that could not be classified as stretch afferents. The stretch afferents
themselves do not fall into a single grouping. Matthews (1933) in the first
single unit study on mammalian muscle afferents divided them into two
main groups, A and B, depending upon how they behaved to a brief muscle
contraction induced by stimulating the ventral roots. During this quick
contraction, the discharge of A fibers tended to decrease whereas the
discharge of B fibers tended to increase. According to Matthews (1933), the A
fibers tended to act as though their end organs were in parallel; and those of
the B fibers, in series with the contracting extrafusal muscle fibers. This type
of behavior suggested that the A fibers were innervating the muscle spindles
and the B fibers were innervating the Golgi tendon organs.

This differentiation of the peripheral connections of the afferent fibers by
B. H. C. Matthews (1933) has been accepted by subsequent investigators,
and his means of distinguishing between spindle fibers and Golgi tendon

organs fibers is still used by investigators. P. B. C. Matthews (1964) adds that the two fiber groups can also be distinguished on the basis of their response to electrical stimulation of efferent fibers that innervate intrafusal muscle, (Golgi tendon organ fibers are unaffected). Although little quantitative data have been presented for distinguishing between spindle and Golgi afferents, workers in the field seem to have little difficulty in making the judgment as to which classification a fiber belongs. Lundberg and Winsbury (1960) and Stuart *et al.* (1970) have measured the response of muscle-stretch afferents to a brief (eighty msec) stretch of the muscle, and find that the thresholds and latencies of Golgi tendon-organ afferents tend to be greater than the large diameter spindle afferents, although there is some overlap. Hunt (1954) classified the stretch afferent fibers to the soleus, and medial gastrocnemius muscles into muscle-spindle fibers and tendon-organ fibers, and measured their conduction velocities. The tendon-organ fibers tended to be larger than 12 microns in diameter, whereas the spindle fibers were of a wide range of diameters (Fig. 8-16).

Investigations subsequent to the Matthews (1933) study have tended to concentrate on the elucidation of the properties of the nerve fibers classified as muscle-spindle afferents, and as a result the properties of the tendon organ afferents have not been fully worked out. The known properties of tendon-organ afferents have been summarized by Jansen (1967): they are large (12 to 20 microns) diameter fibers, the threshold to passive stretch is generally high, and they are excited by muscle contraction. Alnaes (1967) investigated some properties of tendon-organ afferents from the soleus and anterior tibial muscles. He found that 4 of the 27 tendon-organ fibers to the anterior tibial muscle discharged spontaneously with no load on the muscle. No spontaneously firing tendon-organ fibers were found in the nerve innervating the soleus muscle (Alnaes, 1967; Jansen and Rudjord, 1964).

Jansen and Rudjord (1964) compared passive stretch and twitch contraction thresholds of forty-two tendon organ fibers to the cat's soleus muscle. Some fibers were not discharged by passive stretch even at full extension of the muscle. Fibers that did not show a maintained discharge to full extension of the soleus muscle were found to innervate proximal portions of the muscle (Fig. 8-17).

It is apparent from Fig. 8-16 that the diameters of the fibers classified as muscle spindle afferents cover such a wide range that the presence of more than one functional fiber group is suggested. Over the past several years, much effort has gone into determining the nature of the separate fiber groups. The present consensus of opinion is that the spindle fibers can be subdivided into two groups. These two groups of fibers have, in accordance with their presumed peripheral endings, been termed "primary" and "secondary" spindle fibers.

There are various measurements that have been utilized to distinguish between primary and secondary muscle spindle fibers. The distinction most

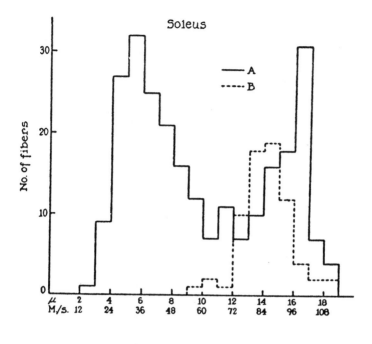

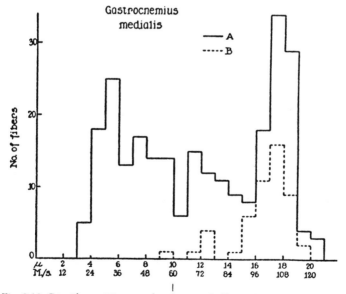

Fig. 8-16. Cat. Above: Diameter distribution of afferent fibers assumed from muscle spindles (A) and tendon organs (B). Soleus nerve. Below: Diameter distribution of afferent fibers assumed from muscle spindles (A) and tendon organs (B). Nerve to medial gastrocnemius. (Hunt, 1954)

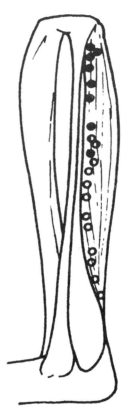

Fig. 8-17. Cat. Localization in soleus of the endings of twenty tendon-organ fibers of two cats. Tendon-organ fibers with a maintained discharge to full physiologic static extension (open circles); tendon-organ fibers without discharge to full static extension (filled circles). (Jansen and Rudjord, 1964)

often utilized is that of conduction velocity. As determined by Hunt (1954), the histograms of conduction velocity estimates for muscle-spindle afferents do not form a simple unimodal distribution (Fig. 8-16). Workers have assumed that the distribution is bimodal and that primary fibers are 12 microns or greater in diameter and conduct at a velocity above 72 meters/sec. Secondary fibers are assumed to be smaller than 12 microns and conduct at velocities below 72 meters/sec. Since there is an overlap in the conduction velocity measurements (Fig. 8-16), fibers with conduction velocities between 60 and 80 meters/sec are often omitted from study. The assumption of bimodality may or may not be valid; the distribution of conduction velocity measurements from medial gastrocnemius spindle fibers looks trimodal to us (Fig. 8-16). The omission of fibers on the basis of

conduction velocity estimates results in incomplete sampling of the population. (It must also be recalled that fibers below 4 microns in diameter are also
not sampled.)

Muscle-spindle fibers classified as primary and secondary muscle-spindle
afferents on the basis of conduction velocity estimates are found to respond
differently to many of the stimulus conditions used. Hunt (1954) found that
the threshold for continuous discharge induced by passive muscle stretch is
higher for slowly conducting afferents (secondaries). Primary fibers tend to
be more responsive to dynamic muscle stretch than secondaries (Cooper,
1961; Matthews, 1963). Secondary spindle afferents are also insensitive to
vibratory stimuli either applied directly to the muscle (Bianconi and van der
Meulen, 1963) or to the muscle tendon (Brown et al., 1967).

Although there are multiple criteria (e.g., vibration sensitive, affected by
efferent stimulation, etc.) for deciding whether a fiber is a primary spindle
fiber, there are not satisfactory multiple criteria for determining whether a
fiber is a secondary spindle fiber or a tendon-organ fiber. Barker, Ip, and
Adal (1962) were unable to relate about 30 percent of the myelinated sensory
fibers to any specific sensory ending such as those found in spindles, tendon
organs, and encapsulated corpuscles. Stacy (1969) found that many sensory
fibers with diameters greater than four microns ended as free nerve endings.
These facts suggest that the fiber categories established by neurophysiologists on the basis of conduction velocity and response to various stimulus
conditions may be "impure" in that fibers forming different types of endings
may be grouped together.

Bessou and Laporte (1962) have succeeded in isolating and recording
simultaneously from a primary and secondary fiber innervating the same
muscle spindle. The locations of the peripheral endings of the isolated
primary and secondary spindle fibers were determined by electrical and
mechanical activation of the fibers near the spindle. The responses of a
primary fiber and a secondary fiber connected to the same spindle to
sinusoidal stretching of the muscle can be seen in Fig. 8-18. The same
stimulus **may or may not** activate the two different afferent fibers to the
same spindle. If both are activated by the same stimulus, the magnitude and
time course of their discharge may be different.

In studying the response of a fiber to different types of stimulation, it is
common for the investigators to present their data in the graphic form of
"frequencygrams" (Bessou et al., 1968b), or as graphs of the "instantaneous
frequency" of discharge (Matthews, 1963). These graphs plot the instantaneous rate of discharge as a function of time (Fig. 8-19). Stimulus onset and
the type of stimulus applied is indicated below the discharge plot. The period
during which stretch is being applied is indicated by a rising stimulus line
and is called the "dynamic" phase of stretch. Once a certain muscle
extension is reached, it is often maintained for a period of time known as the

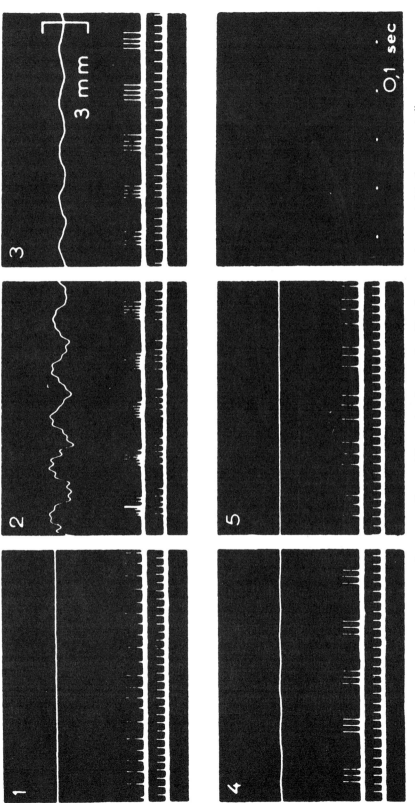

Fig. 8-18. Cat. Discharges of a primary fiber (middle trace) and a secondary fiber (lower trace), connected to the same spindle, produced by sinusoidal stretching of progressively decreasing amplitude (from 1 to 5). The upper trace is the recording of the variations of length of the muscle made with an isotonic lever with a photoelectric transducer. (Bessou and Laporte, 1962)

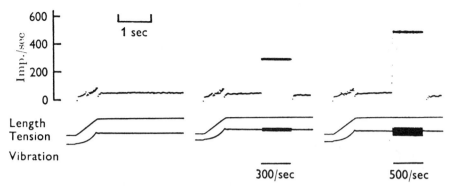

Fig. 8-19. Cat. Response of a primary fiber to vibration of an amplitude sufficient to "drive" it. Top, reciprocal pulse-interval display showing the instantaneous frequency of discharge of the fiber. Bottom, diagrammatic marker showing the period of vibration. The peak-to-peak amplitude of the vibration was 25μ; its frequency was either 300 or 500 Hz. Middle, records of the stretch (labeled length) applied to the muscle to make it taut (6mm applied at 10mm/sec, note typical response of primary ending), and the tension in the muscle (tension increase 60 g wt.). The thickening of the myograph trace (labeled tension) during the vibration is largely the direct response of the myograph to being vibrated, and does not represent a true vibratory tension change. (Conduction velocity of afferent fiber, 114 m/sec.) (Brown et al., 1967)

period of static stretch. Primary endings are more sensitive than secondary endings during the period of dynamic stretch (Matthews, 1963).

The two graphs to the left in Fig. 8-19 illustrate the response of a neuron to vibratory stimuli. Vibratory stimuli are essentially fast sinusoidal stretches of the muscle. As can be seen in Fig. 8-20, primary fibers are extremely sensitive to vibration, whereas secondary spindle fibers are relatively insensitive to it. The sensitivity of primary muscle spindle afferents to vibratory stimuli rivals that of Vater-Pacinian corpuscle fibers (Chapter 9). Like Vater-Pacinian corpuscle fibers, primary fibers can be discharged in phase with the stimulus up to rates of several hundred spikes/sec (Brown et al., 1967). Consideration of Fig. 8-20 forces the conclusion that primary muscle spindle afferents are relatively insensitive to low frequency passive linear stretching; at least as compared to the discharge set up by vibration. Brown et al. (1967) estimate that a sensitive primary fiber can be driven to discharge for every cycle of a two-hundred to three-hundred cycle vibratory stimulus, which produced no more than a four-micron peak-to-peak displacement of the whole muscle. Such sensitivity suggests that much of the responsiveness of primary fibers to different stimuli may be due to tremor transmitted to the muscle via the stimulator. To avoid transmission of vibration to muscle, Matthews and Stein (1969) mounted both preparation and stimulator on a metal table weighing half a ton. It is apparent that the study of muscle-spindle afferents requires stimulus control on the order of that used in the auditory system (Chapter 10).

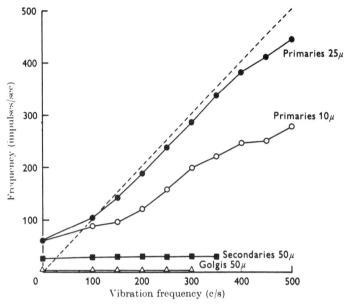

Fig. 8-20. Cat. The average excitatory effect of vibration of certain particular amplitudes at a range of frequencies on a number of primary fibers, secondary fibers, and Golgi tendon organ fibers. The mean frequency of discharge of the fibers (ordinate) is plotted against the frequency of vibration (abscissa) for the stated amplitudes. The frequency of discharge of each fiber was measured over a period of 0.5 sec. There was no fusimotor stimulation, nor was the muscle contracting. The results were obtained from twenty-four primary fibers, twenty-five secondary fibers, and twenty-seven Golgi tendon-organ fibers. The dashed line at 45 degrees shows the frequencies at which the fibers would be discharging if they were all being driven by the vibration. (Brown et al., 1967)

Unlike tendon-organ fibers, most muscle-spindle fibers tend to be spontaneously active even when there is no tension on the muscle. Measures by Hnik et al. (1963) on the spontaneous activity of spindle fibers innervating the gastrocnemius muscle reveal a bimodal distribution of discharge rates with some fibers not discharging at all and the majority of the others discharging between five and forty spikes/sec (Fig. 8-21). The distribution of rates of spontaneous activity of muscle spindle fibers is apparently not affected at all by long term tenotomy (i.e. cutting the tendon attaching the muscle to the bone) as shown in Fig. 8-21.

The discharge patterns of primary and secondary muscle-spindle afferents have been studied in some detail by Matthews and Stein (1969). Although no rate difference was detected between the two fiber types, the discharge of

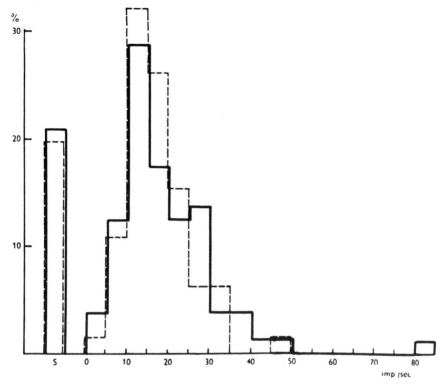

Fig. 8-21. Cat. The distribution of resting frequency values of individual muscle-spindle fibers from the gastrocnemius muscle in a group nine to twenty eight days after tenotomy (broken line) and in the intact control muscle (continuous line). Abscissa - resting discharge frequency in five-sec intervals. Ordinate - number of muscle-spindle fibers exhibiting a given resting frequency expressed as percentage of spindles discharging in the relaxed state. Column S indicates number of silent spindle fibers in the relaxed muscle, expressed as percentage of all spindles (Hnik *et al.*, 1963)

primary fibers tended to be more irregular than that of secondary fibers. The ISI histograms of primary fiber discharge tended to be more variable than those calculated from secondary fiber discharge. At low discharge rates the ISI distributions of primary fibers tended to be positively skewed and sometimes even bimodal.

Cutting the ventral roots and thus eliminating the efferent supply to the spindles produced major changes in the discharge patterns of muscle-spindle afferents, with both a lowering of discharge rate and a decrease in variability, although at low-discharge rates asymmetry of the ISI distributions of primary fiber discharge could still be observed. Matthews and Stein (1969) compared the ISI distributions of de-efferented primary and secondary fibers by

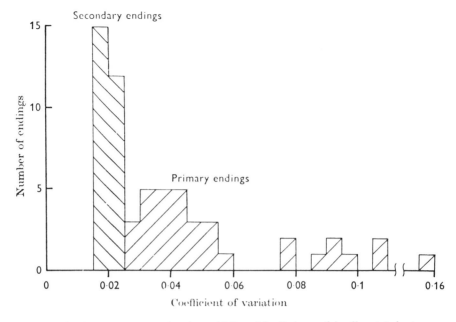

Fig. 8-22. Cat. Histograms comparing the variability of the discharge of de-efferentated primary and secondary fibers. The coefficient of variation was measured when the mean interspike interval was between thirty and forty msec. (Matthews and Stein, 1969)

calculating a coefficient of variation (standard deviation divided by mean interval) for the ISI histograms from all fibers with mean ISI intervals between thirty and forty msec. The resulting distribution of these values is presented in Fig. 8-22. The regularity of the discharge of the secondary afferents is clearly evident in this figure. The coefficients of variation calculated for primary fiber discharge are all greater in value (i. e. more variable) than those calculated for secondary fibers (Fig. 8-22).

Further measures on the effects of sectioning the ventral roots on the discharge patterns can be seen in Fig. 8-23. In this figure coefficients of variation were calculated for the discharge of primary and secondary fibers before and after the sectioning of the ventral roots. The separation between the primary and secondary fiber groups and the effect of the elimination of efferent input are clearly evident. Unfortunately, fibers with conduction velocity estimates between sixty and eighty m/sec were not studied, and therefore it is not known whether these fibers could be identified as primary or secondary on the basis of the coefficient of variation of their ISI distributions.

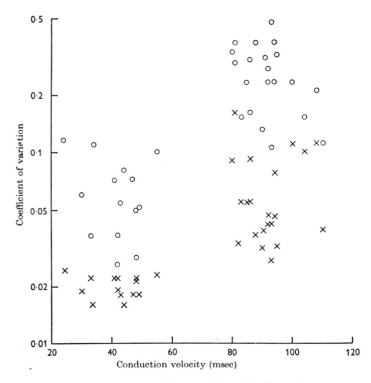

Fig. 8-23. Cat. Comparison of the variability of discharge of twenty-one primary fibers and fourteen secondary fibers that were studied both before and after cutting the ventral roots and that had appreciable fusimotor drive. The coefficient of variation of the interval distribution obtained with the roots intact (open circles), and with the roots cut (crosses), is plotted against the conduction velocity of each individual afferent fiber. (Matthews and Stein, 1969)

EFFERENT FIBERS TO MUSCLE SPINDLES

Although early workers on muscle sensory systems realized that the afferent output was determined in part by the activity of efferent fibers terminating in the muscle spindles, the full complexity of the problem was only revealed when single efferent fibers were isolated and electrically stimulated. It now appears that there are three types of efferent fibers that can affect the discharge of muscle-spindle afferents. Two of these fiber types are of small diameter (gamma efferents) and are called "static" and "dynamic" fusimotor fibers. The third type is of larger diameter (alpha efferent) and may also innervate extrafusal muscle fibers (Bessou et al., 1965).

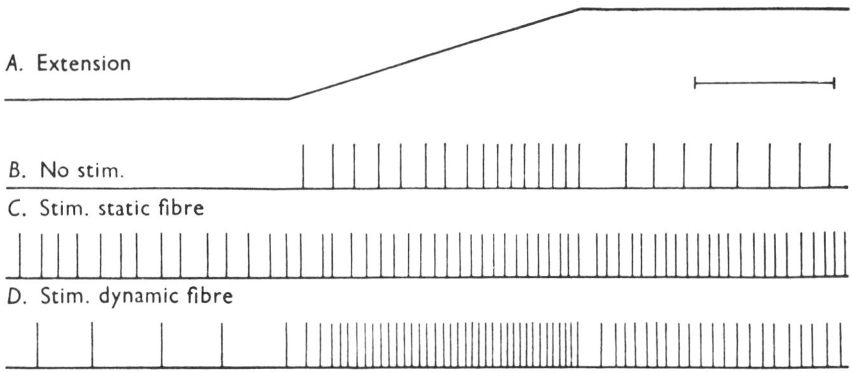

Fig. 8-24. Cat. The effects of stimulating single fusimotor fibers on the response of a primary fiber to stretching the muscle fiber at 30mm/sec. Throughout C a single static fiber was stimulated at 70/sec. Throughout D a single dynamic fiber was stimulated at 70/sec. The action potentials are shown as spikes on a linear time scale. They were not directly recorded but were drawn after comparing their position from measurements of the records of the reciprocal pulse interval. Time marker, 0.1 sec. (Crowe and Matthews, 1964a)

The effects of electrical stimulation of static and dynamic fusimotor fibers on muscle-spindle afferents has been studied in some detail by Bessou and his associates (Bessou, Laporte, and Pages, 1968a; 1968b; Bessou and Pages, 1969) and by Matthews and his associates (Crowe and Matthews, 1964a; 1964b; Brown and Matthews, 1966). The division into static and dynamic fusimotor fibers is based upon the effect on the static and dynamic discharge of spindle afferents when the efferent fibers are electrically stimulated. Electrical stimulation of static fusimotor fibers tends to increase the discharge of primary fibers during rest and during the static stretch, but has little effect on the magnitude of discharge during the phasic part of stretch (Fig. 8-24). Conversely, the electrical stimulation of phasic fusimotor fibers tends to increase discharge of primary fibers during the phasic part of stretch but has little effect during the static phase (Fig. 8-24). Electrical stimulation of phasic fusimotor fibers usually has no effect on the discharge of secondary spindle afferents, but the electrical stimulation of static fusimotor fibers tends to increase the discharge rate of secondary fibers. Both static and dynamic fusimotor fibers innervate more than one spindle, although the effect of electrical stimulation of the parent efferent fiber on the discharge of afferents from the different spindles tends to be similar.

Brown, Crowe, and Matthews (1965) have described quantitatively the effects on primary fiber discharge of electrically stimulating the different types of efferent fibers. From graphs such as those in Fig. 8-25, Brown et al. (1965) obtained a measure that they termed the 'dynamic index," which

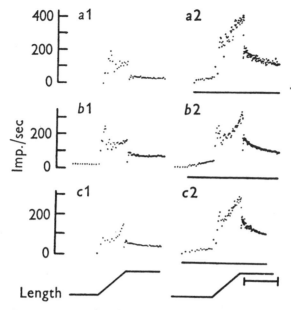

Fig. 8-25. Cat. The effect on three primary fibers of
stimulating the same single fusimotor fiber. This fiber had
a dynamic action on all three primary fibers. a1, b1, c1,
responses of primary fibers to stretching in the absence of
stimulation. a2, b2, c2, responses to similar stretching
applied during stimulation of fusimotor fiber at fifty/sec.
(See bars beneath records.) Each spike potential is
represented by a dot, the vertical displacement of which is
proportional to the reciprocal of the time interval since the
immediately preceding spike potential (i.e., the instantaneous frequency). The 1 sec calibration does not apply to
the periods of dynamic stretching, which are on more open
time scales. (Records untouched.) (Crowe and Matthews,
1964b)

consisted of the spike difference between the rate of discharge at the end of
the dynamic phase of stretching and the rate of discharge when the muscle
had been at the final length for a half second. This dynamic index is plotted
against the change in discharge found when the efferent is stimulated during
the static phase of stretch in Fig. 8-26. The resulting scatter plot clearly
separates the effects of electrically stimulating the static and dynamic
fusimotor fibers. Also included in this figure are measurements for similar
experiments involving electrical stimulation of large diameter (alpha)
fusimotor fibers, which produced effects similar to those produced by

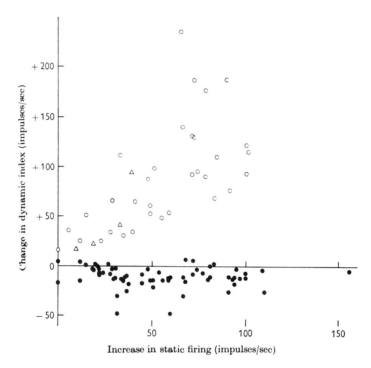

Fig. 8-26. Cat. Scatter diagram relating the effect of stimulating single fusimotor fibers on the "dynamic index" of primary endings to their effect in exciting the same endings under static conditions. Each of the one hundred points represents one combination of a motor fiber with a primary ending. Effects due to fibers classified as dynamic fusimotor fibers (open circles); effects due to alpha motor fibers (open triangles); effects due to fibers classified as static fusimotor fibers (filled circles). Ordinate, the differences between the dynamic index during fusimotor stimulation at 150/sec and that occurring in the absence of fusimotor stimulation; the stretch was three mm applied at five mm/sec. Abscissa, the increase in the discharge of the fiber produced by fusimotor stimulation at 100/sec when the muscle was at the initial length. (Brown *et al.*, 1965)

electrically stimulating dynamic fusimotor efferents. Conduction velocity measurements indicate that although there is much overlap in the two distributions, dynamic fusimotor fibers tend to be of slightly larger diameter than static fusimotor fibers.

9
SENSORY SYSTEMS OF THE SKIN

The external surface of the cat is composed of various specialized areas that come into direct or indirect contact with the external world. Although the external surface is everywhere continuous, for our purposes we may consider it to be composed of a largely furry outside surface and two inside surfaces. The inside surfaces are (1) the mouth-to-anus tubular digestive tract, which is continuous from tip to tail; and (2) the respiratory tract, which consists of a large invagination into the animal. The outside surface and these two inside surfaces show regional differentiations within which specialized processes or measurements take place. For example, the respiratory tract contains places where particles are removed from the air, the air is warmed and humidified, and where the various chemical constituents of the inspired air are analyzed. Each of the specialized regional surface differentiations has specialized sensory systems for measuring the external environment and for regulating the condition of the regional specialized surface; e.g., if the olfactory receptors require mucous for effective functioning, then specialized neural circuits must be established to regulate and control mucous flow and composition. Thus, in studying the afferent nerve supply to a specialized surface, one may encounter two types of sensory systems: those concerned with measuring different aspects of the outside world, and those concerned with the regulation of the sensory surface itself.

In this chapter, only the sensory systems of the outside surface of the cat will be examined. Research on the sensory systems of the inside surfaces is largely in a primitive state of development and is touched on but briefly in this book.

With the exception of the cornea of the eye, the outside of the surface of the cat is covered with skin. The skin is not of uniform composition, however, and it can be further subdivided into distinct areas on the basis of the external appearance of the skin. Thus, hairy and nonhairy areas are distinguished (Figs. 9-1 and 9-2). The nonhairy areas include the anal area, the surface of the vagina and the penis, the nose, the nipples, the eyelids, and nictitating membranes of the eye, the lips, and the foot pads. Although the rest of the cat's external surface is covered with hairy skin, close inspection of the hairy areas reveals that the hair is not of uniform type nor is it uniformily distributed. For instance, the hair on the ear is different from the general body hair. The bridge of the cat's nose is densely covered with short hairs. A section of skin between the eye and the ear is a region of sparse hair cover. Extremely long and stiff hairs project from various parts of the cat's head and from the backside of his forelegs. The testicles of the male cat are covered with short fine hairs.

Histological investigations into the skin of the cat (Strickland and Calhoun, 1963; Creed, 1958) further disclose that the skin at these different parts of the body may be composed of different layers of tissues and that these layers may be of different composition and thicknesses. Examination of the types of structures found in different parts of the skin also discloses large differences in the skin areas. Thus, not only may the hairs be different but exocrine glands and other structures are differentially distributed. As we shall

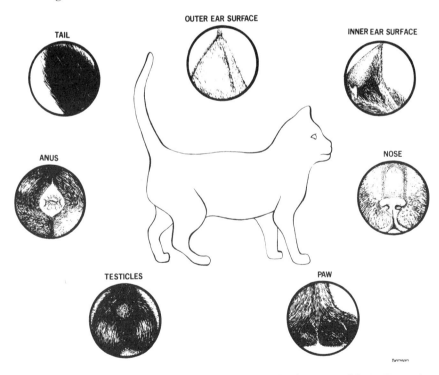

Fig. 9-1. Cat. Close-up views of some of the hairy areas of the skin. (Artwork by M. Berman)

see, the types of sensory end organs found in the different skin regions may vary markedly.

The skin cannot, therefore, be considered a uniform sensory surface; rather, it appears to be a collection of differentiated sensory surfaces. Analysis of the sensory systems of the skin would involve a thorough study of the anatomy and neurophysiology of each region that can be differentiated. At the present time, only a few of these areas have been investigated and these only partially. In some cases, as with the vagina (Poláček, 1968), there is anatomy but no neurophysiology. In other cases, there is some neurophysiology but little comprehensive anatomy. Therefore, our description of the anatomy and neurophysiology of the skin is sketchy and incomplete.

Sensory systems with receptor organs on the external surface of the cat are primarily designed to extract information about the external world. This information is extracted by measuring certain forces or energies that impinge upon the external surface. In many cases, specialized receptor organs, locally placed, have been developed for measuring such things as the light, sound, and chemical composition of the external world. The cat even seems to have a localized area around the nose and face for measuring temperature.

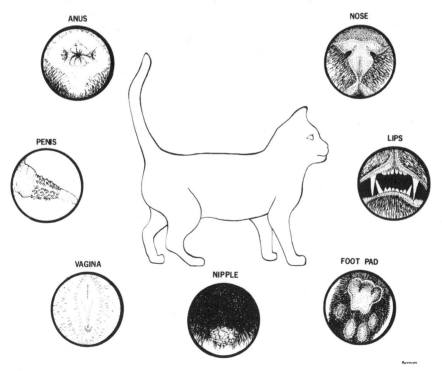

Fig. 9-2. Cat. Close-up views of some of the nonhairy areas of the skin. (Artwork by M. Berman)

Throughout the rest of the cat's outside surface are spread various mechanoreceptors that measure various aspects of physical contact between the cat and various external objects. As we shall see, these mechanoreceptive systems are of a diverse variety as though they were set up to measure different types of object contact (e. g., wind, fleas, or contact of the foot with the earth), and to subdivide the different contact forces from the same object into different aspects such as movement and static contact. Hair systems are provided for measuring objects that need not come into direct contact with the skin.

In studying skin systems, investigators commonly use thermal and mechanical stimulation. Temperature is usually varied by changing the temperature of a metallic surface in contact with the skin, by directing a temperature-controlled water jet onto the skin, or by heating the skin with a radiant heater. Control of the mechanical stimulus is more difficult since there are more ways in which it can vary. The mechanical stimulus used can be a moving one or a stationary one. It can move across the skin or indent the skin from a vertical position or it can be applied to a hair. Some mechanical stimuli commonly used are von Frey hairs, which are hairs of varying thickness and stiffness for exerting different pressures. Various mechanical probes have been designed to provide controlled static displacements, or to produce vibratory stimulation of controlled amplitude and frequency.

Studies on the behavioral reactions of cats to cutaneous stimulation are few in number. Stimulation of the hairs projecting from the inner surface of the pinna is followed by a rapid flicking of the ear and other aversive movements. Stimulation of the short tactile hairs around the cat's mouth and eyes also seems to be particularly irritative to the cat. Schmiedberger (1932) studied the effect of vibrissae removal on the ability of blind and normal cats to find their way around in the dark. He found that cats with vibrissae intact were better at spatial orientation and finding food. Behavioral studies (Kenshalo, 1964; Kenshalo et al., 1967; Brearley and Kenshalo, 1970) have demonstrated that the cat is relatively insensitive to thermal stimulation on the body or foot pads, but can readily detect temperature changes in the skin of the face and upper lip. Tapper (1970) has shown that a cat can detect small pressures on a single tactile pad and that a stimulus to the pad is more readily detectable than one off the pad.

GENERAL DESCRIPTION OF SKIN

Skin envelops the entire outer surface of the body, and its epithelium is continuous with that of the external orifices of the digestive, respiratory, and urigenital systems. Skin is a veneered or stratified tissue that consists of two main layers. At the surface is the epithelium known as the "epidermis," and subjacent is a connective tissue called the "corium" or "dermis." Under the skin is a loose connective tissue layer. the "hypodermis." Below the hypodermis is a flat sheet of skeletal muscle that separates the rest of the body tissues from the integument. The hypodermis binds the skin to the underlying superficial skeletal muscles, deep fascia, aponeurosis, or periosteum. Cutaneous appendages such as hairs, claws, and cutaneous glands grow directly from the epidermis and are integral parts of the skin. The epidermis is composed of from four to five layers of epithelium (Fig. 9-3). The deepest layer is the stratum Malpighii, which is subdivided into two layers: the deep basal layer, stratum basale, or stratum germinativum proper, which is in contact with the dermis; and a layer of variable thickness above it, the stratum spinosum or spinous layer. A granular layer or stratum

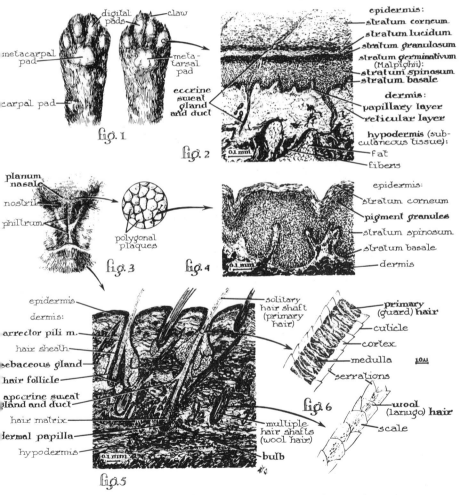

Fig. 9-3. Cat. Histology of a hairy and some nonhairy areas of skin. (Crouch, 1969)

granulosum is formed by the superficial stratum spinosum cells, which are large and readily stainable with most basic dyes. Where the epidermis is very thick, a hyalin layer, the stratum lucidum, is located above the granular layer. This layer is seldom colored with histological stains. The outer layer of the epidermis, the stratum corneum, is composed of flattened cornified cells. The superficial keratinized portion of the epidermis consists of the stratum corneum and stratum lucidum. The epidermis is entirely devoid of blood vessels, but in certain regions contains hair follicles, sweat, and sebaceous glands. The thickness of the epidermis is variable, but is characteristic of the different parts of the body.

The epidermis and cutaneous appendages grow upon the dermis and receive nourishment from it. The epidermodermal junction of skin appears as an irregular line with fingers of dermis extending into the epidermal layer; they form papillary bodies or dermal papillae that interdigitate with epidermal pegs or ridges. The dermis consists of a superficial papillary layer, or stratum papillae, and a deep reticular layer or stratum reticulare that cannot always be clearly separated. The papillary layer consists of loose connective tissue formed by collagenous, elastic, and reticular fibers, enmeshed with superficial capillaries and surrounded by viscous ground substance. The cutaneous appendages that extend into the dermis are covered by the papillary layer, even where they pierce the reticular layer of the dermis. The reticular layer of the dermis is composed of dense, coarse collagenous fiber bundles that form layers in parallel with the body surface. At various levels of the dermis, there are hair follicles, sweat, and sebaceous glands that are epidermal structures extending down into the dermis. There are also blood vessels, nerves, and many nerve endings.

The hypodermis is a subcutaneous layer of loose connective tissue that is the deeper continuation of the dermis. Depending upon the portion of the body, varying numbers of fat cells develop in the subcutaneous layer. The hypodermis is everywhere penetrated by large blood vessels and nerve trunks, and contains many nerve endings.

The character of skin varies from region to region of the body. There are differences in the distribution of skin appendages, e.g., hair, regional differences in the thickness of the epidermis, and regional differences in the character of the epidermodermal junctions.

Two methods that are commonly used in the histological study of skin receptors are the methylene-blue and silver-staining methods. The methylene-blue method is most successful when the skin is stained in vivo. Silver-staining methods are not always successful in coloring the fine terminal processes of nerve fibers. The electron microscope has also been utilized in identifying skin receptors and in characterizing their structural components. The two most commonly observed types of receptors in the skin are similar to receptors observed in the joints, muscles, and tendons; they are the free nerve endings and encapsulated corpuscles. These two types of receptors and the two types of receptors unique to skin, the Merkel cell complex and the hair follicle complex, are formed by the terminals of sensory nerve fibers, their coverings, and in some cases also include specialized epidermal structures, e.g., the inner core of encapsulated corpuscles, the Merkel cell, and the hair follicle.

ANATOMY OF HAIRY SKIN

The epidermis of hairy skin consists of four distinct layers (Strickland and Calhoun, 1963): stratum corneum (320 μ thick); stratum granulosum (one or two cell layers); stratum spinosum (one or two cell layers); and the stratum basale or cylindricum (one layer of cells usually oriented perpendicular to the skin surface). A fifth layer, the stratum lucidum, normally is present in nonhairy skin and is normally absent in hairy skin. In both hairy and nonhairy skin, the dermis is composed of two layers, the stratum papillare and the stratum reticulare. In the hairy skin, there is a definite boundary between these two layers. The stratum papillare is composed of fine collagenous fibers usually parallel to the epidermis. The stratum reticulare has dense, irregularly arrayed collagenous fibers encircling hair follicles and disappearing in the subcutaneous regions. Elastic fibers are present in both the stratum papillare and the stratum reticulare, where they are abundant near the attachment of the arrector pilli muscles. The skin of the cat is thickest on the dorsal neck, lumbar, and sacral regions. It is thinnest on the lateral sides of the lower hindleg, thigh, and lower foreleg (Strickland, 1958). The maximum thickness is 1,900 microns in the dorsal neck region and the thinnest, 375 microns, is on the lower lateral sides of the hindleg. No breakdown of skin structures with respect to the different hairy areas depicted in Fig. 9-1 is available.

Within the hairy skin, various structures have been identified: hair follicles from which the hairs project, sebaceous glands, sweat glands, various blood vessels, subcutaneous fat deposits, and, throughout the various layers, nerve fibers and sensory-end organs of various types. The sebaceous glands are 20 to seventy-five microns in diameter (Strickland and Calhoun, 1963) and empty into the upper portion of the hair follicles. Saccular apocrine sweat glands are found throughout the hairy body skin; the excretory portion of the gland opens into the upper portion of the hair follicle. Innervation of these structures is primarily via the autonomic system (Herxheimer, 1960).

In terms of sensory innervation, the hairy skin of the cat is probably more complex than any other sensory surface. The evidence for the receptor complexity of hairy cat skin derives primarily from neurophysiological investigations and not anatomical studies, which are few in number and often misleading. The receptors in the hairy skin are usually classified as endings on hair follicles and "free" nerve endings. In addition, there are nerve endings on blood vessels and sweat glands. Apparently Vater-Pacini corpuscles (Hunt, 1961) and other encapsulated endings are sparsely present (Malinovský, 1966b; Fitzgerland and Lavelle, 1966; Kuntz and Hamilton, 1938; Ruffini, 1905), but these have not been described in any detail. Malinovský (1966b) on the basis of preliminary observations, in conjunction with investigations on nonhairy skin, cautions that probably each distinguishable hairy area will have to be examined in detail. Since cat cutaneous anatomy is an area currently undergoing rapid redevelopment, only those hairy skin structures that have been described in some detail will be presented here, namely hair systems and tactile pads.

Hair

Hair is a structure unique to mammals and may be used as a defining characteristic. Hair is multifunctional. It is used as a protective and insulating covering and as a sensory device for exploring the outside world. Mammalian hair has been divided into several types on the basis of external appearance, location, and the structure of the hair follicle. The general classifications of mammalian hair types (Danforth, 1925a; 1925b; Noback, 1951) are (1) tactile hairs or vibrissae and (2) body hairs. Body hairs are generally of two types: coarse overhairs, or guard hairs; and fine under hairs, or down hairs. Tactile hairs are located on specialized parts of the body and project out from the body surface. Body hairs cover most of the external surfaces of the body and do not usually project straight out but rather lie down and give the cat's body its streamlined appearance.

Body Hair   Hofer (1914) has classified the cat's body hairs into three types: long guard hairs, or bristles (Leithaar); small guard hairs, or awns (Grannenhaar); and fine down hairs (Woolhaar). These three types of body hair are similar to those found on most nonprimate mammals (Lochte, 1934; Noback, 1951). The bristle guard hairs are the longest and are separately distributed. They can be seen projecting beyond the other hairs of the body of the cat. The smaller awn hairs are shorter and much more densely distributed. The fine down or wool hairs are the shortest and the most densely distributed of the three hair types. The body hair of the cat grows out from clusters of hair follicles. The bristle guard hairs grow out from a central large hair follicle, and the awn guard hairs project from smaller lateral hair follicles. These guard-hair follicles are surrounded by a number of smaller hair follicles from which erupt numerous down hairs, usually with several projecting from a single opening (Fig. 9-4).

Hair is a slender keratinous filament that grows out of the hair follicle. A hair follicle is an invagination of the epidermal epithelium that is continuous

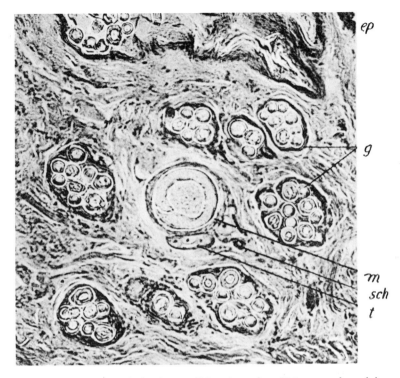

Fig. 9-4. Cat. Section through the skin parallel to the surface. Hair group of an adult cat: ep, epidermis; sch, sweat gland opening; t, sebaceous gland; m, large guard hair; g, bundle of hairs emerging from same follicle opening. (Hofer, 1914)

with the surface epidermis by way of the pilary canal (Fig. 9-5). The hair follicle extends into the dermis, where it is surrounded by connective tissue of the papillary layer. The base of an active follicle is expanded to form a bulb that is invaginated by the connective tissue of a hair or dermal papilla. The upper surface of the hair papilla is covered with epithelial cells, the matrix, that produce the hair root and root sheath. The epithelial wall of the hair follicle is divided into the inner and outer root sheath. The inner root sheath is composed of three concentric layers: the cuticle, an inner layer of kertinized cells; Huxley's layer, a layer of cornified cells; and Henle's layer on the outside closely adherent to the outer root sheath. The outer root sheath is formed of unspecialized epithelium and varies in thickness in proportion to the size of the hair follicle and the hair produced. The hair follicle is surrounded by a dermal connective tissue sheath also made up of two layers: an inner layer of circularly arranged fibers and an outer layer of longitudinal fibers. The glassy membrane, which is part of the dermis, separates the outer root sheath from the connective tissue sheath. The

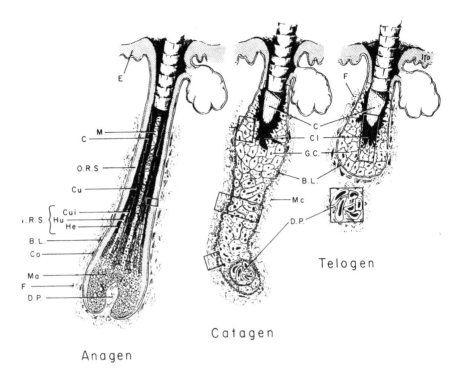

Telogen

Catagen

Anagen

Fig. 9-5. Rodent. Schematic diagram showing anagen (growing), catagen (transition between growing and resting), and telogen (resting) stages of the hair follicle. In anagen, the lower portion of the hair follicle encloses the dermal papilla (DP) and is composed of matrix cells (Ma). They move upward and differentiate into the hair shaft—medulla (M), cortex (C), and cuticle (Cu)—and the three layers of the inner root sheath—Henle (He), Huxley (Hu), and cuticle of the inner root sheath (Cui). The outer root sheath (ORS) surrounds the inner root sheath and is continuous with the epidermis (E). Following the contours of the follicle is the basal lamina (BL) and the layers of collagen fibers (Co). Fibroblasts (F) form a loose layer around the follicles. In catagen a club is formed (Cl), surrounded by a capsule of germ cells (GC). The follicle below the germ cells undergoes degeneration and contains many autophagic vacuoles. The basal lamina (BL) folds extensively. The collagen fibers are actively engulfed and degraded by the macrophages (Mc), which form a layer around the follicle. In telogen the club (Cl) is tightly attached to the cortex (C) of the hair shaft above and to the capsule of germ cells below. The dermal papilla (DP) forms a ball of cells just underneath the hair. (Parakkal, 1970)

connective tissue sheath of a follicle is continuous with the papillary layer of the dermis so that the follicle is not in contact with the dermal reticular layer. The pilary canal occupies the upper end of the follicle and extends from the entrance of the duct of the sebaceous glands to the surface of the skin. Several follicles may share a common pilary canal; the hairs from these follicles pass through the single pilary canal to the surface of the skin. A band of smooth muscle fibers, the hair muscle or arrector pili muscle, is attached at one end to the connective tissue sheath of the hair follicle, just below the level of the sebaceous glands and at the other end to the papillary layer of the dermis. When this muscle contracts, it moves the hair into a vertical position, while depressing the skin in the region of attachement and elevating the region immediately around the hair.

The hair, hair follicle, and sensory terminals within the follicle form a receptor complex involved in detecting contact with external objects. Typically, more than one nerve fiber innervates a hair follicle. These fibers form two bands around the hair follicle: an outer circular band around the dorsal part of the hair follicle within the dermal coat (the circular fibers); and the inner band of fibers oriented parallel to the hair shaft within the outer root sheath, the palisade fibers (Weddell et al., 1955a). Only one type of sensory terminal has been identified in electron micrographs of mouse, rat, monkey, and man hair follicles (Munger, 1971). This terminal type has been described as "lanceolate" endings by Andres (1966), a term describing the shape of the terminal fiber. The terminal has the shape of a flattened cylinder and is encased on its flat sides by flattened discs of Schwann cell cytoplasm (Fig. 9-9). Schwann-cell cytoplasm is absent on the thin edges of the terminal where short processes of the nerve terminal extend to make contact with the outermost layer of the follicle outer root sheath. Lancet endings are arranged in parallel with the hair shaft and form a collar of terminals around the shaft. It is not certain if the lancet endings are terminals of the palisade or circular fibers or of both types of fibers. According to Bonnet (1878), there is wide variety in the number of fibers innervating a hair follicle. The largest follicles receive the greatest number of fibers.

The study of the innervation of hair follicles is yet in its infancy. The study is complicated by the fact that there are different types of hairs on the same region of the body and there are different types of hairs on different parts of the body. In addition, there is evidence that hairs undergo a process of growth followed by a period of quiescence, and structural differences can be observed in the hair follicle during these periods of growth (Danforth, 1925b; Montagna, 1962; Parakkal, 1970). Some recent anatomical investigations have distinguished a hair type (actually the bristle guard hair) on the basis of its association with the tactile pads of the skin, but this close association does not seem to hold for the cat (Iggo, 1968; Burgess et al., 1968).

Vibrissae   On the head of the cat we find long hairs known as vibrissae, sensory hairs, sinus hairs, tactile hairs, or whiskers. Pocock (1914a) has broken down mammalian vibrissae into five categories according to their position on the head: (1) the buccal vibrissae comprise the mystacial vibrissae on the upper lip and the submental vibrissae on the chin and lower lip; (2) the interramal vibrissae on the chin; (3) the genal vibrissae on the cheek; (4) the superciliary vibrissae over the eye; and (5) the subocular vibrissae beneath the eye present mainly in large herbivores. In the cat the subocular and interramal vibrissae are missing and the genal tuft is double (Fig. 9-6). The mystacial vibrissae in the cat are arranged in five rows over the upper lip. The vibrissae on the bottom row are the shortest and finest. Danforth (1925a) has shown in the mouse that the vibrissae are remarkably constant in number and position.

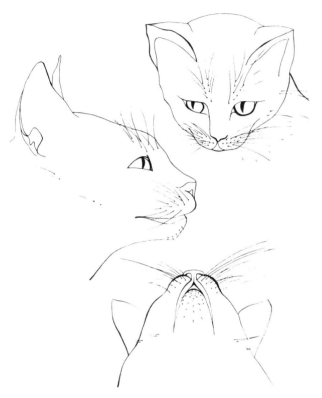

Fig. 9-6. Cat. Vibrissae of the cat. The vibrissae of the cat are classified according to their position on the head into: the superciliary vibrissae over the eye, the genal vibrissa on the cheek, the mystacial vibrissae on the upper lip, and the submental vibrissae on the chin. (Artwork by M. Berman)

The cat is able to direct these vibrissae. When inspecting an object with the head, the vibrissae are directed forward and fan out to cover an extensive area around the face. The vibrissa system is a specialized perceptual system related to the life style of the animal. Animals that use the mouth to grasp food (especially moving food) have them well developed. They are probably used for the perception of objects too close to the face to be clearly viewed with the eyes. They are lacking in only a few mammals, among them anteaters and man (Van Horn, 1970). Vibrissa systems are relatively undeveloped in the higher primates (where, according to Pocock (1914a), their development is negatively correlated with the development of the hand as a grasping instrument), and in large aquatic herbivores, and in sloths.

The follicles of the vibrissae are similar to the body-hair follicles except for certain distinguishing characteristics. The follicles of vibrissae are surrounded by a thick fibrous capsule (ausserer Haarbalg), which is attached to the dermal papilla (Haarpapille) at the bottom of the follicle (Fig. 9-7). At the top of the follicle the capsule forms a ring of fibrous tissue, the outer conical body *(ausserer Konus)* around the neck of the follicle. Between the follicle and capsule, there is a large blood sinus that is divided into a lower, cavernous sinus *(spongioser Sinus)* and an upper, ring sinus *(Ringsinus)*. The outer sheath of the follicle is thickened markedly in the region of the cavernous sinus to form the superior enlargement *(obere Wurzelscheiden-anschwellung)* and less markedly thickened in the region of the ring sinus to form the inferior enlargement *(untere Wurzelscheidenanschwellung)*. The glassy membrane *(Glashaut)* is also thickened in the region of the superior and inferior enlargements. The mesenchymal sheath *(innerer Haarbalg)*, a network of fibroblasts, collagen, and elasten, surrounds the follicle and adheres to the glassy membrane. The cavity of the cavernous sinus is traversed by delicate, anastomosing trabeculae and by plexuses of nerve fibers and capillaries that connect the mesenchymal sheath to the capsule wall. The *Ringwulst,* an umbrella-shaped shelf, is formed by the mesenchymal sheath and nerve fibers that extend laterally and hang down into the lower part of the ring sinus. The mesenchymal sheath does not form trabeculae within the ring sinus. The mesenchymal sheath lining the roof of the ring sinus forms a spongy tissue, the inner conical body *(innerer Konus)*, which contains numerous small veins and venules. Arterial blood enters the lower sinus, passes up through the cavernous meshwork of trabeculae and blood vessels into the ring sinus and is drained by a plexus of veins in the inner conical body.

Nerve trunks from branches of the trigeminal nerve enter the capsule of the sinus follicle in more than one locus. The nerve fibers travel through the cavernous sinus and enter the mesenchymal sheath; most of the nerve fibers form a dense plexus around the follicle. The sensory terminals found in the sinus follicles of the rat, rabbit, and cat have been described in detail by Andres (1966b). The sinus follicles of vibrissae contain Merkel-type end organs, lanceolate endings, and corpuscular endings. Nerve fibers terminating in the basal cell layer of the superior enlargement are associated with Merkel cells (A in Fig. 9-7). Nerve fibers pass through the outer-sheath basement membrane and between the cells of the outer root sheath. Within this sheath the fibers bend, course parallel to the long axis of the hair shaft,

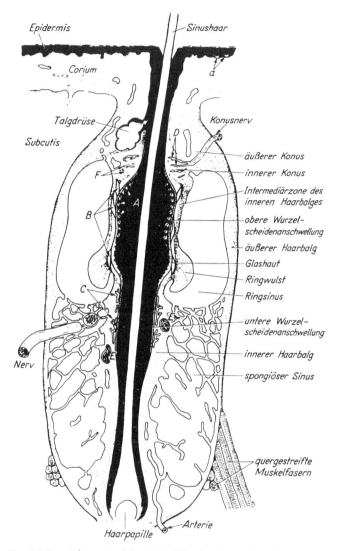

Fig. 9-7. Rat. Schematic of the hair follicle of a vibrissa from the upper lip. For clarity, the outer root sheath is colored black. A, Merkel cell complex; B, straight lanceolet nerve endings; C, branched lanceolet nerve endings; D, circular lanceolet nerve endings; E, encapsulated corpuscle; F, free nerve endings. (Andres, 1966b)

and terminate as flattened, disclike expansions. The terminal disc is enveloped by a Merkel cell (Fig. 9-8), a specialized epithelial cell found only in stratified squamous epithelium (epidermis and hair). The Merkel cell is

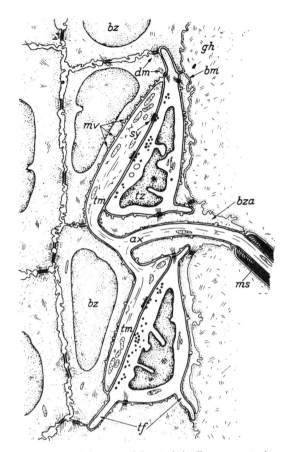

Fig. 9-8. Rat. Schematic of the Merkel cell apparatus in the
sinus hair follicle seen in Fig. 9-7. Tactile (Merkel) cell (tz),
tactile feeler (tf), tactile meniscus (tm), sensory-nerve fiber
(ax) with myelin (ms). Synapses (sy) between the tactile
cells and the menisci; basal cells (bz) with surface-
membrane vesiculations (mv), basal-cell processes (bza)
functioning as terminal-axon coverings, desmosomes (dm),
glassy membrane (gh). (Andres, 1966)

oval and contains a lobulated nucleus. Ultrastructurally, it is easily distinguished from other epidermal cells by the accumulation of "secretory"
granules in the cytoplasm subjacent to the nerve terminal. Short cytoplasmic
processes, the tactile feelers (Fig. 9-8) project from the Merkel-cell surface
into the basal-cell layer. Within the connective tissue lining of the
hair follicle, we find both lanceolate and lamellated receptors. The lancet
receptors are similar to those found in the follicles of body hair (Fig. 9-9).
Finger-shaped processes arise from the edges of the terminal and project into

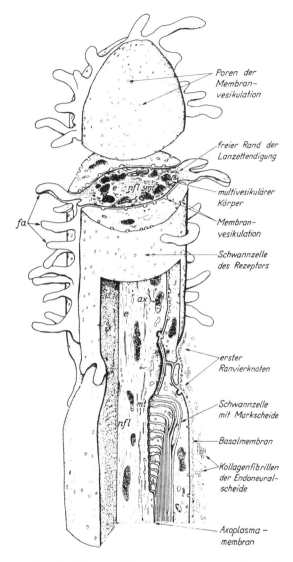

Poren der
Membran-
vesikulation

freier Rand der
Lanzettendigung

multivesikulärer
Körper

Membran-
vesikulation

Schwannzelle
des Rezeptors

erster
Ranvierknoten

Schwannzelle
mit Markscheide

Basalmembran

Kollagenfibrillen
der Endoneural-
scheide

Axoplasma –
membran

Fig. 9-9. Schematic of the straight lanceolet ending of the
sinus hair follicle in Fig. 9-7 (B). The terminal fiber (ax)
loses its myelin (Schwannzelle mit Markscheide) at the
first node of Ranvier (erster Ranvierknoten). Short
processes (fa) of the nerve terminal extend out from the
Schwann cell covering (Schwannzelle des Rezeptors) into
the connective tissue surrounding the hair follicle. Open
structures shows pores of the vesiculated membrane (Pore
der Membranvesikulation), free edge of the Lanceolet
endings (Freier Rand der Lanzettendigung), collagen
fibrils of the endoneunal border. (Kollagenfibrillen der
Endoneuralscheide), axoplasmic membrane (Axoplasma
membran). (Andres, 1966b)

the connective tissue space. Within the sinus hair follicle, three different types of lancet receptors can be distinguished: straight, branched, and circular lancet receptors. The straight lancet receptors (B in Fig. 9-7) are found in the connective-tissue lining of the upper portion of the superior enlargement of the outer root sheath and within the connective tissue forming the *Ringwulst*. They are oriented parallel to the hair shaft and abut the glassy membrane. The branched lancet receptors (C in Fig. 9-7) are found in the connective tissue lining the inferior enlargement of the outer root sheath. The circular lancet receptors (D in Fig. 9-7) are found in the connective tissue of the inner conical body. Small lamellated end organs (E in Fig. 9-7) occur in the connective tissue surrounding the inferior enlargement of the outer root sheath. Free nerve endings (F in Fig. 9-7) were observed in the connective tissue of the inner conical body of the rat's sinus follicle, but not in the sinus follicles of the cat or rabbit.

Carpal Hairs   In addition to the long vibrissal hairs projecting from his head, the cat possesses a small group of long hairs on the back of his foreleg (Fig. 9-10). According to Beddard (1920), most mammals that use their front legs for grasping as well as locomotion are endowed with these hairs, and in nearly all orders of mammals he could find species that had them. They were absent from all ungulates except Hyrax, and from the higher primates. In groups where the hairs were generally present, certain species did not have them; thus, they were found in the lion but not in the tiger.

Like the vibrissae, the hair follicles of these carpal hairs (Ksjunin, 1901) are characterized by a large blood sinus. According to Nilsson (1969b), the structure and innervation of the hair follicles of the carpal hairs are similar to the vibrissae hair follicles of the mouse as described by Andres (1966), except that no encapsulated corpuscles were seen in them. Nilsson (1969a) has observed that these carpal hairs are associated with a number of Vater-Pacinian corpuscles and some tactile pads. The carpal hairs are innervated by a branch of the ulnar nerve (Fig. 9-10).

Other Hair Systems   It is evident in Fig. 9-1 that the hairy skin of the cat can be subdivided into different areas. With the exception of the body hair and vibrissae hairs, the sensory receptors of these regions have been little studied. Weddell and his associates have studied in some detail the innervation of the dorsal surface of the rabbit's ear (Weddell and Pallie, 1955; Weddell *et al.*, 1955a; 1955c). The structure and innervation of the hairy systems of the inner surface of the pinna, the bridge of the nose, and the testicles have not been described in any detail for the cat.

In addition to the vibrissa systems on the head, the cat is endowed with eyelashes and a small number of hairs projecting at right angles from the skin around the eyes, nose, and mouth. The cat is extremely sensitive to

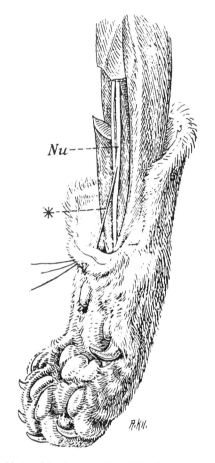

Fig. 9-10. Cat. The carpal hairs of the foreleg. A branch (*) from the ulnar nerve (Nu) innervates these sinus hair follicles. (Fritz, 1909)

movement of these hairs, which constitutes an irritative stimulus. The location of some of these hairs is shown in Fig. 9-11.

Tacile Pads

If the hairs are removed from a portion of the body of a cat, a series of small, fairly evenly spaced bumps can be seen projecting from the surface of the skin (Fig. 9-12). These small prominences are known by various names; e.g., *Haarscheibe*, Pinkus discs, tactile pads, touch corpuscles, etc. Because of the obvious sensory nature of these protuberances, we shall refer to them with the term "tactile pad." Although "touch corpuscle" carries the same connotation, it could be confused with the encapsulated sensory receptors of

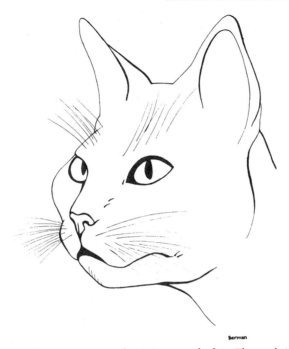

Berman

Fig. 9-11. Cat. Some accessory hair systems on the face. The two hairs
near the nose are long, thin, and wispy and may be part of the vibrissa
system. The location and number of the other hair systems near the eye
and corner of the mouth are approximate only. (Artwork by M.
Berman)

the skin. The neutral term "Pinkus disc" is also acceptable. According to
Pinkus (1904; 1927), these tactile pads are of widespread occurrence in
mammals, including humans (Smith, 1970). Pinkus described them as
Haarscheibe because of their close association with the large guard hairs or
bristles; but this association of hair and pad does not exist in the cat (Iggo and
Muir, 1969).

Tactile pads are approximately 0.15 to 0.35 mm in diameter (Burgess *et al.*,
1968; Kasprzak *et al.*, 1970) and can be recognized by the smooth covering of
epidermis and their bright red color due to high vascularization (Iggo and
Muir, 1969). There are approximately 7 pads/sq. cm in the skin of an adult
cat's thigh and 20 to 25 pads/sq. cm on the ankle (Burgess, 1971). The
epidermis of the pad is thicker than that covering the surrounding dermis,
although the stratum corneum covering the pad is thinner (Fig. 9-13). The
dermal core of the pad is thicker than the surrounding dermis and contains
very fine collagen bundles, closely woven, with little extracellular fluid space.
At the base of the epidermis of the central area of a pad, there is a single layer
of modified epidermal cells that differ in appearance from the rest of the

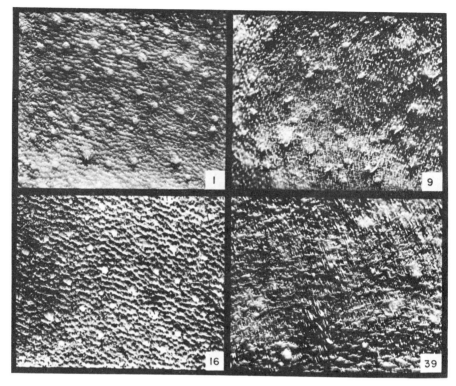

Fig. 9-12. Cat. Illustration of tactile pad density in cats of one day, nine days, sixteen days, and thirty-nine days of age. (Courtesy of D. Tapper)

epidermal cells. Because these cells resemble tactile cells first described by Merkel (1875), they are called "tactile" or "Merkel cells." These cells are located immediately above the basal layer of the epidermis. They are almost spherical in shape and invest the flattened, disclike expansion of a nerve terminal. The Merkel cell contains a lobulated nucleus, and numerous electron-opaque "secretory" granules are present in the cytoplasm adjacent to the nerve terminal. Merkel cells possess desmosomes that attach them to adjacent epithelial cells. The superficial surface of the Merkel cell gives rise to rodlike processes that are embedded in the overlying epidermis (Fig. 9-14). The deep half of the cell sends thin lamellae around the edge of the nerve terminal, thus separating it from the dermis below. Two types of nerve fibers innervate the structures of the pad. One of these is a single large myelinated fiber that branches as it enters the pad and terminates on the Merkel cells in the manner shown in Fig. 9-14. Fine nonmyelinated fibers also enter the pad but their mode of termination has not been described. The pads are functional at birth (Kasprzak *et al.*, 1970).

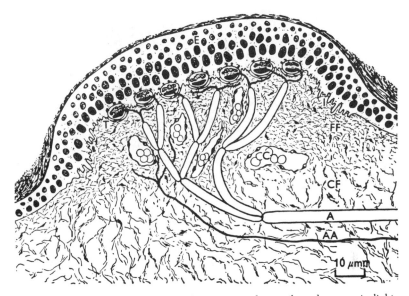

Fig. 9-13. Cat. A diagram showing the structure of a tactile pad as seen in light microscope sections: A, single myelinated axon; AA, nonmyelinated axons; E, thickened epidermis of the tactile pad; FF and CF, fine and coarse bundles of collagen fibers of the dermis; I, extensive indentations of the dermis by epidermis at the periphery of the pad; T, tactile cell and its associated nerve plate; C, capillary. (Iggo and Muir, 1969)

ANATOMY OF NONHAIRY SKIN

There are several distinct nonhairy portions of skin that can be distinguished on the outer surface of the cat (Fig. 9-2): the nose, the lips, the eyelids, the nictitating membrane, the nipples, the anal area, the genitals, and the foot pads. In addition, the surface of the ear drum and part of the external auditory canal are nonhairy (Strickland and Calhoun, 1960; Wilson, 1907). The general structure of some of these areas has been described (Ashino *et al.*, 1960; Sekigushi, 1960; Strickland and Calhoun, 1963; Wilson 1907). The different types of encapsulated nerve endings in the lip have been studied by others (Malinovsky, 1966a; Malinovsky and Matonoha, 1968). We shall describe only the anatomy of the foot pads and the nose, since the anatomy and physiology on these two structures are the most complete.

The Nose

The nose of the cat consists of a rough patch of moist, tough, bumpy skin known as the "planum nasale" (Fig. 9-2). A cross section (Fig. 9-3) through the structure reveals that it is composed of several layers of tissue (Strickland

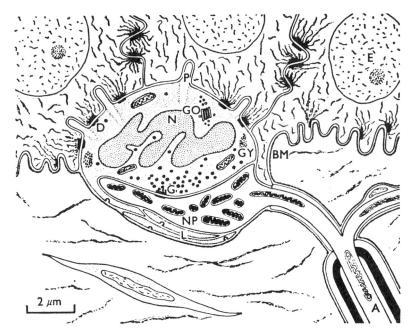

Fig. 9-14. Cat. A diagram showing the structure of a tactile (Merkel) cell and its associated nerve plate: A, myelinated axon; BM, basement membrane; D, desmosome; E, epithelial cell nucleus; G, granular vesicles in the tactile cell near a junction with the nerve plate (NP); GO, Golgi apparatus; GY, glycogen; L, lamellae underlying the nerve plate; p, cytoplasmic process from the tactile cell. (Iggo and Muir, 1969)

and Calhoun, 1963). The epidermis is as thick (nine hundred microns) as that found on the foot pads and is composed of five distinct layers of cells: the stratum corneum (15 to thirty-five microns thick); the thin stratum lucidum; the stratum granulosum (three to four layers of cells containing dark cytoplasmic granules); the stratum spinosum, containing several layers of cells; and the stratum basale. Large amounts of pigment are contained in the epidermis. The underlying dermis is composed of collagenous, elastic, and reticular fibers; nerve fibers and receptors; and blood vessels. Two layers of dermis, the stratum papillare and stratum reticulare, are recognized. Papillary bodies, fingers of dermal connective tissue, extend into the epidermal layers (Fig. 9-3). No sweat glands or sebaceous glands are present in the planum nasale (Gylek, 1912; Strickland and Calhoun, 1963).

Two different types of receptor end organs have been described in the planum nasale of the cat: nerve fiber Merkel cell complexes in the epidermis, and encapsulated corpuscles in the dermis. According to Halata (1970), the only type of receptor end organ found in the epidermis consisted of the Merkel cell-nerve fiber complex in the basal layers of the epidermis. These

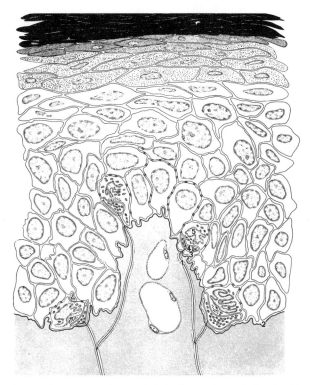

Fig. 9-15. Cat. Schematic representation of Merkel cell complex in the basal epidermal layer
of the planum nasale: 1. myelinated nerve fiber; 2, basal membrane; 3, cytoplasmic process
of Merkel cell; 4, disclike terminal of the nerve fiber; 5, Merkel cell. (Halata, 1970)

receptors were observed in two forms: single Merkel complex in the basal
epidermal layer above the papillary bodies (Fig. 9-15), and groups of these
complexes are in interpapillary pegs of the epidermis (Fig. 9-16). Merkel end
organs are found in the epithelial lining of the vibrissa follicle (Fig. 9-8), in
the epidermis of tactile pads of hairy skin (Fig. 9-14), and in the epidermis of
the planum nasale (Figs. 9-15 and 9-16) and foot pads. Because Merkel cells
have only been observed in stratified squamous epithelium (epidermis and
hair) and because they are attached to adjacent squamous cells by dermo-
somes, they are considered to be of epidermal origin. Because they contain
what appears to be secretory granules, they are believed to be receptor cells
that excite nerve terminals by secreting unknown neurotransmitter substances (Munger, 1971).

The encapsulated corpuscles in the planum nasale have been investigated
by Malinovský (1966b) as part of a continuing series of investigations on the
variability and distribution of receptors in different parts of the skin of the cat

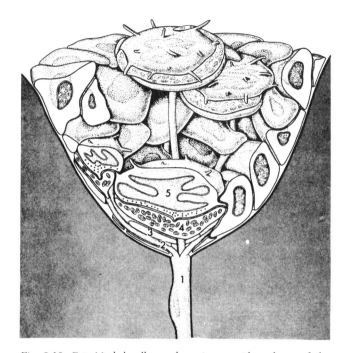

Fig. 9-16. Cat. Merkel cell complexes in an epidermal peg of the planum nasale. Only the cells of the epidermal peg are illustrated. The cells of the overlying epidermis (clear area) and the surrounding dermis (dark area) are not drawn. A nerve fiber (1) is seen entering the epidermal peg from below. It divides and sends its branches to Merkel cells, which are modified epithelial cells characterized by their peglike processes extending from their surfaces. 1, nerve fiber with Schwann cell; 2, nerve fiber without Schwann cell; 3, cytoplasmic process; 4, terminal disc; 5, Merkel cell. (Halata, 1970)

and other animals (Malinovský, 1967; 1970). Encapsulated corpuscles are found in large numbers in many nonhairy parts of the skin and in the tongue (Malinovský, 1966a); and they resemble the encapsulated corpuscles found in the cat's vagina (Poláček, 1968) and in the joints (Poláček, 1966). Examples of encapsulated corpuscles can be seen in Fig. 9-17. In the nose, encapsulated corpuscles are found in large numbers in the superficial layers of the papillary bodies adjacent to the epidermis. Malinovský (1966b) found a total of 756 of these corpuscles in the noses of five cats. In the majority of corpuscles, the terminal nerve fiber or its branches were situated either in a clearly visible inner core or in a darkly stained substance containing nuclei. The capsules of these corpuscles were thin and formed of a small number of lamellae. The majority of the corpuscles were of the paciniform type, that is, each corpuscle contained a single nerve terminal fiber that did not branch. Most of the paciniform corpuscles contained a simple, straight or bent

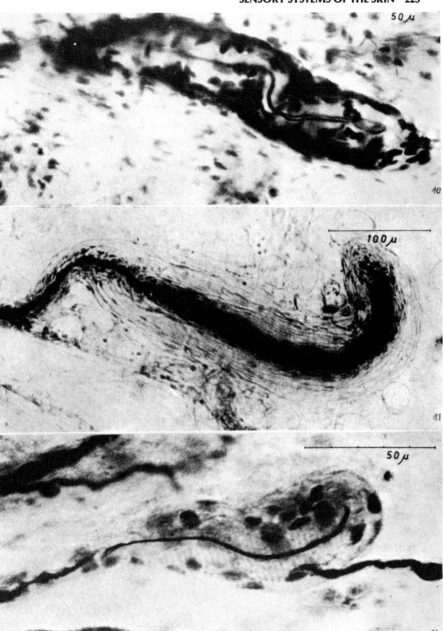

Fig. 9-17. Cat. Top: Encapsulated corpuscle with ramified axon and simple capsule from the vagina. Silver impregnation. Middle: Encapsulated corpuscle in the mesentary. Silver impregnation. A paciniform type. Bottom: Encapsulated corpuscle with simple capsule. The tongue, near the muscle, the fibers of which cover the corpuscle. Silver impregnation. (Poláček, 1966)

terminal fiber, while a few contained a fiber that formed different types of loops. The Golgi-Mazzoni type of corpuscles contained a terminal fiber that branched within the capsule of the corpuscle. This type of corpuscle was further subdivided on the basis of the number of terminal branches formed (Fig. 9-18). The third type of corpuscle found in the planum nasale were the "branched" corpuscles. This type of receptor was distinguished by the accompaniment of the division of the terminal fiber by the division of the inner core of the corpuscle or by the division of the entire corpuscle. The

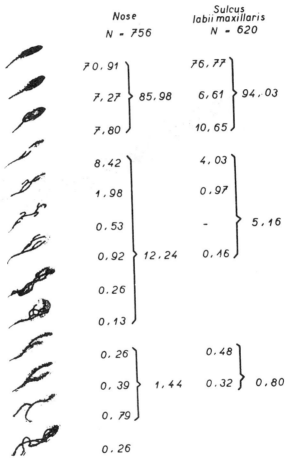

	Nose N - 756	Sulcus labii maxillaris N - 620
	70,91 ⎫	76,77 ⎫
	7,27 ⎬ 85,98	6,61 ⎬ 94,03
	7,80 ⎭	10,65 ⎭
	8,42 ⎫	4,03 ⎫
	1,98	0,97
	0,53	- ⎬ 5,16
	0,92 ⎬ 12,24	0,16 ⎭
	0,26	
	0,13 ⎭	
	0,26 ⎫	0,48 ⎫
	0,39 ⎬ 1,44	0,32 ⎬ 0,80
	0,79 ⎭	
	0,26	

Fig. 9-18. Cat. Comparison of the variability of sensory corpuscles from the planum nasale and the area of the sulcus labii maxillaris. The first group of three are paciniform type of corpuscles, the second group of six are Golgi-Mazzoni type of corpuscles, the third group of three are branched corpuscles, and the last one is a polyaxonal corpuscle. Numbers give the percentage of occurrence. (Malinovský, 1966)

smallest group of corpuscles, the polyaxonal corpuscles, contained the terminals of two or more nerve fibers. The appearance of these different types of encapsulated corpuscles and the relative frequency with which they are found are presented in Fig. 9-18. This figure contains also, for comparison purposes, the corpuscles found in the adjoining region of the groove in the upper lip, the sulcus labil maxillaris. These encapsulated corpuscles develop postnatally (Malinovský, 1970; Polacek and Halata, 1970).

Foot Pads

The cat is a digitigrade animal; i.e., it walks on its toes. On the bottom of the foot the hairy skin gives way and there is a group of smooth, though tough-skinned, surfaces known as the foot pads (Fig. 9-19). Similar foot pads are also found in other animals (Frei, 1928; Pocock, 1914b). The large central pad is known as the metacarpal foot pad. Distal to the metacarpal foot pad are a group of smaller digital foot pads. There are five digital foot pads on the front feet and four on the hind feet (the "heel" pad is located some distance up the leg). Like the nose, the foot pads are composed of a thickened epidermis and the dermis. According to Strickland and Calhoun (1963), the epidermis and dermis of the foot pads are composed of the same cell layers as is the planum nasale (Fig. 9-3). Sweat glands are present in large numbers in the foot pads.

The different types of receptor end organs found in the skin of the cat's foot pad have been reviewed by Jänig (1971). These end organs are located in the epidermal, dermal, and subcutaneous layers of the foot pad. While Malinovský (1966c) reports that only free nerve endings are found in the epidermis of the foot pad, Jänig (1971) reports that Merkel end organs were observed in epithelial ridges of the foot pad. The parent nerve fibers forming the terminals in Merkel end organs were myelinated and from five to 12 microns in diameter. According to Malinovský (1966c), the dermal layers of the foot pad contain free nerve endings and a large number of small encapsulated end organs. These end organs or corpuscles were located in the papillary bodies or in the connective tissue between the papillary bodies near the epidermis. The longitudinal axis of orientation of a corpuscle was usually vertical or oblique to the surface of the foot pad. Encapsulated corpuscles are formed by one or more nerve terminals, an inner core of fine grained material that surrounds the nerve terminal and a capsule that surrounds the terminal and inner core of the corpuscle (Malinovský, 1966c). The capsule is usually formed by a small number of lamellae that appear to be continuous with the coverings of the nerve fiber.

The encapsulated corpuscles found in the foot pads of the cat are of greater morphological variety than those described in any other tissue. Malinovský (1966c) classified encapsulated corpuscles in the cat foot pad into twelve

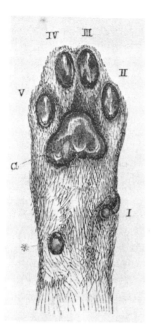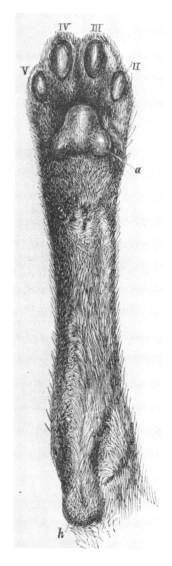

Fig. 9-19. Cat. Left: Under-surface of forepaw. I-V: the five toes, I being the pollex. a, metacarpal trilobed pad that lies beneath the distal ends of the metacarpal bones*, pisiform pad. Right: Under-surface of hind paw. II-V: the four toes. a, metacarpal pad. h, heel. Reproduced with permission from Mivart, G. (1881), *The Cat*, John Murray, London.

types on the basis of the form of the encapsulated nerve fiber (Fig. 9-20). Paciniform corpuscles (receptors one and two in Fig. 9-20) contain a single

Different animals joints	Foetus Newborn joints	Cat joints	Dog joints	Cat foot pads
69.3	F 82.13 / N 84.00			40.32
		74.5	46.7	
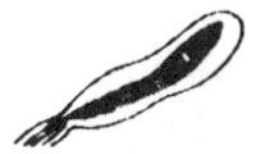 12.05	F 0.43 / N 5.00			11.04
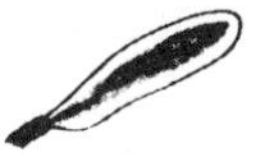 8.7	F 9.36 / N 5.00	3.2	13.3	13.08
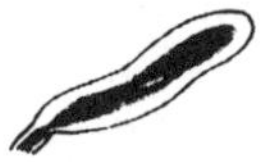 2.3	F 1.70 / N 2.00		23.4	7.68
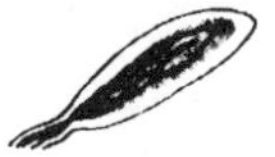 0.4	F 0.85 / N –			4.20
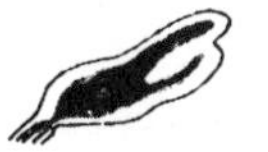 0.3	F – / N 2.00	1.1		0.72
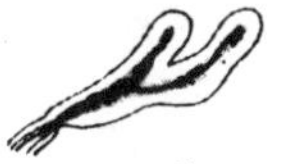 3.1	F 1.26 / N –	9.6		3.24
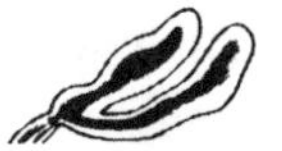 1.9	F 1.85 / N –	7.5		
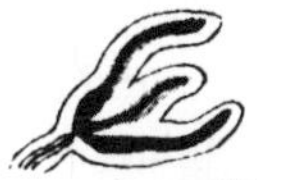 0.15		2.1		0.12
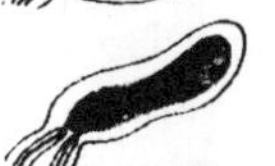 0.15			3.3	2.88
				2.76
			10.0	
				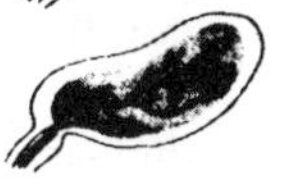 8.76

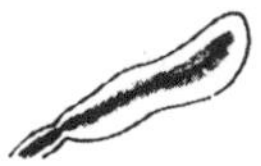

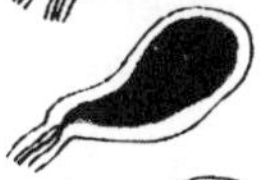

Fig. 9-20. Mammals. Comparison of variability of the main types of terminal encapsulated corpuscles of different animals in summary, in joint capsules of a human foetus and newborn, in joint capsules of a cat and a dog and in foot pads of a cat. The numbers give the percentage of occurrence. (Malinovský, 1966c)

terminal fiber that is either straight or bent. The Golgi-Mazzoni type of corpuscles are characterized as containing a terminal fiber that divides to form two to four or more branches within the capsule of the corpuscle (third, fourth, and fifth receptors in Fig. 9-20). A small number of these corpuscles contained a terminal fiber that divided into several branches that rolled together in a clew (eleventh receptor in Fig. 9-20). In only one case was there no apparent inner core surrounding the terminal fiber and its branches in this type of Golgi-Mazzoni corpuscle. Another group of Golgi-Mazzoni corpuscles contained a terminal fiber that divided into primary branches, and then divided further into secondary and tertiary branches to form spraylike endings (twelfth receptor in Fig. 9-20). A small number of the corpuscles containing spraylike endings were devoid of darkly staining inner-core material. The third group of end organs, the branched corpuscles, (sixth, seventh, eighth, and ninth receptors in Fig. 9-20) were formed by a terminal fiber that divided and maintained a separate inner core for each of the branches. A fourth group of corpuscles, the polyaxonal corpuscles, contained more than one terminal fiber (tenth receptor in Fig. 9-20). In addition a single end organ similar to the Meissner corpuscle was observed directly under the epidermis of the cat's foot pad. The nuclei of the cells forming the inner core of the Meissner type of corpuscle were aligned perpendicular to the long axis of the corpuscle.

Vater-Pacinian corpuscles were found primarily in the subcutaneous tissue of the foot pad (Jänig, 1971). They were found between fat lobules deep under the skin, and were frequently found in association with tendons (Jänig, 1971). Lynn (1969) has conducted a thorough investigation of the distribution of Vater-Pacinian corpuscles in the foot pads of the cat and his findings are presented in Fig. 9-21. As can be seen, these corpuscles tend to be found in groups in specific locations deep below the surface of the foot pads.

The Vater-Pacinian corpuscle consists of an outer lamellated capsule and a complex cellular inner core in which a single unmyelinated nerve ending is situated (Fig. 9-22). The capsule, consisting of seven or eight lamellae of epithelium of perineural origin, encloses the contents of the corpuscle (Munger, 1971). A dense mesh of connective tissue envelops the entire corpuscle and is segregated from the contents of the corpuscle by the capsule. The inner core of the corpuscle is composed of successive layers of simple cellular lamellae divided into a middle zone and a central zone. The middle zone of the corpuscle is formed by alternating fluid-filled spaces and cellular lamellae that number from thirty to sixty. In the central zone the lamellar cells form numerous concentric sheets of thin cytoplasm separated by collagen fibers. The most central sheets are in close contact with the connective-tissue covering of the nerve terminal. A Vater-Pacini corpuscle is supplied by a single myelinated fiber and occasionally corpuscles are found strung out on a single nerve fiber like beads (Goglia, 1965). The fibers

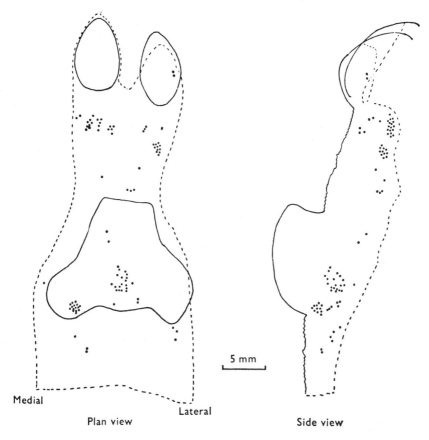

Medial

Lateral

Plan view

Side view

5 mm

Fig. 9-21. Cat. The distribution of Vater-Pacini corpuscles in and around the foot pads. Locations of Vater-Pacini corpuscles found during post-mortem dissection of the foot (filled circles). Limits of dissection (broken line). (Lynn, 1969)

innervating Vater-Pacini corpuscles are larger than those innervating the smaller encapsulated corpuscles (Poláček *et al.*, 1969). Vater-Pacini corpuscles are of widespread occurrence and are found in the cat mesentery, the genitals (Poláček, 1968), the bladder (Shehata, 1970), and elsewhere.

NEUROPHYSIOLOGY OF SKIN

The complexity of the skin senses has for years posed a formidable obstacle for neurophysiological investigators. Not only were their tools inadequate to solve many of the technical difficulties involved in stimulating the skin and recording from an adequate sample of viable single units, but they also faced the task of acknowledging that one of the Aristotelian five senses is divisible

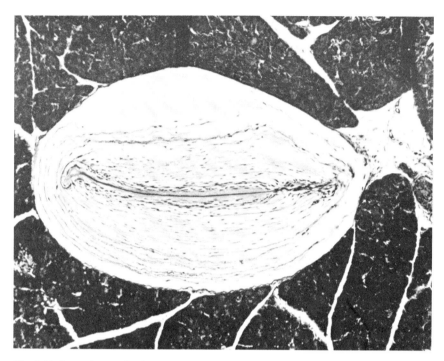

Fig. 9-22. Cat. A longitudinal section through a Vater-Pacini corpuscle from cat pancreas (light microscopy). There has been some shrinkage of the capsule and outermost lamellae away from the surrounding tissue, but the longitudinal arrangement of the lamellar envelopes of the middle zone, the general disposition of the inner zone, and the full extent of the nerve terminal are well depicted (overall length of corpuscle = 1500 μ approx.). From "Non-Auditory Vibration Receptors," *International Audiology*, (1968), *I*, 311, by courtesy of Dr. T.A. Quilliam, Department of Anatomy, University College, London.

into a myriad of subsystems. In the cat the epidermal surface can be divided into a large number of anatomically distinguishable surfaces, and there is also the incontrovertible evidence that the sensory systems of each surface are divisible into many subsystems on the basis of receptor end-organ morphology and single unit studies of their innervation. Recent neurophysiological measurements indicate that in the hairy body skin of the cat there may be ten or more separate myelinated fiber systems responsive to mechanical stimulation, as well as several unmyelinated mechanically sensitive fiber systems.

Early neurophysiological investigators were unprepared for the complexity of the sensory systems subserving the outside surface of the animal. Impediments to investigation were in part perceptual and philosophical. Philosophical and psychological concepts of human skin functioning did not sharply delineate different skin areas, nor were the sensory systems within an area clearly separable into diverse functioning systems. As we shall see, both thermal and mechanical stimulation of the skin surface excite fibers belonging to a variety of sensory systems, and with the primitive response measures at their disposal, psychophysical investigators had no way of determining whether their stimulus was activating one or more sensory systems, or to what degree they were being activated.

Hairy Body Skin, Myelinated Fibers

The difficulties faced by neurophysiological investigators on the skin are nowhere more apparent then in the long series of investigations on the hairy body skin of the cat. The nerves innervating the skin are composed of fibers of diverse diameters indicative of complex neural populations. In addition to the philosophical and procedural problems alluded to above, neurophysiologists studying the cat's body skin were largely unaided by neuroantomical studies. In fact, many cutaneous neuroanatomists have insisted on a Spartan simplicity of receptor types that simply does not exist. In spite of these handicaps, neurophysiologists have worked out in some detail the different types of sensory systems that exist there and some of their characteristics. The present picture is one of incredible complexity, and one that promises reevaluation of many of the current concepts in cutaneous anatomy and physiology.

The present understanding is due in part to the quantitative studies by Zotterman (1939) and Werner and Mountcastle (1965), although mainly to the studies of Hunt and McIntyre (1960a; 1960b) and to the continuous series of investigations by Iggo and his associates and more recent studies by Burgess and Perl and their co-workers. Since the present understanding of the skin senses took a long period of development (and even now is subject to modification), we shall present a recent and complete breakdown as compiled by Burgess, Petit, and Warren (1968). In many cases, earlier workers lumped together units that we now know to belong to distinct neural categories. Allusion will be made to other workers only when their distinctions between units correspond to those of Burgess et al., (1968).

The preparation chosen by Burgess et al. (1968) for most of their work was the sural nerve that innervates the skin on the hind leg. Recordings were made with glass pipettes inserted into the whole nerve. Units were activated by electrically stimulating the sural nerve, a procedure that enabled the investigators to measure conduction velocities for each fiber. Like most cutaneous nerves, the sural nerve contains fibers of a wide range of diameters (Fig. 9-23). This technique of recording does not sample unmyelinated fibers and is somewhat biased in favor of the larger myelinated fibers. As we shall see, however, there is still more than enough diversity to keep several investigators occupied.

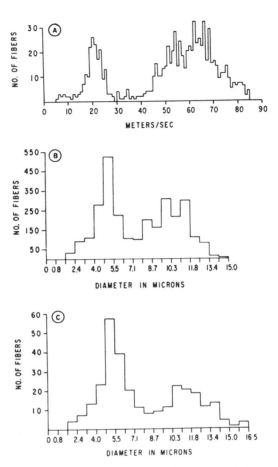

Fig. 9-23. Cat. A: sural nerve microelectrode sample (841 fibers). Conduction velocities of all sural fibers studied with microelectrodes. This population is unselected in the sense that every fiber providing a stable potential was included. B: diameters of the 2,864 fibers found in four sural nerves as determined with the light microscope. An effort was made to measure all the fibers in the four nerves. C: diameters of 294 randomly selected fibers from two sural nerves as measured from electron micrographs. (Burgess *et al.*, 1968)

The stimuli used by Burgess *et al.* (1968) were a vibrator with controlled rate and amplitude of movement used to determine velocity and amplitude thresholds, various devices for indenting and grabbing the skin (von Frey hairs, brush, etc.), tuning forks for testing vibratory stimuli, and devices for heating and cooling the skin. In addition, the projection of the fibers to cervical levels of the spinal cord was studied by electrically stimulating the dorsal columns to elicit antidromic spikes at the peripheral recording site (Petit and Burgess, 1968).

The myelinated fibers present in the sural nerve (other nerves were studied to a limited extent) were divided into eleven separate fiber types. Criteria for classification included: conduction velocity or fiber size; type of stimulus activating a unit; characteristics of receptive field; and response chacteristics of the unit (phasic or tonic, spontaneous activity, threshold, etc.). The eleven fiber types identified by Burgess *et al.* (1968), their frequency of occurrence, and conduction velocity measurements are presented in Table 9-1.

Hair Fibers   Three types of fibers responding to hair movements were distinguished: G1 hair fibers, G2 hair fibers, and D hair fibers. D hair fibers were excited by small movements of down hairs as well as movements of bristles and awns. G1 and G2 hair fibers were discharged by movements of the longer stiffer bristles and awns, with G1 hair fibers discharging preferentially to bristles. All three fiber types were discharged by moving a number of hairs within a skin receptive field. G2 hair fibers and D hair fibers typically had smaller receptive fields than G1 hair fibers. All three fiber types exhibited no spontaneous activity and discharged only while the hairs were moving. Discharge ceases after the movement ceases; static dislocations of hair is not an adequate stimulus for discharge. There were wide differences in the thresholds to hair movement of the G1 fibers and the G2 and D hair fibers (Table 9-2). G1 fibers required hair movements of 5-20 microns/msec for discharge whereas movements from 0.5 to 1.5 microns/msec and 0.1 to 1.0 microns/msec were sufficient to discharge G2 hair fibers and D fibers respectively. Measurements of the conduction velocities of the three separate fiber groups disclose that the different groups are composed of different-sized fibers (Fig. 9-24). The D hair fibers are the smallest of the three fiber groups. The study by Petit and Burgess (1968) also revealed that the D hair fibers, unlike the other two fiber groups, do not project to the cervical level via the dorsal columns as do most fibers from the other two fiber groups (Table 9-3).

Type I and Type II Fibers   Two types of fibers exhibiting tonic discharge to gentle punctate mechanical stimulation were distinguished by Burgess *et al.* (1968). These two fiber groups are identical to those distinguished by Iggo (1966a; 1968), who has designated them type I and type II fibers.

The discharge patterns of type I fibers in the cat have been investigated in some detail by Werner and Mountcastle (1965), Tapper (1965), Iggo and Muir (1969), and Burgess *et al.* (1968). In the main, these accounts agree although in describing the discharge of type I fibers, we shall draw mainly from the latter three reports, since Werner and Mountcastle may have

Table 9-1. Frequency of Occurrence and Conduction Velocities of Sural Nerve Fibers (Burgess et al, 1968)

Receptor Type	Number of Fibers Observed	Percent of Sural Sample	Mean Conduction Velocity	Conduction Velocity Range (95% of fibers fall from range shown)
G¹ hair	106	12.8%	75m/sec	66 t0 83 m/sec
G² hair	72	8.7%	53m/sec	41 to 62 m/sec
D hair	130	15.7%	21m/sec	16 to 27 m/sec
Type I	156	18.8%	65m/sec	54 to 72m/sec
Type II	85	10.2%	54m/sec	45 to 65 m/sec
Field	103	12.4%	55m/sec	40 to 70 m/sec
Pacinian corpuscle	34	4.1%	65m/sec	54 to 74 m/sec
Tap	16	1.9%		50 to 76 m/sec
High threshold	108	13.9%	27m/sec	6 to 60 m/sec
Insensitive hair	13	1.6%		60 to 77 m/sec
Subcutaneous	5	0.6%		

Table 9-2. Sural nerve fiber properties (Burgess et al, 1968)

Receptor type	Receptive field dimensions (mm²)	Discharge	Velocity threshold (p/msec)	Amplitude threshold (p)	Von Frey hair threshold (mg)	Response to cooling[1]
G₁hair	11±4.5 x 6±2.2	Phasic	5-20 (a) 60 (b)	-	-	0
G₂hair	7±2.9 x 5±1.6	Phasic	0.008-0.05 (a) 0.5-1.5 (b)	5-15	10-25	+
D hair	7±2.1 x 6±2.3	Phasic	0.1-1.0 (b)	3-6	5-8	++
Type I	Punctuate (several) (foci)	Tonic (irregular) (discharge)	-	5-10	8-20	++
Type II	Punctuate (one) (focus)	Tonic (regular) (discharge)	-	10-15	10-25	++
Field	12±4 x 7±2.5	Variable	0.1-1.0 (a)°	10-80	15-70	Variable
Pacinian corpuscle	2 to 4 mm focus	Phasic	0.02-10 (a)	-	-	0

[1] Number of plus signs shows relative magnitude of response. (a), determined on the skin. (b), determined by moving hair.

° Applies only to rapidly adapting field receptors.

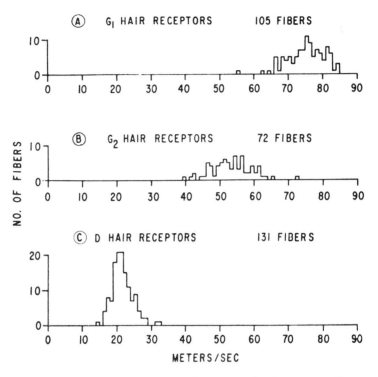

Fig. 9-24. Cat. Conduction velocities of G1, G2, and D hair receptor fibers. (Burgess *et al.*, 1968)

recorded from some type II fibers. Type I units are discharged by mechanical stimulation of the tactile pads. Only one fiber innervates each pad although each fiber usually innervates more than one pad (Fig. 9-25). The pads innervated by a single fiber are close together and form a receptive field. Receptive fields of different fibers are non-overlapping. Type I fibers exhibit either no spontaneous activity, or extremely low levels of resting discharge (1-5/sec). When present, this resting activity is irregular and can be influenced by the temperature of the skin and previous history of stimulation (Burgess *et al.*, 1968). The effective stimulus for discharge is one that deforms a tactile pad; indentation or stretching of the skin adjacent to the pad or bending nearby hairs are not effective stimuli for discharging a fiber, provided the pad itself is not deformed. The most effective stimulus is the movement of a probe across the surface of a pad, such a procedure eliciting bursts of spikes at transient rates greater than one thousand spikes/sec.

These tactile pad units are also sensitive to deformation produced by a probe indenting the surface of the pad from a vertical direction. Discharge

Table 9-3. Dorsal column projection of sural nerve fibers (Petit and Burgess, 1968)

Fiber type	No. of fibers observed	% of sural sample	No. tested from cervical-dorsal columns	No. activated from cervical-dorsal columns	% of peripheral primary afferent fibers found at cervical level
G¹ hair	106	12.8	56	54	96
G² hair	72	8.7	36	28	78
D hair	130	15.7	59	1	2
Type I	156	18.8	66	0	0
Type II	85	10.2	29	29	100
Field	103	12.4	48	38	79
Pacinian corpuscle	34	4.1	9	9	100
Tap	16	1.9	9	6	67
High-threshold	108	13.0	39	0	0
Insensitive hair	13	1.6	11	11	100
Subcutaneous	5	0.6	3	1	33

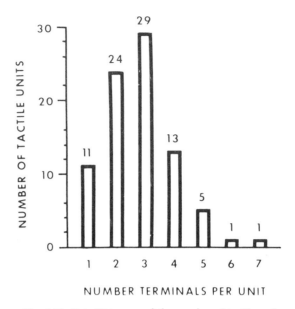

Fig. 9-25. Cat. Histogram of the number of tactile pads
(terminals) innervated by each type I fiber. (Tapper, 1965)

can be elicited by forces of less than 1.0 mg or displacements of 1-5 microns
(Iggo and Muir, 1969). The thresholds estimated by Burgess *et al.* (1968)
are 8-20 mg, with von Frey hairs and rapid displacements of 10-15 microns. If
a probe is pressed into the pad the neuron fires tonically during the period of
active indentation (the dynamic period) and while the indentation is
maintained (the static period). The discharge of a neuron during the periods
of dynamic and static stimulation is shown in Fig. 9-26. Discharge from the
neuron is greatest during the dynamic phase of stimulation and may achieve
transient rates of fifteen hundred spikes/sec (Iggo and Muir, 1969). During
the static phase of stimulation, discharge falls off, first rapidly and then
slowly. With a sufficient degree of static displacement, discharge has been
observed for as long as thirty minutes (Iggo and Muir, 1969).

Discharge of these units to the type of stimulation applied by the
investigators (displacements by a vertically oriented probe) was characterized
by irregular discharge; i.e. long and short intervals could occur together.
Thus, interval distributions of activity elicited during static stimulation and
following the major declines in spike output (Fig. 9-26) tend to be skewed
(Fig. 9-27). Short interspike intervals are represented even at low discharge
rates and this feature of the interspike interval distribution of elicited
discharge from type I units clearly distinguishes them from type II units,
where the intervals are often extremely regular.

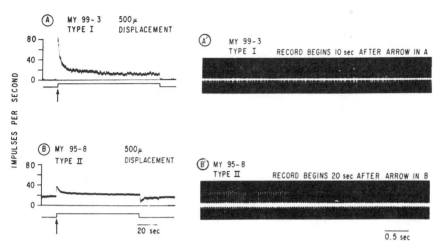

Fig. 9-26. Cat. Mechanically evoked activity in type I and type II fibers. A: PST histogram illustrating the magnitude and duration of discharge evoked by 500-micron displacement of a single tactile pad. Lower trace indicates the duration of the displacement. A′: a portion of the discharge occurring in A to illustrate the pattern of activity. B and B′: PST histogram and spike train of a type II fiber. (Burgess *et al.*, 1968)

Conduction-velocity estimates by Burgess *et al.* (1968) on type I fibers range between fifty and eighty meters/sec (Fig. 9-28). The estimates in Fig. 9-28 are in agreement with those of Brown and Iggo (1967) but not with those of Tapper (1965), who estimated conduction velocities by electrically and mechanically stimulating the skin rather than the fiber itself. The conduction-velocity estimates in Fig. 9-28 indicate that type I fibers are nine to twelve microns in diameter. No anatomical measurements exist on the diameter of the fibers innervating tactile pads.

Besides being responsive to mechanical stimulation of the tactile pads, type I fibers are responsive to skin temperature changes. The effect of skin temperature on resting discharge and mechanically evoked discharge has been studied by Tapper (1965), Iggo and Muir (1969), and Casey and Hahn (1970). These studies indicate that the magnitude of both evoked and resting discharge is in part dependent upon skin temperature. Rapid cooling of the skin may elicit discharge from type I fibers, but the maximum number of spikes elicited is less than 10 percent of that elicited by gentle mechanical stimulation. Similarly, Casey and Hahn (1970) demonstrate that the response to mechanical stimulation can be diminished by cooling the skin.

Lindblom and Tapper (1966) studied the effect on type I fiber discharge of stimulating simultaneously two pads connected to the same fiber. They found that the effects of the two stimuli are not additive, but rather the pad with the strongest stimulus determines the discharge rate.

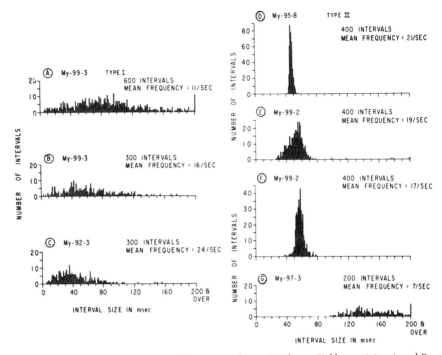

Fig. 9-27. Cat. Interspike interval histograms of type I and type II fiber activity. A and B: portions of type I discharge illustrated in Fig. 9-26. C: activity from another type I fiber responding at a somewhat higher frequency. D: taken from the type II fiber discharge shown in Fig. 9-26. E and F: part of a type II response with E starting 5 sec and F starting 30 sec after stimulus onset. G: some of the most irregular type II activity observed. (Burgess *et al.*, 1968)

Type II units, like type I units, are responsive to gentle mechanical stimulation of the skin, and they are maximally sensitive to mechanical stimulation of a small locus on the skin. Unlike type I units, however, the peripheral terminations of type II units cannot be identified with an external structure such as tactile pads. According to Burgess *et al.* (1968), almost all fibers identified as type II units possess a single focal region in their receptive field of one to two millimeters within which the threshold to mechanical stimulation is lower than that of the surrounding skin. Only a few fibers identified as type II units have been reported to have more than one focal region; and three fibers out of eighty-five units identified as type II units seemed to terminate in domes similar to tactile pads (Burgess *et al.*, 1968). Unlike type I units, more than half the type II units exhibited a resting discharge up to 20 spikes/sec. This resting discharge tends to be extremely regular. Conduction-velocity estimates on type II fibers range between forty-five and seventy meters/sec (Fig. 9-28) indicating large fibers between eight

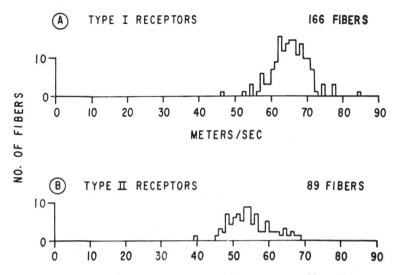

Fig. 9-28. Cat. Conduction velocities of type I and type II receptor fibers. (Burgess *et al.*, 1966)

and eleven microns. On the average, type II fibers tend to be slightly smaller than type I fibers (Fig. 9-28). Type II fibers are sensitive to static and dynamic deformation of the skin surface. This mechanical stimulation need not be applied to the focal point since stretching of the skin is sufficient to discharge type II fibers (Iggo 1966, 1968; Brown and Iggo, 1967; Burgess *et al.*, 1968). The discharge patterns of resting and evoked activity of type II fibers tend to be regular, with long intervals predominating (Fig. 9-27). Petit and Burgess (1968) have demonstrated that type II fibers project to cervical levels via the dorsal columns whereas type I fibers do not (Table 9-3).

Pacinian Corpuscle and Tap Fibers   Two types of sural nerve fibers were observed by Burgess *et al.* (1968) to be sensitive to high-frequency vibratory stimuli: "Pacinian corpuscle (Vater-Pacini corpuscle) fibers" and tap fibers. These fibers had similar characteristics except that tap fibers were much less sensitive than corpuscle fibers to vibratory stimuli of five hundred Hz or greater. No resting discharge was shown by either type. Conduction-velocity estimates for the two fiber types were also similar (Table 9-1 and Fig. 9-29). All Vater-Pacini corpuscle fibers projected to cervical levels of the spinal cord and 67 percent of the tap fibers did also.

Some of the characteristics of fibers innervating Vater-Pacini corpuscles have been examined by Hunt (1961), who studied fibers in the interosseous nerve and the sural nerve. Vater-Pacini corpuscle fibers are relatively insensitive to low-frequency vibration but can be set into continuous nonde-

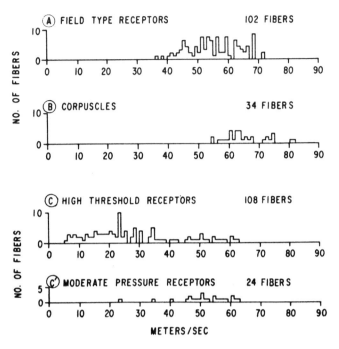

Fig. 9-29. Conduction velocities of field. Vater-Pacini corpuscle, and high-threshold receptor fibers. C′shows conduction velocities for the most sensitive of the high-threshold group. (Burgess *et al.*, 1968)

cremental discharge by high-frequency vibratory stimuli (Fig. 9-30). A spike for every stimulus cycle is observable to 650 Hz. Large-amplitude low-frequency stimulation was ineffective at eliciting discharge. The lower limit of effective stimuli varied between forty and ninety Hz, depending on the

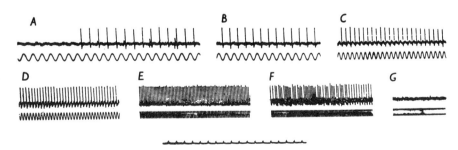

Fig. 9-30. Cat. Discharge, in response to vibration, recorded from a single afferent fiber from a Vater-Pacini corpuscle located adjacent to the tibia. Upper trace, nerve impulses; lower trace, frequency of vibration applied to corpuscle. Final frequencies Hz A 90, E 102, C 180, D 550, E 650, F 700, G 1000. Time marker, 10 msec. (Hunt, 1961)

corpuscle. Upper limits varied between six hundred and eight hundred Hz. Hunt (1961), recording from more than one Pacinian corpuscle fiber simultaneously, demonstrated that the different fibers may discharge in phase with the vibratory stimulus. Sato (1961) has studied the response of fibers innervating the Vater-Pacini corpuscles of the cat's mesentery and he found that these, too, were sensitive to high-frequency vibratory stimuli (Fig. 9-31). Sato also studied the response of the fibers to short-duration mechanical stimuli delivered to the corpuscle.

High-Threshold Fibers About 13 percent of the myelinated fibers of the sural nerve were classified by Burgess *et al.* (1968) as high-threshold fibers. This group was extremely heterogeneous and was broken down into three subgroups on the basis of the fiber sensitivity to mechanical stimulation. The least sensitive fibers only discharged to mechanical stimuli that damaged the skin. Conduction velocities ranged from six to sixty-five m/sec (Fig. 9-29) with the least sensitive fibers being the slowest conducting. None of the high-threshold units were found to project in the dorsal columns of the cervical

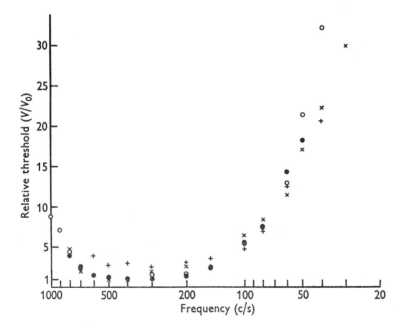

Fig. 9-31. Cat. The relation between vibration frequency and threshold of fibers innervating undissected Vater-Pacini corpuscles with intact blood supply. Four different sets of experiments are shown (x, +, open circles, filled circles). x, +: Vibration was suddenly applied. Open circles, closed circles: Slowly increasing vibration to finite amplitude was applied. Semi-log. scale. (Sato, 1961)

levels of the spinal cord (Table 9-3). High-threshold units were also studied in the posterior femoral cutaneous nerve by Burgess and Perl (1967). These high-threshold fibers were found to have large receptive fields of punctate representation.

Fibers that only discharge to mechanical stimulation that produces tissue damage are frequently referred to as "nociceptive" fibers (Burgess and Perl, 1967; Burgess *et al.* 1968), with the implication that these fibers belong to a sensory system that measures tissue damage. The difficulty with this interpretation is that these fibers may have only responded to tissue-damaging stimuli simply because the appropriate stimulus had not been applied. Assuming that a fiber group is nociceptive implies that it only responds to tissue-damaging stimuli and that all other alternatives have been tried. The high-threshold units do respond to tissue-damaging stimuli, but each stimulus elicits fewer and fewer spikes (Burgess and Perl, 1967), suggesting that part of the tissue being damaged is the receptor itself. A sensory system erected to measure tissue damage should be itself resistant to destruction.

The readiness with which neurophysiologists and neuroanatomists attribute nociception to many fiber groups is attested to by the ubiquity of "pain" fibers. Pain is a sensation and as such is a central interpretation of peripheral neural events. Rather than being a natural attribute of the normal functioning state of any neural group, it is most likely that the sensation of pain is a signal of severe irregularity in a sensory system. If part of a neural sensory system is functioning abnormally due to injury, population discharge patterns will be set up that have no probability of occurrence were the system functioning within normal limits. Thus, "pain" may in many cases be the sensational reaction to paradoxical sensory inputs. Some such provisional interpretation seems likely in lieu of the widespread occurrence of "pain" fibers.

Other Fiber Types in Hairy Body Skin　As can be seen in Table 9-1, Burgess *et al.* (1968) distinguished eleven different types of myelinated fibers in the sural nerve. Two of these, subcutaneous fibers and insensitive hair fibers, were not studied in any detail. All the other fiber types except field fibers have been discussed above. Field fibers were activated by vigorous movements of skin within large oval areas of the skin, or by multiple hair movements. Wide variations occurred in most measures taken from field fibers. Some responded tonically (although not beyond five or six seconds) to skin indentation, others phasically. A wide range of conduction velocities were found for field fibers (Fig. 9-29). No resting discharge was shown by field fibers.

In summary, there are several different myelinated fiber types that have been observed to be responsive to mechanical stimulation of the skin. These different fiber types tend to respond to different aspects of the same mechanical stimulus and are differentially sensitive to different types of mechanical stimulation. The precise mode of mechanical stimulation to which each fiber is responsive has not been fully determined. Because of their different response properties, the units will respond differently to the same mechanical stimulus. A summarizing diagram from Iggo (1970) showing the typical discharge from four different fiber types to the same mechanical stimulus is presented in Fig. 9-32. Iggo (1966, 1968, 1970) and Brown and Iggo (1967) have determined by quantitative measurements in other species that some of the unit types found in cutaneous nerves in the cat are also found in rabbits, dogs, and in some primates.

Hairy Body Skin, Unmyelinated Fibers

Although unmyelinated cutaneous sensory fibers outnumber the myelinated cutaneous fibers about 16 to one (Barker, 1967), they have received much less attention from neurophysiologists. This tradition will be continued here since the existing studies only crudely describe the unmyelinated fiber types found

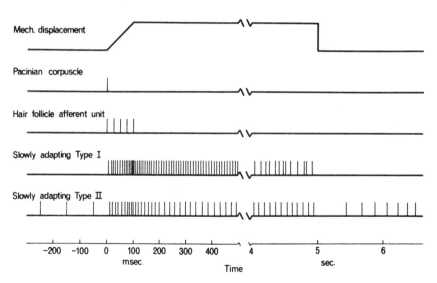

Fig. 9-32. Cat. Diagram to show the differences in the responses of cutaneous afferent units to an identical mechanical stimulus. The movement of the mechanical probe is indicated in the upper trace, and the unit responses are: Pacinian corpuscle, phasic; hair follicle afferent unit, phasic; type I unit, tonic with no resting discharge; type II unit, tonic with a resting discharge. The time scales for the left- and right-handed sides of the figure are different. (Iggo, 1970) Reprinted from *Dukes' Physiology of Domestic Animals*, edited by Melvin J. Swenson, copyright 1933 by H.H. Dukes; copyright 1935, 1937, 1942, and 1947 by Comstock Publishing Co., Inc.; copyright 1955 by Cornell University; copyright © 1970 by Cornell University. Used by permission of Cornell University Press.

to respond to cutaneous stimulation. Iggo (1960) separated the unmyelinated fibers in the saphenous nerve into two groups: mechanically sensitive, and temperature sensitive. The sensitivity of the mechanical fibers varied widely. Discharges following cessation of stimulation were observed frequently. Repeated applications of the same stimulus elicited fewer and fewer spikes from a fiber. Maximum discharge rates were less than one hundred spikes/sec. Receptive fields were usually small (a few millimeters square).

Bessou and Perl (1969) studied 147 unmyelinated fibers supplying the cat's hairy skin. They divided the fibers into low-threshold and high-threshold fibers on the basis of response to thermal and mechanical stimulation. The most commonly encountered low-threshold units were discharged by both mechanical and thermal stimulation of the skin. The commonest high-threshold units (polymodal nociceptors) responded to moderate to intense mechanical stimulation and discharged vigorously to noxious heat. These high-threshold units also responded to acid applied to the skin. A breakdown of the unmyelinated fiber types as classified by Bessou and Perl (1969) is presented in Table 9-4.

Bessou et al. (1971) have recently studied unmyelinated mechno-responsive fibers in greater detail. They report that these fibers form a relatively homogeneous population and can be distinguished from other unmyelinated fibers by their vigorous discharge to gentle mechanical stimulation. Most discharge to a force of 15 mg applied to the receptive field by a von Frey hair. A smooth probe moving across the surface of the skin only excites the cells to any degree if it is moving slowly, rapid movements being ineffective. Repeated stimuli often gave diminishing responses. Discharge was not synchronous with oscillatory stimuli beyond one Hz. Rapid cooling of the skin discharged the fibers at frequencies about 20 percent of the maximum discharge shown to mechanical stimulation.

Neurophysiology of Other Hair Systems

Vibrissae Single unit recordings from trigeminal nerve fibers innervating the cat's mystacial vibrissae have been briefly described by Iggo (1968) and at somewhat greater length by Fitzgerald (1940), whose work we shall report in detail. According to Fitzgerald, about 5 percent of the units examined exhibited spontaneous activity. Spontaneous activity rates were less than forty/sec and were regular. The majority of the vibrissa units studied responded to sideward movements of the hairs. In general, only one hair was found to be effective in discharging a single unit, but more than one unit could be discharged by moving a single hair. The response of a unit

Table 9-4. Classification of Fibers in a Survey of 131 Unmyelinated Fibers of Cutaneous Nerves* (Bessou and Perl, 1969)

	No.	%	Mechanical Threshold	Noxious Heat	Cooling	Chemical Irritants
Low-threshold mechanoreceptor	47	36	0.01 to 0.045 g	--	+	-
Thermal	8	8	0.2 to unre-	Variable		
Warm	1		sponsive		-	?
Cool	7			Variable	+	?
Polymodal nociceptors	39	30	0.2 to 45 g	+	-+	+
High-threshold mechanoreceptor ? cold	18	14	0.6 to 45 g	- (or delayed)	-(>10C)	-
High-threshold subcutaneous	3	2	High with (intact skin)	-	-	- (intact skin)
Unclassified°° or inexcitable	16	12				

*Data from 31 experiments considering every unit whose discharge was successfully isolated. † For punctate stimulators of the von Frey type. ‡None down to 10 C prior to activation by heat or irritant chemicals. °° Inadequate data collected for classification.

apparently depended upon which direction the hair moved, since the degree of discharge depended upon the direction of movement. Units with spontaneous activity could be inhibited by movements in one direction and excited by movements in the opposite direction. Most units exhibited tonic discharge to static displacements of hair, but some only responded phasically during movement.

The cat's vibrissa systems have recently been investigated by Hahn (1971). He found that 77 percent of the forty-four units investigated displayed some level of spontaneous activity, although two thirds of these had rates less than one spike/sec. All units were relatively insensitive to static displacements of the vibrissae, but were quite responsive to small sinusoidal oscillations of the whiskers. Threshold for discharge varied with the frequency of stimulation. The units were maximally sensitive to vibrations above one hundred Hz. Hahn divided the units into two groups on the basis of their response to sinusoidal stimulation: those that seemed to be responding to the velocity of the stimulus, and those that responded to both the velocity and magnitude of the deflection. These two groups, however, did not differ with respect to several other measuring variables (i.e., location, latency, rate of spontaneous activity, etc.). Units responding to vibrissa movements have also been examined in rats by Zucker and Welker (1969).

Carpal Hairs   The discharge of fibers in the ulnar nerve responding to movements of carpal hairs have been described by Nilsson (1969b). Over 50 percent (17 out of twenty-two) of the units displayed a measurable degree of spontaneous activity (up to 20/sec). Each unit could be discharged by moving only one hair. Pushing the hairs in was more effective at eliciting discharge than sideward movements (a transient rate of eight hundred/sec as opposed to a rate of five hundred/sec). All of the units were sensitive to directional movements of the hairs, in that movements around the long axis of the hair in some directions tended to elicit a large discharge, movements in the opposite direction elicited no discharge or inhibited the spontaneous discharges. Discharge of all units was apparently greater during movement than during static displacement. Units were divided into those that discharged to static displacements and those that discharged only to the dynamic phase of stimulation. Responses of a unit with spontaneous activity and another without it can be seen in Fig. 9-33. Conduction velocity measurements on the two types of fibers disclosed that the phasic units were more slowly conducting than the tonic units (Nilsson, 1969b).

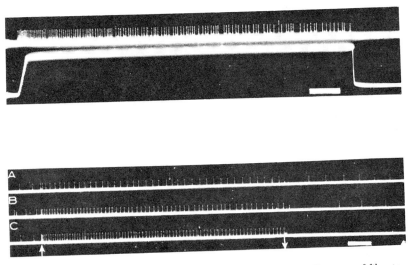

Fig. 9-33. Cat. Response of two fibers to movements of carpal hairs. Top: Response of fiber to movement of hair to a plateau of 450 microns. Bottom: Response of a fiber with spontaneous activity to static displacement of a hair at three different amplitudes: 150, 350, and 500 microns. Onset and end of stimuli at arrows. Time bar 100 msec. (Nilsson, 1969b)

Ear Hairs   The hair cover on the inner surface of the pinna is clearly distinct from that covering the rest of the body. This portion of the external surface of the head developed independently of the skin cover on the rest of the face, which is innervated primarily by the trigeminal ganglion. Reptiles and birds have no outer pinna. Thus, when an ear was needed, special sensory systems had to be developed to innervate this inner surface of the pinna. The cutaneous sensory systems for the inner surface of the pinna are apparently supplied by cells in the jugular ganglion of the vagus and the cells in the geniculate ganglion of the facial nerve. The cells in the dorsocaudal portion of the geniculate ganglion have been shown to innervate the hairs in the inner surface of the pinna (Boudreau *et al.*, 1971). Each cell innervates a number of hairs in a small patch of skin several millimeters square (Fig. 9-34). The cells exhibit no spontaneous activity and are discharged by

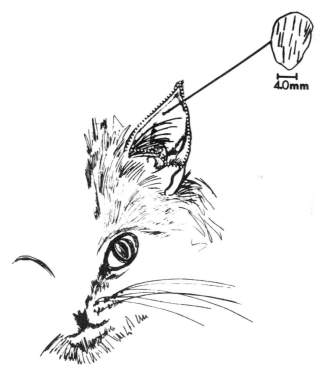

Fig. 9-34. Cat. Geniculate ganglion ear units could be discharged by moving hairs on the inner surface of the pinna. The area within which hair movements were effective is outlined with a dotted line. Geniculate ganglion ear units had small receptive fields, an example of which is shown in this figure (inset). (Boudreau *et al.*, 1971)

moving hairs within the innervated area in any direction. Discharge occurs only during hair movement and is greater when more than one hair is moved. Only one hair emerges from a single follicle.

Hairs on the dorsal surface of the ear of the rabbit have been studied by Weddell and his associates (Weddell and Pallie, 1955; Weddell et al., 1955a; 1955b). According to Brown et al. (1967), the types of hair systems found on the rabbit ear correspond to the D fibers and G2 fibers innervating the body skin.

Neurophysiology of Nonhairy Skin

Foot Pads, Mechanically Sensitive Units Jänig, Schmidt, and Zimmerman (1968) recorded from large myelinated fibers in the medial and lateral plantar nerves. In these fibers they examined spontaneous activity rates, conduction velocities as estimated from latencies to electrical stimulation of the dorsal roots, and various discharge properties in relation to mechanical stimulation of the skin of the foot pad and surrounding regions. Three different types of mechanical stimulation were used: short square-wave pulses, sinusoidal stimulation, and constant-force stimulation. On the basis of their measurements, they divided their fiber population into three groups: PC fibers, phasic fibers, and tonic fibers. PC fibers were considered to innervate Vater-Pacinian corpuscles on the basis of the resemblance of their discharge characteristics to fibers innervating Vater-Pacinian corpuscles elsewhere in the body (Hunt, 1961; Sato, 1961). We use the terms "tonic" and "phasic" fibers in accordance with standard terminology as discussed in Chapter 4 of this book. Jänig et al. (1968) used "RA" and "SA" in place of "phasic" and "tonic."

PC fibers had conduction-velocity estimates between forty and sixty-five m/sec. PC fibers were the fibers most sensitive to mechanical pulse stimulation, with 90 percent of the thresholds below 4.0 microns of skin indentation. These units could be discharged by pulse stimulation over a fairly wide area as indicated by plots of receptive fields; i.e., measures of the points at which stimuli could elicit discharge (Fig. 9-35). Although the points of maximum sensitivity to pulse stimuli tended to be on the edges of the pads, PC fibers could be discharged when pulse stimuli of sufficient magnitude were applied to large areas of the pad or to the surround. PC fibers were extremely sensitive to any transient mechanical stimulus and could even be discharged by clapping hands. Sinusoidal mechanical stimuli could drive the discharge of PC fibers to synchronized discharges of several hundred spikes/sec. The application of constant pressure on the other hand only elicited an initial phasic discharge.

Phasic and tonic fibers were similar in most respects. They were differentiated from PC units on the basis of their discharge to constant

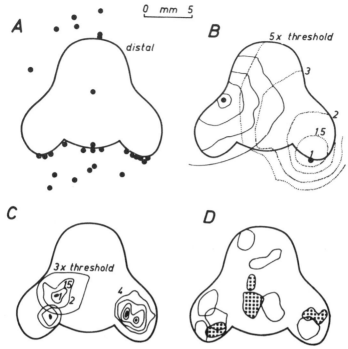

Fig. 9-35. Cat. The spatial distribution in the foot pads of the receptive fields of PC-, phasic and tonic fibers. A. Sites of maximum sensitivity of 28 PC-fibers explored in three experiments. The solid line gives the contour of the large pad. B. Receptive fields of 2 PC-fibers with thresholds of 2.6 μ (proximal unit) and 2.1 μ (distal unit). The lines border areas from which skin indentations of 1.5, 2, 3, and 5 times threshold evoked a response of the fiber. For both fibers the fields were constructed from 30 individual measurements. C. Receptive fields of one phasic fiber (medial unit, threshold 6.5 μ) and 2 tonic fibers (distal unit 9 μ, proximal unit 15 μ threshold) explored and plotted as in B. D. The 2 times threshold receptive fields of 4 phasic (dotted areas) and 7 tonic fibers. (Jänig et al., 1968)

mechanical stimulations: PC units discharged only at the onset of stimulation, phasic fibers discharged for a few hundred milliseconds, and tonic units discharged throughout the stimulus period. The thresholds of phasic and tonic units to pulse stimuli tended to be higher than those of PC units and the receptive fields tended to be smaller (Fig. 9-35). Conduction velocity measurements for phasic and tonic units ranged between forty and eighty m/sec. Phasic units had no resting discharge whereas 80 percent of the tonic units had a low (less than one spike/sec) level of resting discharge. Unlike phasic fibers, the tonic fibers were frequently discharged by the application of a few drops of ethyl chloride, a procedure that resulted in a rapid change in skin temperature.

Lynn (1969) recorded from dorsal root fibers that innervated the foot pad and that were sensitive to mechanical stimulation. He attempted to determine the peripheral terminations of twenty-two of these units by dissecting away portions of the pad until the unit stopped discharging to mechanical stimulation. Eleven of the twenty-two fibers were determined to end within or immediately below the skin on the plantar surface, eight ended deeply within the pad, and three ended on the digits. All of the fibers that ended on deep structures could be classified as PC (Vater-Pacinian) corpuscle fibers according to the physiological criteria of Jänig et al. (1968). Five of the fibers ending superficially were of the phasic type described by Jänig et al. (1968). In some cases the units could not be defined on the basis of the criteria established by Jänig et al. and in two cases there was clear overlap of response properties. Single sensory fibers innervating the nonhairy skin of the hands of monkeys have been studied by Talbot et al. (1968).

Nose Skin, Temperature Sensitive Units Temperature-sensitive units have been studied in the hairy body skin of the cat and in the tongue of the cat. These studies are in part complicated because some of the thermosensitive units to the hairy skin and tongue are responsive to other forms of stimuli also. Thus, it has been shown that the myelinated fibers to the cat's hairy body skin are preferentially responsive to mechanical stimulation, and that the discharge elicited by temperature changes is usually less than 10 percent of that elicited by thermal stimulation. As we have seen, there exists in the hairy skin unmyelinated fibers that are discharged by thermal stimuli and not mechanical stimuli. Nagaki et al. (1964) have demonstrated that the response of chemoreceptive fibers in the chorda tympani can be affected by the temperature of the chemical solution applied to the tongue.

One part of the cat's skin that is innervated by large numbers of thermo-responsive fibers is the nasal region in and around the nonhairy portion of the skin. Single units have been isolated from the infraorbital nerve, a branch of the trigeminal nerve. Two different types of fiber groups have been identified in this nerve; they have been termed "warm" fibers and "cold" fibers. Units, apparently large myelinated fibers, responsive to mechanical stimulation of the nose can also be seen in this nerve (Hensel, 1952), but these have not been reported on in detail in the cat. Barker and Welker (1969) have described three types of mechanoresponsive units innervating the nose of the coati and raccoon.

Warm fibers in the infraorbital nerve have been described by Hensel and Kenshalo (1969). The warm fibers were found to innervate the nose-skin area distinguished by its short thin fur. The fibers were discharged by the application of heat in the form of radiant energy. Units were distinguished as warm fibers on the basis of the following criteria: (1) tonic discharge at constant temperatures between thirty degrees and forty degrees centigrade

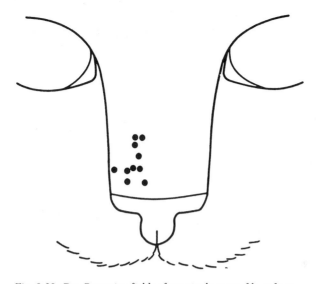

Fig. 9-36. Cat. Receptive fields of ten single warm fibers from the right infra-orbital nerve in various cats. (Hensel and Kenshalo, 1969)

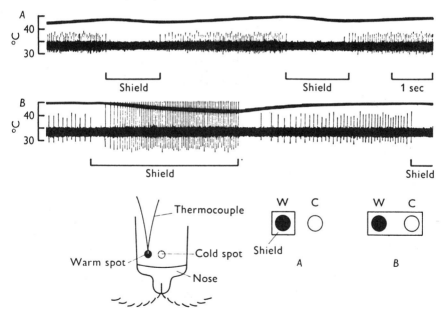

Fig. 9-37. Cat. Afferent impulses from a preparation containing a single warm fiber (small spike) and a single cold fiber (large spike): A, when the warm spot is shielded from heat radiation, the warm fiber discharge stops: B, simultaneous shielding of warm (W) and cold (C) spots causes inhibition of warm fiber and excitation of cold fiber. (Hensel and Kenshalo, 1969)

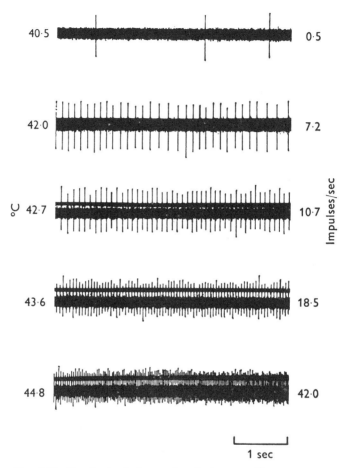

Fig. 9-38. Cat. Static discharge of a single warm fiber at various constant temperatures of the skin, using constant heat radiation as the stimulus (Hensel and Kenshalo, 1969)

and temperature dependence of frequency of discharge; (2) increase in frequency of discharge on sudden warming; (3) no response on sudden cooling, if the fiber was silent, or a decrease in frequency of the steady discharge; (4) no response to mechanical stimulation. By interposing shields in the path of the heat beam, Hensel and Kenshalo (1969) were able to determine that each fiber was affected by stimulation of a small patch of skin one or two mm in diameter (Fig. 9-36).

The degree of spike activity depended upon skin temperature. The application of heat elicited a tonic regular discharge from the units (Fig. 9-37). Stimulation with a constant temperature elicited a train of spikes

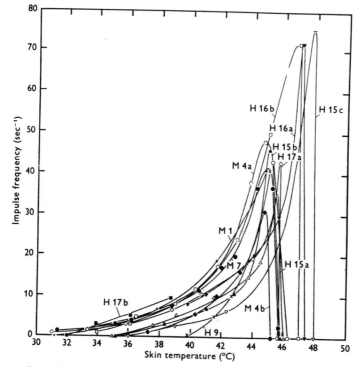

Fig. 9-39. Cat. Static impulse rates of single warm fibers as a function of skin temperature using constant heat radiation (H) or water-circulated metal thermodes (M) of constant temperature as the stimulus (Hensel and Kenshalo, 1969)

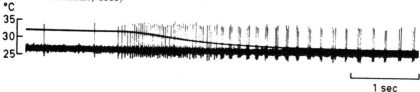

Fig. 9-40. Cat. Afferent impulses of a single cold fiber from the infraorbital nerve and temperature of thermode when cooling the nose from 32 to 27 C. (Hensel and Wurster, 1970)

characterized by a dynamic response (i. e., initial high discharge) and a static response (i. e., a tonic maintained discharge). Examples of spike discharge at different skin temperatures can be seen in Fig. 9-38. During the dynamic response, spike frequencies as high as two hundred/sec were seen. The static response was quite stable and was dependent solely upon skin temperature and not upon whether the final temperature was reached from an ascending or descending direction. Plots of the static impulse frequencies obtained for twelve fibers are shown in Fig. 9-39. As can be seen, impulse frequencies increase in a monotonic fashion, with skin temperature increases up to forty-

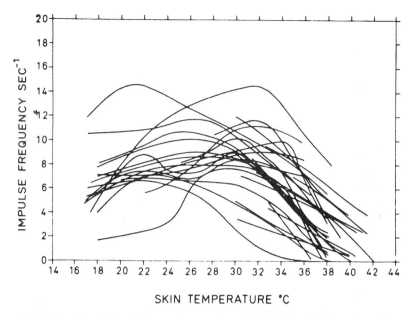

SKIN TEMPERATURE °C

Fig. 9-41. Cat. Static discharge frequencies of 32 single cold fibers from the infraorbital neve as a function of constant temperatures of the nose (Hensel and Wurster, 1970)

four degrees to forty-eight degrees centigrade (peak apparently depends upon the fiber), and then decline precipitously. No conduction velocity estimates have been made of either warm or cold fibers to the cat's nose, although on the basis of spike shape and amplitude, Hensel and Kenshalo (1969) state that warm fibers are both small myelinated and unmyelinated fibers.

Reports by other investigators on "warm" fibers responsive to thermal stimuli tend in general to agree with the preceding description by Hensel and Kenshalo (1969), although Hensel and Huopaniemi (1969) report on a fiber that tended to discharge in bursts during the dynamic phase of heating.

Units innervating the cat's nose and responding to a decrease in skin temperature have been studied by Hensel and Wurster (1970). These units innervated spots in a narrow strip between the hairy skin and nonhairy skin of the nose. These units were thought to be small myelinated fibers. At body temperatures these units exhibited regular spontaneous activity. An increase in skin temperature decreased unit discharge. A decrease in skin temperature produced an increase in discharge with bursting in the low temperature ranges (Fig. 9-40). Quite low rates were obtained when discharge rate was measured to maintained temperatures. Peak static discharge was eight to 10/sec in the most sensitive temperature region (thirty to thirty-four degrees centigrade). Static discharges from thirty-two units as a function of skin temperature are plotted in Fig. 9-41. Temperature-sensitive units have also been studied in primates (Iggo, 1969; Poulos and Lende, 1970a, 1970b). Unlike temperature-sensitive units in the body skin of cats, units in the hairy skin of primates tend to be myelinated.

It is apparent from the above studies that the cat has a thermometer on its nose. That a cat utilizes this sensory system can be demonstrated by offering a cat a hot piece of meat. The cat will inspect this tidbit by sniffing the air and approaching it with its head outstretched. When the head is still some inches away from the hot food, the cat will wrinkle its nose and withdraw. The relative insensitivity of the body skin to temperature follows from the fact that the surface of the body skin is heavily insulated from the outside by the dense hair covering. It is only on the bridge of the nose where hairs are extremely short and on nonhairy areas that the skin is not thermally insulated.

10

THE AUDITORY SYSTEM

Much as fish live in the sea, the cat is immersed in an ocean of air. Disturbances in the air produced in one place are transmitted decrementally to other parts of the environment. Sound in air is the vibratory motion of air particles propagated longitudinally from a sound source. The sound source is a vibrating body that first strikes out, then pulls away from air particles adjacent to it. When the vibrating body strikes the air particles, it produces a condensation of particles. When it pulls away, it produces a rarefaction of particles. Although the movement of individual air particles is exceedingly small, the alternate compressions and rarefactions are propagated longitudinally because the moving air particles strike adjacent particles, setting them into motion.

The alternating condensations and rarefactions of air particles can be described in the terms of the frequency and amplitude of their motion. The frequency of sound is expressed as the rate of repetition of the condensation and rarefaction motion, usually in units of one thousand cycles/sec (kc) or one thousand Herz (kHz). The amplitude of sound is usually measured in terms of the pressure exerted by the vibrating air molecules upon a surface in the path of their propagated motion, in units of dynes/sq. cm. However, because the extent of the dynamic range of the human ear is so great (0.001 dynes/sq. cm. to one thousand dynes/sq. cm.), it is found more convenient to condense this range into a logarithmic or decibel scale. The decibel formula is:

$$dB\text{–}SPL = 20 \log (Pi/Po).$$

Where dB-SPL is the stimulus level in decibels sound pressure level, Pi is the sound pressure in question, and Po is the reference level, usually 0.0002 dynes/sq. cm.

The auditory system is concerned with the measurement of sound waves in air. The basic functions of the auditory system are the identification and localization of sounds in space. The cat, like all other mammals, is sensitive to only a small part of the sound-wave spectrum. The cat audiogram (a plot of the behavioral thresholds at which certain sound frequencies are just detectable) as determined by a number of investigators demonstrates that the cat is maximally sensitive to sound frequencies between 1.0 kHz and 20 kHz, with frequencies above or below these values requiring greater stimulus levels for detection (Fig. 10-1). The upper limit of detection is above sixty kHz.

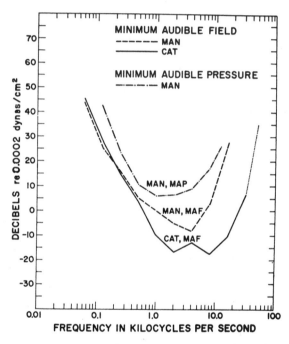

Fig. 10-1. Audiograms for cat and man (Miller et al., 1963)

GROSS ANATOMY OF THE EAR

The auditory portion of the ear of mammals can be divided into three segments: the outer, middle, and inner ear (Fig. 10-2). The outer ear consists of the pinna and the external auditory canal. The middle ear is an air-filled bony chamber located within the mastoid portion of the temporal bone of the skull. The external ear is partitioned from the middle ear by a membranous wall called the "tympanic membrane" or "eardrum." Attached to the tympanic membrane are the middle-ear ossicles, a chain of three small bones

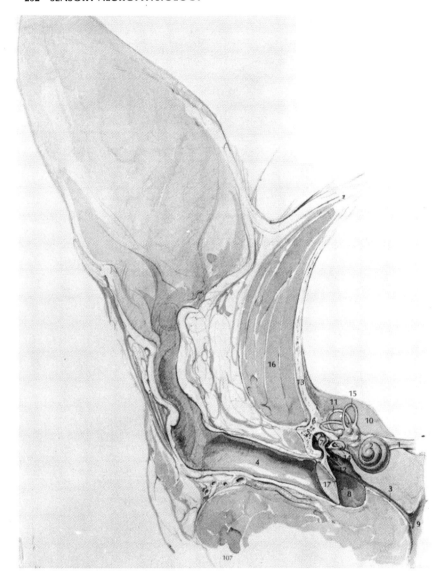

Fig. 10-2. Cat. Gross anatomy of the ear.
1. Cochlear nerve
2. Cochlea
3. Eustachian tube
4. External auditory
   canal
5. Incus
6. Lateral semicircular
   duct

7. Malleus
8. Middle-ear cavity
9. Nasopharynx
10. Petrous bone
11. Posterior semicircular
    duct
12. Round window
13. Squamous part of temporal
    bone

that conduct sound energy from the tympanic membrane to the cavity of the inner ear. The middle-ear cavity communicates with the fluid-filled inner ear at two openings: the oval window that is normally closed off by a segment of the middle-ear ossicles, and the round window that is normally closed off by the round window membrane. The middle-ear cavity is also connected to the pharynx by way of the auditory or Eustachian tube.

The inner ear, which consists of the vestibule, the cochlea, and the semi-circular canals, is enclosed in the petrous portion of the temporal bone. The auditory portion of the inner ear consists of an osseous or periotic cochlea and a membranous cochlea, also called the cochlear duct or cochlear partition. The oval window opens into the vestibule of the inner ear, an irregularly ovoid cavity located medial to the tympanic cavity. The bony cochlea is anteromedial to the vestibule (Fig. 10-2).

The bony cochlea is a narrow fluid-filled canal that coils like a snail shell into a spiral of three turns around an axis formed by a conical pillar of spongy bone called the modiolus. The cell bodies of the cochlear nerve fibers, collectively called the "spiral ganglion," are located within the modiolus along the inner wall of the cochlear canal. The cochlear canal, the chamber of the osscous cochlea, is approximately 23.5 mm long. It is widest in the basal coil and narrows toward the apex or tip of the cochlea.

The gross structure of the cochlea is best visualized if one pictures the cochlea uncoiled and sectioned longitudinally as in Fig. 10-3. The cochlear canal is divided longitudinally by the cochlear partition into an upper and lower chamber. The cochlear partition does not extend the entire length of the cochlea, but at its apex leaves a small opening, the helicotrema, through which the upper and lower chambers communicate. The upper chamber, the scala vestibuli, extends from the oval window, through the vestibule to the helicotrema. The lower chamber, the scala tympani, extends from the helicotrema to the round window whose membrane separates it from the tympanic cavity. The scala tympani and scala vestibuli are perilymphatic spaces in communication with the vestibule and bony semicircular canals.

When the cochlea is viewed in cross section, as in Fig. 10-4, it can be seen that the cochlea actually contains three chambers: the scala vestibuli, the scala media or cochlear duct, and the scala tympani. The middle triangular-shaped chamber, the cochlear duct, is contained within the cochlear partition that divides the bony cochlea into the scala vestibuli and scala tympani. The cochlear duct, which is also called the "membranous cochlea," is a closed tube that ends blindly both at the apex and at the basal end of the cochlea at the vestibular caecum. The cochlear duct contains the fluid endolymph and

---

14. Stapes in oval window
15. Superior semicircular duct

16. Temporal muscle
17. Tympanic membrane

(Gilbert, 1968)

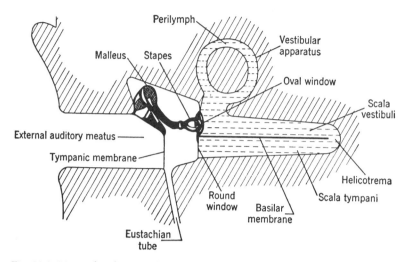

Fig. 10-3. Mammal. Schematic drawing of the ear with the cochlea uncoiled. Sound waves entering the external canal displace the tympanic membrane setting the three ossicles in motion. (Bekesy, 1935)

communicates with the saccule by a slender ductus reuniens that arises at its basal end. The receptor cells of the cochlea are located in the organ of Corti, which is contained within the cochlear duct.

The receptor cells are innervated by afferent fibers whose cell bodies are located in the spiral ganglion and by efferent fibers whose cell bodies are located within the brain stem. The central processes of the spiral ganglion cells travel in the cochlear division of the eighth cranial nerve to the cochlear nuclear complex, where they all terminate. Most of the cochlear nuclear complex neurons send their axons to the superior olivary complex (Fig. 10-5). Axons of other cochlear nuclear cells bypass the superior olivary complex to terminate in the nuclei of the lateral lemniscus, the inferior colliculus or medial geniculate body.

Those cochlear nuclear fibers terminating in the superior olivary complex either remain uncrossed and terminate in the homolateral superior olivary complex or cross in the trapezoid body to terminate in the contralateral superior olivary complex. Thus, the neurons of the superior olivary complex receive homolateral, contralateral, or bilateral inputs from the cochlear nuclei. The axons of most superior olivary complex neurons (crossed and uncrossed) form the lateral lemniscus, along with cochlear nucleus fibers that bypass the superior olivary complex. Fibers of the superior olivary complex and some of the cochlear nuclear fibers terminate in the nuclei of the lateral lemniscus. The axons of the nuclei of the lateral lemniscus join the superior olivary complex and the cochlear nuclear fibers that bypass this nuclear

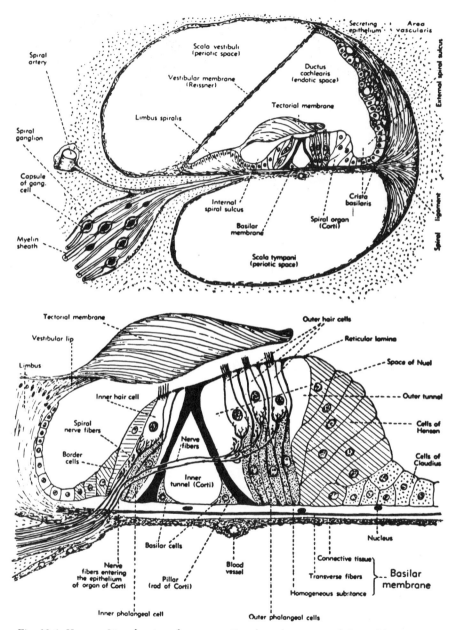

Fig. 10-4. Human: Line drawing of a cross section through one turn of the cochlea. Upper: Section through the organ of Corti and adjacent structures. Lower: The organ of Corti and basilar membrane in greater magnification. (Rasmussen, 1943)

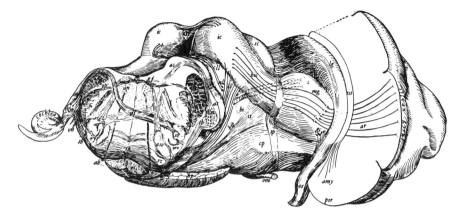

Fig. 10-5. Cat. Diagrammatic section through the region of the superior olive of the cat representing the arrangement of fiber tracts in this region and showing the course of the olivocochlear bundle.
The abbreviations are as follows: ab, abducens nerve; an, abducens nucleus; ar, auditory radiation; as, dorsal acoustic stria; aso, medial superior olivary nucleus; at, dorsal cochlear nucleus; bic, brachium of the inferior colliculus; dt, spinal trigeminal tract; ic, inferior colliculus; ll, lateral lemniscus; mg, medial geniculate body; nc, cochlear nerve; nll, nuclei of the lateral lemniscus; nt, spinal trigeminal nucleus; op, olivocochlear bundle; pro, lateral nucleus of the trapezoid body; rb, inferior cerebellar peduncle; so, lateral superior olivary nucleus; tb, trapezoid body; tz, medial trapezoid nucleus; vcn, ventral cochlear nucleus. (Papez, 1929)

group and continue on as the lateral lemniscus to terminate in the inferior colliculus.

THE OUTER EAR

The pinna or auricle of the external ear is a curved plate of cartilage attached to numerous muscles and covered with skin (Fig. 10-2). The auricular cartilage is thin and pliable, and is curved at its proximal (cranial) end so that its edges overlap, enclosing a funnel-shaped chamber, the concha or orifice of the external auditory canal. Normally the apex of the concha is directed 45° from the mid-sagittal line. The most proximal end of the auricular cartilage is connected to the annular cartilage of the external auditory canal. Six muscles connect various parts of the auricular cartilage with one another and fifteen muscles attach the pinna to the skull. These muscles and the elastic nature of the auricular cartilage permit the ear to be turned to locate the source of sound or even folded down to close off the ear canal. The pinna of the cat may be swept through an anterior-posterior azimuth of approximately 180°. The pinnae are used actively by the cat in his exploration of the environment. Sounds of interest are focused upon by directing one pinna or both pinnae so that the concha is pointed toward the source of the queried sound.

The external auditory canal is an L-shaped tube extending from the pinna to the tympanic membrane (Fig. 10-2). The external canal consists of a lateral cartilaginous meatus and a medial osseous meatus. The auricular cartilage of the pinna forms the lateralmost portion of the cartilaginous canal. The annular cartilage is interposed between the auricular cartilage and the osseous external auditory meatus, a tunnel through the temporal bone. The discontinuities between the auricular and annular cartilage and between the annular cartilage and bone permit the freedom of movement of the pinna. The entire external canal is approximately two cm long and terminates cranially at the tympanic ring to which the tympanic membrane attaches (Wiener *et al.*, 1965).

Wiener, Pfeiffer, and Backus (1965) have investigated the sound-pressure transform characteristics of the external ear of anesthetized cats. They compared sound-pressure levels measured in free field, at the entrance of the auditory canal and at the eardrum. In most cases the sound source was directed with its axis horizontal with and pointed at the center of the cat's head. The position of the sound source was measured in degrees azimuth from a mid-sagittal reference line. Thus at 0° the speaker is directed toward the cat's nose, at +45° toward the concha, at +90° toward the side of the head of the test ear, and at −90° toward the side of the head opposite to the test ear.

The pinna increases the sound pressure at the eardrum for frequencies above 1 kHz when the speaker is directed toward the concha of the pinna (from 0° to +90° azimuth). However, when the speaker is directed from an angle of −90° (directed toward the opposite ear), the pinna of the test ear shields the external auditory canal and produces a loss in sound pressure for frequencies greater than 3.0 kHz.

Because the auditory canal is a tube closed off at one end by the tympanic membrane, it has resonating characteristics that result in the amplification of certain frequencies of sound. The resonating characteristic of the external canal results in the amplification of frequencies between one to 12 kHz, with a broad maximum of 14 dB between four and six kHz.

The combined action of the pinna and external canal results in a sound-pressure transformation, the magnitude of which is dependent upon the direction and frequency of the sound source. When the sound source is directed toward the nose or test ear (0° and 90°), there is an increase in pressure at the test ear for frequencies above 300 Hz that reaches a maximum of 20 dB around 4 kHz (Fig. 10-6). When the sound source is directed toward the ear opposite the test ear (−90°), pressure at the test ear increases for frequencies above approximately six hundred Hz, reaches a maximum of about eight dB near three kHz, and decreases and produces a loss above approximately five kHz. At a negative azimuth, sound diffraction and shielding by the head and pinna result in a decrease in the pressure ratio at the high frequencies where these effects are greatest. The sound diffraction

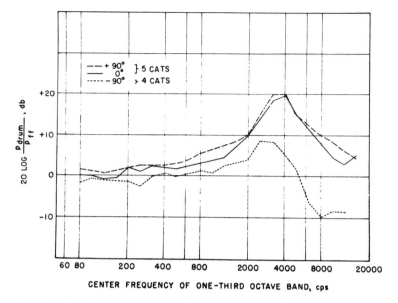

Fig. 10-6. Sound-pressure transform of combined action of pinna and auditory canal. The ratio, in decibels, of the sound pressure at the eardrum to the free-field pressure as a function of frequency, with azimuth as the parameter. (Wiener *et al.;* 1965)

produced by the head and pinna and the resonance in the external auditory canal produce binaural pressure differences. The result is a pressure difference at the two eardrums of approximately 15 dB at four kHz and 20 dB at eight kHz, with little difference below approximate two hundred Hz.

THE MIDDLE EAR

The tympanic membrane is an oval, semi-transparent membrane attached at its margin to the tympanic sulcus of the temporal bone. The ring formed by the tympanic sulcus is incomplete superiorly, forming the tympanic incisure or tympanic notch. On the medial surface of the tympanic membrane, the handle or manubrium of the malleus attaches radially from the approximate center of the membrane nearly to its outer edge (Fig. 10-2). The handle of the malleus draws the center or umbo of the tympanic membrane inward, giving the membrane a somewhat conical shape. Near the superior tip of the manubrium, two ligaments form faint ridges, the anterior and posterior malleolar folds. The area of the tympanic membrane superior to the folds is called the "pars flaccida" or "Shrapnell's membrane." It is thin and lax, and is attached directly to the petrous bone at the tympanic notch. The larger part of the tympanic membrane, the pars tensa, is inferior to the malleolar folds and appears to be tightly stretched. The border of the pars tensa is attached to the tympanic sulcus by a fibrocartilaginous ring.

The tympanic membrane consists of four layers of tissue. The outermost layer is a thin continuation of the skin lining the external auditory canal. The second layer is composed of connective tissue whose collagenous fibers attach to the manubrium and radiate outward to the fibrocartilaginous ring. The circular fibrous layer is a connective tissue layer in which the collagenous fibers are arranged concentrically. The innermost layer is formed by the mucous membrane of the tympanic cavity. The two fibrous layers are absent in the pars flaccida area of the tympanic membrane. The total area of the tympanic membrane is approximately 41.8 sq. mm. (Wever *et al.*, 1948).

The tympanic cavity contains the auditory ossicles, the chorda tympani nerve, muscles and ligaments, and the Eustachian or auditory tube, which communicates with the nasopharynx. The tympanic cavity is located within the temporal bone, partly within the tympanic bulla, a large, hollow, egg-shaped bone located on the ventral surface of the skull. The tympanic cavity is divisible into three segments: a dorsal portion, the epitympanium, which is occupied almost entirely by parts of the middle-ear ossicles; a middle portion, the tympanic cavity proper, which is located between the tympanic and round windows; and a ventral portion, the cavity of the tympanic bulla. A bony septum separates the cavity of the tympanic bulla from the tympanic cavity proper. The two cavities communicate through a small ellipitical opening in the bony septum at its dorsocaudal margin. On the medial wall of the tympanic cavity, there is a bony prominence, the promontorium, of the petrous bone that houses the cochlea. The oval or vestibular window, which is closed by the base of the stapes, is located on the dorsolateral surface of the promontory. The round window, which is covered by the delicate round-window membrane, is located ventral to the promontory. The ostium of the auditory or Eustachian tube is the anterior extremity of the tympanic cavity proper.

The auditory ossicles form a chain of three small bones across the dorsal part of the tympanic cavity, extending from the tympanic membrane to the oval window (Fig. 10-2). The most lateral and largest of the three bones is the malleus. The smallest and most medial is the stapes. The handle of the malleus attaches to the tympanic membrane, and the base of the stapes to the margin of the oval window. Interposed between the malleus and stapes is the incus. The middle-ear ossicles are connected to one another by means of articular ligaments.

Two small striated muscles are associated with the malleus and stapedius bones (Blevins, 1963; 1964). The larger, the tensor tympani, issues from the fossa tensor tympani, a depression in the petrous bone dorsal to the vestibule. Its tendon emerges from the muscle and gradually tapers to its point of insertion on the handle of the malleus. The smaller muscle, the stapedius, lies in a narrow cavity in the posterior wall of the tympanic cavity. Its tendon inserts upon the neck of the stapes. Contraction of the tensor tympani, which is innervated by a branch of the mandibular division of the fifth cranial nerve, draws the handle of the malleus inward and tends to restrict the outward movement of the tympanic membrane. Contraction of the stapedius muscle, innervated by small branches of the facial nerve, pulls the neck of the stapes backward, tilting the anterior edge of the footplate outward, thus reducing its inward movement against the fluid in the cochlea.

Air-borne sound energy in the external auditory canal is absorbed and reflected by the tympanic membrane. The absorption of energy results in the deflection and motion of the tympanic membrane. Movement of the tympanic membrane results in movement of the manubrium of the malleus, which rotates around an axis passing through the lateral process of the malleus. The inward movement of the manubrium results in an outward movement of the malleus head, which is attached to the body of the incus. The incus rotates around an axis passing through its short process so that the long process of the incus moves inward with the outward motion of the malleus head and incus body. The inward motion of the incus long process, which articulates with the stapes head, results in the inward movement of the stapes footplate through the oval window into the vestibule of the bony cochlea. Thus, sound energy applied to the tympanic membrane is transmitted to the cochlear fluid surrounding the auditory receptor organ.

The amount of air-borne sound energy reflected and absorbed by the tympanic membrane depends in part upon the acoustic impedance of the middle-ear structures and of the inner ear. The greatest amount of resistance encountered by sound energy traveling from the air in the external canal to the fluid-surrounded auditory receptor is that of the inner ear. Wever and Lawrence (1954) calculate that at an air-sea water interface, where the volume of water is vast and essentially unbounded, the amount of air-borne sound energy absorbed by the water would be 0.1 percent of the applied energy. Thus, over 99 percent of the applied energy is reflected back from the fluid surface, resulting in a loss of thirty dB. Cochlear fluid is of small volume and is enclosed within a bony canal bounded by the stapes footplate at one end, and the round-window membrane at the other end.

The middle ear acts as a mechanical transformer, matching the impedances of air in the external auditory canal and the bounded fluid of the cochlea. Helmhlotz (1873) suggested that three separate middle ear-mechanisms combine to produce the middle-ear transfer function: (1) the lever action of the curved tympanic membrane; (2) the lever action of the middle-ear ossicles; and (3) the hydraulic action resulting from the difference in the area-size of the tympanic membrane and stapes footplate. The contribution of the first mechanism is considered by some to be minimal. Most workers agree that the second mechanism makes a small contribution to the transform function and that the third mechanism is the major contributor in impedance matching.

Helmholtz postulated that the tympanic membrane behaves as a conical lever so that a small pressure, acting on the surface of the tympanic membrane, displaces the center of the membrane, increasing its curvature and displacing the manubrium with lesser amplitude but greater force. According to his theory, the distribution of displacement amplitude along the tympanic membrane should be minimal at the extreme periphery and center and maximal in between. Békésy (1960), using a mechanical capacitance probe, observed the displacement pattern of human cadaver tympanic membranes to pure tone stimuli. Below a stimulus frequency of 2.4 kHz, the membrane vibrated essentially as a stiff plate around an axis located at the superior edge of the membrane, with maximal displacement near the inferior edge of the membrane below the manubrium and minimal displacement near the outer and superior edge of the membrane. Békésy postulated an elastic area inferiorly, the "lower fold," which would enable this pattern of displacement. Above 2.4 kHz the pattern of displacement became complex, with different sections of the membrane vibrating at different phase. More recently Tonndorf and Khanna (1970) observed the vibration pattern of the tympanic membrane of cat cadavers using time-averaged holography. The main advantage of this method is that it does not appreciably load the tympanic membrane as a capacitance probe might. The vibration pattern observed using this method differed considerably from that observed by Békésy. Namely, for low stimulus frequencies the membrane vibration pattern was more complex with two peaks of maximal displacement amplitude, one located anterior to and a second located posterior to the manubrium. The manubrium, located between the two maximas, vibrated with an amplitude less than either maxima. The flaccidity of the superiorly located pars flaccida was important in maintaining the mobility of the membrane and malleus and not a lower fold, as postulated by Békésy.

Because the amplitude of displacement of the manubrium was less than that of maximum tympanic-membrane displacement, and because the maxima appeared between the center and outer edges of the membrane, Tonndorf and Khanna (1970) conclude that the conical lever effect of the tympanic membrane does contribute to the middle-ear transfer function. From their measures of amplitude displacement, they calculated the conical lever ratio of the membrane to be approximately 2.0 for the cat. Actually, to prove the postulated conical lever effect, one would have to demonstrate that the manubrial force exceeds the product of membrane pressure and area of the membrane. Since Tonndorf and Khanna measured displacement amplitude differences only, their proof is only indirect.

The second middle-ear mechanism Helmholtz postulated as contributing to the middle-ear transfer function was that of the ossicular lever system.

Investigators agree that the ossicular chain produces a small contribution to the middle-ear transform. Guinan and Peake (1967) observed the direction, amplitude, and phase of ossicular motion with respect to sound-pressure level (SPL) at the eardrum in live, anesthetized cats. They report that below 140 dB-SPL the ossicles move as a single rigid body with an axis running from the posterior ligament of the malleus through the short process and posterior ligament of the incus. The stapes moves in and out of the oval window like a piston along a line passing through the center of the head and footplate of the stapes. At higher SPL the stapes shows some rocking motion due to slippage at the incudostapedial joint. At high frequencies (above three khz), there is a phase lag in the displacement of the incus and stapes with respect to the malleus.

The displacement of the stapes is linearly related to SPL at the tympanic membrane up to 130 dB-SPL for frequencies below 2.0 khz and to higher SPL's for frequencies above 2.0 khz. Above these levels the relationship between stapes displacement and SPL becomes nonlinear.

The ossicular lever ratio, the ratio of manubrium displacement to stapes displacement, is approximately two for frequencies below 7kHz and is frequency dependent at higher frequencies (Fig. 10-7). The cavities of the middle ear also appear to play a role in determining the middle-ear transfer

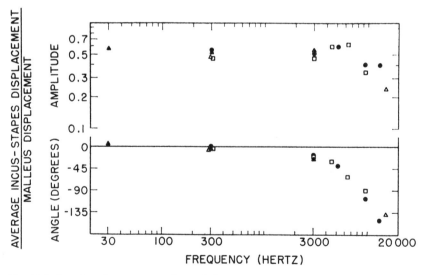

Fig. 10-7. Cat. Sound-pressure transform of the middle-ear ossicles. Displacement of the incus and stapes relative to the malleus displacement. The average of stapes and incus measurements have been divided by (amplitude) or subtracted (angle) from the corresponding malleus measurements. The different symbols represent data from different cats. From Guinan, J.J. and Peake, W.T. (1967), "*Middle-Ear Characteristics of Anesthetized Cats,*" *J. Acoust. Soc. Amer.* 41 1237-1261.

function. Guinan and Peake (1967) caution experimenters using anesthetized animals with closed middle-ear cavities that their preparations may have reduced middle-ear sensitivity. They note that opening the tympanic bulla and the bony septum separating the bulla cavity from the tympanic cavity increased transmission for frequencies around 4.0 kHz.

The third and most influential middle-ear mechanism contributing to the middle-ear transfer function is the hydraulic effect of the difference in area-size of the tympanic membrane and footplate of the stapes. Namely, the force applied to the larger area of the tympanic membrane, 41.8 sq. mm., is concentrated on the smaller area of the stapes footplate, 1.15 sq. mm. (Wever et al., 1948). There is some dispute as to the area-size of the effective area of the tympanic membrane; i.e., that area of the tympanic vibrating in phase as a whole to a low-frequency stimulus. According to Bekesy's observations in the human cadaver (1960), there is a central cone constituting two thirds of the total area that moves as a unit to frequencies below 2.4 kHz. According to Wever and Lawrence's observations on displacement of the membrane to static pressure in the cat cadaver (1954), the effective area of the cat's membrane is between sixty to 72 percent of the total area. Tonndorf and Khanna (1970), on the basis of their time-averaged holograms of tympanic-membrane vibration patterns in cat cadavers, report that the full area of the cat membrane rather than the "effective area" should be used to calculate the areal ratio. Using the total area of 41.8 sq. mm. the areal ratio would equal approximately 36.3. Using two-thirds of the total area (27.9 sq. mm.) would result in an areal ratio of approximately 24.3.

According to Wever and Lawrence (1954), a transform ratio of sixty-three is required to overcome the impedance mismatch between air and an essentially unbound sea of water. They suggest that the magnitude of the transform ratio required to overcome the impedance mismatch between air and cochlear fluid may be of the same magnitude. The total transform ratio of the middle ear for frequencies below 7.0 kHz with ossicular lever ratio of two and an effective areal ratio of 24.3 is approximately fifty and is over seventy when total areal ratio is used. According to Tonndorf and Khanna (1970), three factors — the tympanic membrane lever ratio, an adjusted ossicular lever ratio, and the total area ratio — determine the total transform ratio, which they calculate to be approximately one hundred.

THE INNER EAR

The membranous cochlear duct is approximately 23.5 mm long and makes three turns around the bony modiolus within the osseous cochlea. The extreme basal end of the cochlear duct forms a large hook that twists in a direction opposite to the rest of the cochlea. The cochlear duct or scala media is a triangular-shaped chamber whose walls are formed by the basilar membrane, vestibular membrane, and stria vascularis (Fig. 10-4). The spiral lamina, which divides the cochlear canal in half, consists of the osseous spiral lamina, a bony ledge projecting into the canal from the modiolus, and the membranous spiral lamina or basilar membrane. The radial extent of the osseous spiral lamina decreases from base to apex of the cochlea, with the result that the basilar membrane is wider at the apex than at the base (Fig. 10-8). The periosteal connective tissue on the upper surface of the osseous spiral lamina forms a ridge called the spiral limbus. The tympanic lip of the spiral limbus is continuous with the fibers of the basilar membrane. The basilar membrane extends across the cochlear canal to attach to a fibrous band called the "spiral ligament," a thickening of the periosteum lining the cochlear wall. The basilar membrane is composed of radially arranged

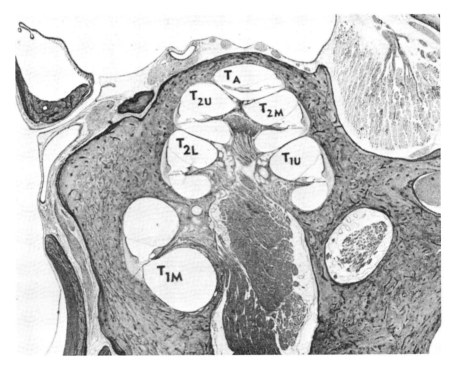

Fig. 10-8. Cat. A mid-modiolar section through a cat's cochlea showing the different turns with the exception of the lower or basal portion of the first turn. T1m, middle of first turn; T1u, upper part of first turn; T2l, T2m, T2u, lower, middle, and upper parts of second turn; Ta, part of the small apical turn. (Miller *et al.*, 1963)

collagenlike fibers embedded in a dense ground substance. The pars tecta (arcuate) portion of the membrane extends from the osseous spiral lamina to approximately one third the width of the membrane. The pars pectinata portion comprises the outer two thirds of the membrane. As the osseous spiral lamina decreases its extent apically, the width of the basilar membrane increases from approximately 0.2 mm in the upper basal coil to 0.37 mm at the apex, as measured from the base of the inner pillar cell of the organ of Corti (Keen, 1939). The cochlear canal is further divided by a delicate membrane, the vestibular (Reissner's) membrane, which extends obliquely from the spiral lamina to the spiral ligament of the outer wall of the bony cochlea. The region of attachment of the vestibular membrane to the spiral ligament forms the vestibular crest, the region of attachment of the basilar membrane to the spiral ligament, the basilar crest.

The outer wall of the cochlear duct is formed by the stria vascularis, spiral prominence, and the outer sulcus cells that line the spiral ligament between the vestibular and basilar crests. The stria vascularis, a highly vascularized, pigmented cell layer, extends from the vestibular crest to the spiral prominence. The spiral prominence is formed by a richly vascularized thickening of the periosteum. The outer sulcus cells line the external spiral sulcus, the concavity formed by the portion of the spiral prominence facing the basilar membrane.

The organ of Corti, the neuroepithelial receptor surface of the cochlea, rests upon the basilar membrane within the cochlear duct and extends the entire length of the cochlear duct. The organ of Corti consists of sensory hair cells and various supporting cells (Fig. 10-4). There are two types of receptor cells, the inner and outer hair cells, and several types of supporting cells. The supporting cells containing filaments (the pillar and outer phalageal cells) are believed to give stability to the organ of Corti. These cells extend from the basilar membrane to the free surface of the organ of Corti. They are in contact with one another and with the receptor cells at their free surface, where they fuse to form the reticular lamina. Supporting cells that do not contain filaments are the border cells, inner phalangeal cells, and the cells of Hensen, Claudius, and Boettcher (Fig. 10-4).

A prominent feature of the organ of Corti is the tunnel of Corti (inner tunnel), which is formed by the supporting inner and outer pillar cells, or rods of Corti. The inner and outer pillar cells have slender conical cell bodies that extend into the scala media. At the apex of the cell, the cell expands into a flat flange that contacts neighboring inner and outer pillar cells and receptor cells. The inner and outer pillar cells meet at their apexes to form the tunnel of Corti. The pillar cells contain darkly staining microtubules that course from the base of the cell up to the apex, where they form junctional complexes. There are approximately forty-seven hundred inner pillar cells and thirty-three hundred outer pillar cells in the cat (Retzius, 1884). The outer pillar cells are taller (ninety microns) than the inner pillar cells (fifty-five microns). In man the lengths of the outer and inner pillar cells appear to increase from the basal coil of the cochlea to the apical coil, inner pillar cells from forty-eight to seventy microns and outer pillar cells from sixty-two to one hundred and three microns.

A single row of inner hair cells is arranged on the inner side of the tunnel, closely parallel to the inner pillar cells. There are approximately twenty-six hundred inner hair cells in the cat (Retzius, 1884). The inner hair cells appear to be structurally similar along the extent of the cochlear duct. The inner cells are pear shaped with a thickened cuticular layer at their upper end that bears approximately sixty hairs or stereocilia. Except at the cochlear apex, the inner hair cells are inclined radially, with their upper hair-bearing pole directed outward. The hairs or stereocilia of the inner hair cells are budlike in shape and are anchored with a rootlet in the cuticular plate. The cilia form a flattened W-shaped pattern, with the upper portion of the W facing the modiolus. The outer two rows of stereocilia are longer than those of the innermost row. There also appear to be differences in length of stereocilia from the basal to apical turn of the cochlea. Unlike the vestibular receptor cell, there does not appear to be a basal body or kinocilium in the inner hair cells of adult cats.

The supporting cells associated with the inner hair cells are the inner phalangel and border cells. The inner phalangeal cells form a row of cells between the inner pillar and the inner hair cells. The border cells form a row of cells on the opposite side of the inner hair cell, toward the modiolus. The inner hair cell is completely surrounded by the supporting cells, and nerve fibers innervating the inner hair cells must travel through and are supported by them.

There are three or more rows of outer hair cells on the lateral side of the outer pillar cells. The outer hair cells number ninety-nine hundred in the cat (Retzius, 1884). The outer hair cells are rod shaped, with from one hundred to one hundred twenty stereocilia extending from the cuticular plate of the cell. The stereocilia of outer hair cells are arranged in three rows forming a W, which faces the modiolus with its upper side. The lengths of the cilia vary from two microns in the basal turn to six microns in the apical turn. The cilia in the outer limbs of the W are longest and the cilia of the outer rows are longer than the innermost row. As in the inner hair cells, there appear to be no basal bodies in the cell.

Outer phalangeal cells rest upon the basilar membrane and surround only the inferior third of the outer hair cell. The outer phalangeal cells send stiff phalangeal processes containing microtubules upward between the hair cells. These processes expand at the surface of the organ of Corti to form a flat plate that appears to be fused at its edges to the apexes of adjacent hair cells. The upper two thirds of the outer hair cells are surrounded by fluid spaces, the spaces of Nuel, that are in communication with the tunnel of Corti. The fluid within the spaces of Nuel and tunnel of Corti is believed to differ from endolymph and perilymph and is called cortilymph. The cells of Hensen are located adjacent to the outermost row of outer phalangeal cells. Beyond Hensen's cells, the cells of Claudius line the basilar membrane and extend toward the cochlear wall to join the cells of the external sulcus. In the basal turn of the cochlea, Boettcher's cells are interposed between the cells of Claudius and the basilar membrane. The size of the cells of Hensen and Claudius vary from base to apex (Fig. 10-9). In the basal turn they form a thick mass on the basilar membrane, whereas in the apex the cells of Claudius are shorter. The cells of Hensen form a dome-shaped structure apically.

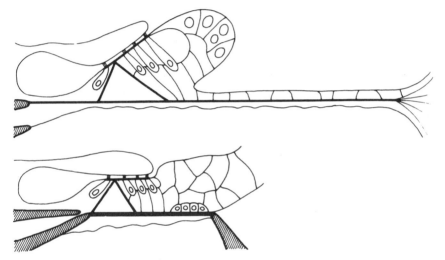

Fig. 10-9. Schematic representation of the different structural features of the cochlear partition in basal (lower) and apical (upper) turn. (Spoendlin, 1970)

The tectorial membrane extends from the vestibular lip of the spiral limbus over the organ of Corti to the cells of Claudius (Fig. 10-4). This membrane has a fibrous structure and is composed primarily of protein. The cilia of the outermost row of both outer and inner hair cells are embedded superficially in shallow grooves in the tectorial membrane.

Stapes footplate displacement results in displacement of cochlear fluid near the oval window and in stimulation of the auditory receptors. The mode of passage of sound energy from the cochlear fluid near the oval window to the auditory receptor is not known. Wever and Lawrence (1954) suggest three possible modes of propagation of sound energy in the cochlea: (1) propagation in cochlear fluid; (2) propagation over the basilar membrane; or (3) interaction between fluid and membrane. The first possible mode, fluid propagation, requires displacement of the fluid contents of the cochlea from the oval window to the round window, in response to stapes footplate displacement. However, Evans (1970), recording single unit responses of auditory nerve fibers in guinea pig to pure tone stimulation, reports that opening the cochlea and draining it of perilymph fluid had no effect on the thresholds and frequencies to which a nerve fiber responded. The results of the Evans' (1970) study also appear to rule out mode 3, interaction of fluid and membrane, since removal of the fluid had no effects.

The second mode, propagation of sound energy along the cochlear partition, has been observed in human cadavers by Békésy (1960), utilizing high level stimulus intensities. However, alteration of the stiffness of the basilar membrane near the oval window appears to have little effect upon hearing and upon the generation of cochlear slow potentials further along the membrane (Wever, 1964). Furthermore, there is ample evidence to indicate that sound conduction is a molecular phenomena, not one requiring displacement of large masses of solids or liquids. For stimulus frequencies above one hundred Hz, displacement of the cat stapes of less than 10^{-9} cm is sufficient to elicit a behavioral response from a trained cat.

Measurements of cochlear partition motion by Békésy (1960), and more recently by Johnstone and Boyle (1967), indicate that a frequency-to-place transformation occurs in the auditory signal at the cochlea. Depending on the frequency of the auditory signal, different parts of the cochlear partition are maximally vibrated. High frequencies vibrate regions at the base of the cochlear partition, while tones lower in frequency preferentially vibrate areas located more and more apically. Experiments involving restricted lesions of different parts of the organ of Corti produce partial impairments in the ability of a cat to detect certain frequencies as measured by the audiogram. By correlating locus of cochlear destruction with audiogram changes, Schuknecht (1960) was able to determine the tonotopic organization of the organ of Corti and the spiral ganglion. His calculations and reconstructions are presented in Fig. 10-10.

The frequency-to-place transformation of sound in the cochlea appears to be related to the mechanical properties of the basilar membrane and the cochlear partition. The static elasticity of the basilar membrane increases one hundred fold from base to apex in the human cadaver (Békésy, 1960). The width and the mass of the basilar membrane increase gradually from base to apex (Fig. 10-9). The longitudinal coupling of the radial filaments in the pars pectinata, which is provided by the ground substance surrounding the filaments, becomes increasingly looser toward the apex as the membrane gets thinner. The basilar membrane is attached to the osseous spiral lamina near the base of the inner pillar cells in the basal turn, whereas in the apical turn it is attached to the osseous spiral lamina halfway under the spiral limbus. Within the organ of Corti the distance between the bases of the pillar cells

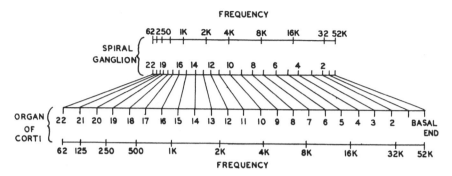

Fig. 10-10. Cat. Tonotopic organization of the organ of Corti and spiral ganglion of cat based upon audiograms of cats with selected lesions in the cochlea. Frequency has been spatially oriented along an organ of Corti of average length (22 mm). (Schuknecht, 1960) From Rasmussen, G.L. and Windle, W.F., *Neural Mechanisms of the Auditory and Vestibular Systems*, 1960, Courtesy of Charles C. Thomas, Publisher, Springfield, Illinois.

increases, the height of the outer hair cells increases, and the inclination of the reticular lamina increases toward the apex. Whereas in the basal turn the cells of Hensen, Claudius, and Boettcher form a large mass on the basilar membrane, apically the cells of Hensen form a dome-shaped structure, the cells of Claudius grow smaller and form a thin layer on the basilar membrane, and the Boettcher cells disappear. All of these structural features appear to result in a graduation in the stiffness of the basilar membrane from base to apex that determines the longitudinal resonating characteristics of the basilar membrane.

INNERVATION OF THE ORGAN OF CORTI

The afferent and efferent innervation of the auditory receptors of the cat organ of Corti have been described by Spoendlin (1966; 1968; 1969; 1970). The afferent innervation arises from the cells of the spiral ganglion, the efferent from cells within the brain stem superior olive complex. Both afferent and efferent fibers pass through small channels in the osseous spiral lamina and enter the organ of Corti through small openings in the basilar membrane called the "habenula perforata" (Fig. 10-11). From less than 10 to over sixty fibers pass through each habenula opening, with an average of 20 to thirty fibers per opening. All fibers lose their myelin sheaths prior to entering the organ of Corti, and once within take either a spiral or radial course. There are three groups of radial fibers: the short radial fibers that pass directly to the inner hair cells; the basilar tunnel fibers that travel along the floor at the tunnel at Corti to the outer hair cells; and the radial tunnel fibers that pass suspended in the tunnel to the outer hair cells. There are three groups of spiral fibers, the inner spiral fibers that travel beneath the inner

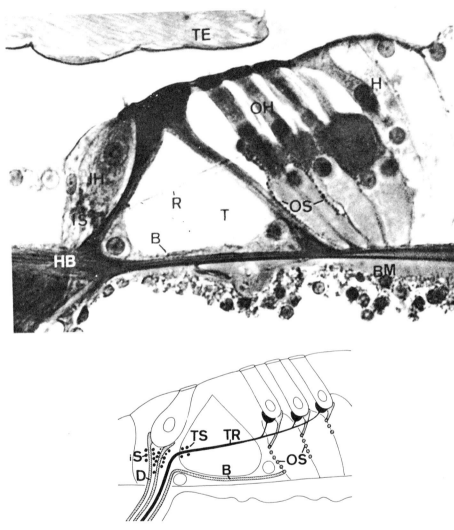

Fig. 10-11. Cat. Top: Light microscopic picture of the organ of Corti in osmium-fixed un-decalcified material. The nerve fibers are better visible than after decalcification and the usual light microscopic tissue preparation techniques. The upper tunnel radial fibers (R) and the outer siral fibers (OS) are clearly outlined. The inner spiral fibers (IS) and the basilar fibers at the bottom of the tunnel (B) are more difficult to distinguish. The nerve fibers penetrate the organ of Corti at the habenula perforata (HB). Basilar membrane (BM), inner hair cells (IH), outer hair cells (OH), Hensel cells (H), space of the tunnel of Corti (T), tectorial membrane (TE). (Spoendlin, 1966.) Reproduced with the permission of the publishers S. Karger, Basel.

Bottom: Schematic representation of different groups of nerve fibers in the organ of Corti. The efferents are drawn in black. D: short radial fibers to inner hair cells; iS: inner spiral fibers; TS: tunnel spiral fibers; TR: tunnel radial fibers; B: basilar tunnel fibers; OS: outer spiral fibers. (Spoendlin, 1970.)

280

hair cells; the tunnel spiral fibers that course within the tunnel of Corti along the inner pillar cells; and the outer spiral fibers that take a spiral course near the outer hair cells.

THE SPIRAL GANGLION

The cells of origin of the afferent innervation of the organ of Corti are the bipolar cells of the spiral ganglion. These cells are 9-19 microns in length according to Alexander (1901) and 18-22.5 microns in length according to Scharf (1950b). Most of the cell bodies of spiral ganglion cells are myelinated (Scharf, 1950b) as are cell bodies of the vestibular ganglion (Scharf, 1950b; 1958). The spiral ganglion of the cat consists of approximately forty thousand (Schuknecht and Woellner, 1953) to fifty thousand (Howe, 1935) bipolar cells. Wolff (1936) reports that, in the kitten, the spiral ganglion cells are oriented with their long axes parallel to the osseous spiral lamina and are arranged in rows of threes and fours within the spiral (Rosenthal's) canal of the modiolus. This bony spiral canal is located along the perimeter of the modiolus and extends apically to the lower half of the apical turn. Thus the ganglion cells form two and one-half spirals around the modiolus, as compared to the three full spiral turns formed by the organ of Corti. The ganglion cells first appear basally approximately four mm from the vestibular caecum and form a reduced hook in the basal end of the cochlea.

Groups of 20 to thirty ganglion-cell dendritic fibers travel through small channels in the osseous spiral lamina. These fibers pass through the habenula perforata and enter the organ of Corti. The dendritic fibers lose their myelin and satellite cell sheaths prior to entering the organ of Corti and are reduced in diameter from 3-5 microns within the bony channels to from 0.25 to 0.7 micron within the habenula (Spoendlin, 1966). Spoendlin (1966) estimates that a total of seventy-five thousand spiral ganglion fibers enter the organ of Corti. The dendritic processes of the spiral ganglion cells are divided into the short radial fibers, which innervate the inner hair cells and the basilar tunnel fibers (long radial fibers), which cross the tunnel of Corti, turn in a spiral direction, and form three rows of outer spiral bundles, which innervate the outer hair cells (Fig. 10-11).

THE AFFERENT FIBERS

The fibers innervating the inner hair cells pass radially from the habenula perforata directly to the inner hair cells (Fig. 10-11). The short radial fibers are relatively large, with an average diameter of 0.5 to 1.0 micron. According to Spoendlin (1966), most of the fibers of a nerve bundle passing through a habenula opening supply only one inner hair cell. There does not appear to be much branching of radial fibers, even at the level of the hair cell. Thus, each short radial fiber appears to innervate only one inner hair cell and each inner hair cell makes contact with terminals of approximately 10 to 20 radial fibers. The short radial fibers terminate as small end bulbs around the lower two thirds of the inner hair cells. Spoendlin (1969) estimates that 90 percent of the spiral ganglion fibers terminate upon inner hair cells and that only 10 percent pass these cells to innervate the outer hair cells.

The fibers traveling to the outer hair cells pass from the habenula to the inner pillar cells, where they take a short spiral course before passing between the pillar cells into the tunnel of Corti. Within the tunnel they course along the bottom of the tunnel, usually embedded in deep folds of the pillar cells (Fig. 10-11). Spoendlin (1966) calls these fibers "basilar tunnel fibers." The fibers (approximately 0.3 micron in diameter) travel in a spiral direction and cross the tunnel obliquely. Upon contacting the outer phalangeal cells, the fibers bend basalward and take on a spiral course forming the outer spiral bundles. These outer spiral fibers are arranged in three columns: the first, between the outer pillar and first phalangeal cell; the second, between the first and second phalangeal cells; and the third column, between the second and third phalangeal cells (Fig. 10-11). The outer spiral fibers appear to travel a considerable distance, approximately 0.6 mm, before terminating. The outer spiral fibers do not appear to give off collaterals along most of their spiral course, but branch near their termination. They give off numerous short collaterals to hair cells, where they terminate as small bouton-type enlargements. Each outer spiral fiber innervates up to 10 hair cells and each outer hair cell, in turn, appears to receive terminals from at least three different outer spiral fibers.

THE EFFERENT FIBERS

The receptor cells of the organ of Corti also receive efferent innervation via the olivocochlear bundle. The origin and course of the fibers of the olivocochlear bundle in the cat have been described by Rasmussen (1946; 1960). The olivocochlear bundle arises bilaterally from cells located in the superior olivary complex of the brain stem. Approximately 80 percent are of contralateral origin and 20 percent of homolateral origin (Rasmussen, 1960). The uncrossed component, the uncrossed olivocochlear bundle (UOCB), arises from cells located in the homolateral dorsolateral periolivary nucleus, which is situated dorsal to the lateral superior olive (Fig. 10-12). The crossed component, the crossed olivocochlear bundle (COCB), arises from the contralateral retro-olivary or dorsomedial periolivary nuclear group, which is situated dorsomedial to the medial superior olive. The input to the cells of origin of the olivocochlear bundle fibers have been described in some detail for the cat by Warr (1969). Both the dorsomedial and dorsolateral periolivary nuclei received input from the homolateral posteroventral cochlear nucleus.

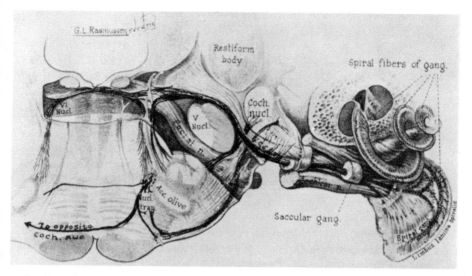

Fig. 10-12. Cat. Drawing of the efferents of the cochlear nerve and cochlear nucleus in the cat. The efferents of the dorsal acoustic stria are not shown. The medial nucleus of the trapezoid body (Nucl. trap.) is located medial to the medial superior olive (Acc. olive). The lateral superior olive is the s-shaped nucleus located lateral to the medial superior olive. The dorsomedial periolivary nucleus or retroolivary nucleus is located dorsal to the medial trapezoid nucleus and medial superior olive. The dorsolateral periolivary nucleus is located dorsal to the lateral superior olive. (Rasmussen, 1966) From Rasmussen, G.L. and Windle, W.F., *Neural Mechanisms of the Auditory and Vestibular Systems*, 1960. Courtesy of Charles C. Thomas, Publisher, Springfield, Illinois.

In addition, the dorsomedial periolivary group receives inputs from the contralateral posteroventral cochlear nucleus (Warr, 1969) and inputs from the ipsilateral medial nucleus of the trapezoid body (Morest, 1968).

The olivocochlear fibers leave the superior olivary complex dorsally with the fibers of the dorsomedial periolivary nucleus located medial to the fibers of the dorsolateral periolivary nucleus. Beneath the facial genu the dorsolateral periolivary fibers form a compact bundle that decussates to form the COCB. The fibers of the COCB join the fibers of the UOCB near the lateral surface of the descending facial root and travel as a compact bundle laterally over the spinal tract and nucleus of the trigeminal nerve. The olivocochlear bundle (OCB) contains approximately five hundred fibers, ranging in diameter from three to five microns. The fiber population of the uncrossed component has been estimated to number approximately one fourth that of the crossed component. Lateral to the spinal tract of the trigeminal nerve, the OCB consists of from two to four fascicles that join the vestibular root. Fine fibers of the OCB traverse the glial portion of the vestibular root and enter and terminate within the cochlear nuclear complex. The rest of the OCB emerges from the brain stem with the vestibular nerve root and travels to the internal auditory meatus within the vestibular nerve. The OCB fibers traverse the ganglion of the vestibular nerve and join the cochlear nerve at the vestibulocochlear anastomosis of Oort.

Within the spiral canal the OCB fibers branch and form the intraganglionic spiral bundles. These branches are one micron or less in diameter (Rasmussen, 1960). The degeneration pattern of these intraganglionic spiral fibers following brain stem transection of the COCB between the facial genu indicates that branches of COCB fibers are distributed to all turns of the cochlea, with a greater number of UOCB fibers distributed to the apical and middle turns of the cochlea (Rasmussen, 1953). Unlike the rat, in which COCB fibers are distributed only to outer hair cells (Iurato, 1964), the COCB fibers of cat are distributed to both inner and outer hair cells (Spoendlin, 1969; 1970).

Within the osseous spiral lamina, there is branching of the olivocochlear fibers so that an estimated twenty-five hundred to three thousand olivocochlear fibers emerge into the organ of Corti through the habenula perforata (Spoendlin, 1966). The olivocochlear fibers entering the organ of Corti are unmyelinated and have diameters ranging from 0.1 to 1.5 microns. Within the organ of Corti the olivocochlear fibers form three bundles (Fig. 10-11): (1) the inner spiral bundle, which is located below the inner hair cells; (2) the tunnel spiral bundle, which is located in the tunnel near the inner pillar; and (3) the upper tunnel radial fibers, which cross the tunnel at a median level surrounded only by the fluid of the tunnel.

The inner spiral bundle consists of about two hundred fibers in the upper turns of the cochlea and less in the lower basal turn. The diameters of these fibers range from 0.1 to 1.0 micron with the majority not exceeding 0.2 micron. Fernández (1951) reports that these fibers appear to extend apicalwards and basalwards. Spoendlin (1966) noted that inner spiral fibers gave rise to vesiculated enlargements that appeared to make contact with the radial fibers of the afferent terminals and not with the inner hair cells directly. These enlargements were also observed to make contact with supporting cells.

Other olivocochlear fibers pass to the tunnel of Corti and form the tunnel spiral bundle and radial tunnel fibers. The tunnel spiral bundle runs along the inner pillars within the tunnel of Corti, entirely surrounded by the tunnel fluid. The tunnel spiral bundle is absent or consists of a few fibers in the lower basal turn of the cochlea. In the more apical turns the bundle contains about forty fibers with diameters usually below 0.2 micron. Fernández (1951) reports that in the guinea pig the tunnel spiral fibers eventually cross the tunnel to terminate on outer hair cells. Spoendlin (1966) reports that in the cat the majority of tunnel spiral fibers appear to terminate in the area under the inner hair cells.

The radial tunnel fibers cross the tunnel of Corti at a median level and appear suspended in the fluid of the tunnel of Corti like telephone lines

(Fig. 10-11). The radial tunnel fibers cross in small fascicles of from one to six fibers, usually numbering from two to four fibers in the basal turn and from one to two in the higher turns. A total of eight thousand olivocochlear fibers with diameters ranging from 0.3 to 1.5 micron appear to cross the tunnel in the radial tunnel bundles. Some of these radial fibers pass directly to the base of the first row of outer hair cells, while others pass beween the phalangeal cells to the second and third row of outer hair cells. At the level of the outer hair cells the radial tunnel fibers branch to produce an estimate of forty thousand efferent nerve endings. The spiral distribution of the radial tunnel fibers appears to be less extensive than that of the outer spiral bundles and their distribution appears to be predominantly radial. The radial tunnel fibers appear to be restricted to the regions around the hair cell base and are separated from most of the outer spiral (afferent) fibers. The radial tunnel fibers terminate as large, vesiculated endings on the bases of the outer hair cells.

AFFERENT AND EFFERENT TERMINALS

The afferent terminals have been described to be small bouton-type enlargements that contain few inclosures (Spoendlin, 1966). The efferent terminals are larger and contain a large number of inclosures believed to be synaptic vesicles. The efferent terminals also appear to differ histochemically and can be selectively stained for acetylcholinesterase (AChE) activity (Ishii and Balogh, 1968). The afferent terminals are often referred to as type I or nonvesiculated endings and the efferent terminals, as type II or vesiculated endings.

Most of the outer hair cells make contact at their bases with afferent and efferent terminals. The innermost row of outer hair cells makes contact with efferent terminals throughout most of the length of the cochlea. The number of efferent terminals in contact with the bases of the outer two rows of hair cells decreases apically. All outer hair cells in the basal turn make contact with 6 to 10 efferent and five to eight afferent endings per hair cell, according to Spoendlin (1966). In the middle turn of the cochlea, there are no efferent terminals in contact with the outermost row of outer hair cells. The inner two rows of outer hair cells make contact with a reduced number of efferent terminals, with an average of three efferent to eight afferent endings per hair cell. In the apical turn of the cochlea, efferent terminals are usually found only in contact with the innermost row of hair cells. The extreme basal and apical ends of the cochlea appear to contain very few efferent terminals (Ishii and Balogh, 1968). The majority of the efferent terminals to the outer hair cells arise from crossed olivocochlear fibers and only a small portion from uncrossed olivocochlear fibers (Spoendlin, 1970). The average innervation ratio of outer hair cells is approximately one efferent fiber to twenty-two hair cells and one afferent fiber to two to three hair cells.

286 SENSORY NEUROPHYSIOLOGY

The inner hair cells appear to make direct contact only with afferent terminals. These terminals are larger and contain more inclosures than the afferent terminals of outer hair cells. The afferent terminals form a basket around the lower two thirds of the inner hair cells. Direct contact between inner hair cells and efferent terminals is extremely rare. However, efferent terminals appear to make contact with afferent fibers beneath the inner hair cells. Throughout all turns of the cochlea, the fibers of the inner spiral bundle show strong signs of AChE activity (Ishii and Balogh, 1968). According to Spoendlin (1970), equal numbers of fibers in the inner spiral bundle arise from the crossed and uncrossed components of the olivocochlear bundle. The average innervation ratios of inner hair cells are approximately twenty-three afferent fibers per hair cell and one efferent fiber per thirty hair cells.

THE COCHLEAR NERVE

The central (axonal) processes of the spiral ganglion cells pass through the central core of the modiolus, form the cochlear nerve, and join the vestibular and facial nerve within the internal auditory meatus. These nerves share a common dural sheath that lines the internal auditory canal. The Schwann sheath coverings of the spiral ganglion cell central processes are replaced by neuroglia prior to the entry of these nerve fibers into the cranial cavity. Cell bodies of cochlear nucleus neurons have not been observed in the non-glial portion of the cochlear nerve in the cat (Kiang et al., 1965b; Osen, 1969a; van Noort, 1969). However, the glial portion of the cochlear nerve of the cat has been reported to contain cell bodies of cochlear nuclear neurons (Galambos and Davis, 1948). The cochlear nerve fibers appear to be compactly arranged and evenly distributed within the cochlear nerve trunk. Myelinated nerve fibers one micron or greater in diameter number approximately 51,700 in myelin-stained and protargol silver-stained cat nerves (Gacek and Rasmussen, 1961). Fiber diameters range from one micron to eight microns and have a unimodal distribution, with a peak at three microns (Fig. 10-13). Electron microscopy has not been utilized to determine if small, unmyelinated nerve fibers are present in significant numbers within the cat cochlear nerve. Less than 10 percent of squirrel-monkey cochlear nerve fibers are unmyelinated, with diameters between 0.4 and 1.0 micron (Alving and Cowan, 1971).

Because of the spiral development of the spiral ganglion, the central processes of these ganglion cells take a twisted course within the cochlear nerve trunk (Lorente de Nó, 1933a; Sando, 1965). The nerve fibers arising from ganglion cells within the apical and middle turns of the cochlea form the core of the nerve trunk. The fibers arising from the most apical turn twist approximately one and three-fourths turns about the axis of the nerve trunk. The fibers from the middle turn of the cochlea make one full turn, while

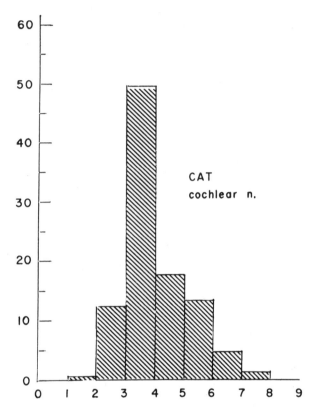

Fig. 10-13. Cat. Distribution of fiber diameter of the cochlear nerve in cat. Ordinate, percentage composition; abscissae, fiber diameter in microns. (From Gacek and Rasmussen, 1961)

fibers innervating more basal segments of the cochlea display progressively less twisting. The fibers innervating the basal turn and basal hook region join the nerve trunk inferiorly and maintain this inferior position.

NEUROPHYSIOLOGY OF COCHLEAR NERVE

The most extensive and systematic analysis of discharge patterns of cat cochlear nerve fibers comes from Kiang and his associates of the Eaton-Peabody Institute and Massachusetts Institute of Technology in Boston. There have been carefully planned attempts by members of this group to investigate the sensory functions of the auditory system from the outer ear to the central nervous system. The sound-conducting characteristics of the external and middle ears have been investigated and described by members of this group (Wiener *et al.*, 1965; Guinan and Peake, 1967) to provide as accurate a description as they could obtain of the auditory input to the nervous system. Rigorous stimulus and experimental controls, which are required in the study of information processing by the nervous system, are constantly emphasized by members of the Eaton-Peabody group. Under Kiang's influence the emphasis of neurophysiological investigations has been on the quantitative description of the response characteristics of populations of units sampled. Where anatomical evidence points to morphological subpopulations within a nucleus or nuclear complex, attempts are made to localize histologically the units studied. Thus, the response characteristics of units within an anatomical subpopulation and differences in response characteristics of different subpopulations can be described.

In the Eaton-Peabody group studies of the cochlear nerve, single unit recordings are made with glass micropipettes. Cats are anesthetized with Dial-urethane and placed in a sound-isolating chamber. Standard response measures recorded are spontaneous activity, responses to continuous pure tones, to tone and noise bursts, and to clicks (Kiang, Watanabe, Thomas, and Clark, 1962; 1965b; Kiang, Sachs, and Peake, 1967; Kiang, Moxon, and Levine, 1970) and responses to monaural two-tone, tone-noise, or click-noise combinations (Kiang, Watanabe, Thomas, and Clark, 1965b, Sachs and Kiang, 1968; Goldstein and Kiang, 1968).

SPONTANEOUS ACTIVITY

Spontaneous activity (unit activity in the absence of experimenter-controlled sound stimuli) is observed in all cochlear nerve fibers (Kiang et al., 1965b). Spontaneous activity rates vary widely from fiber to fiber and range from less than 6 spikes/min to 130 spikes/sec (Fig. 10-14). The spontaneous discharge rate of each fiber is stable over time and appears to be unrelated to the stimulus frequencies to which the fiber is sensitive. Fibers with widely differing rates were observed in any one cat, indicating that differences in rate are not related to the cat or to day-to-day differences in experimental conditions. The frequency distribution of spontaneous activity rates presented in 1965 (Fig. 8-10 in Kiang et al., 1965b) indicated a slight tendency toward grouping of fibers at certain preferred rates. In addition, examples of data from individual cats (Fig. 8-3 in Kiang et al., 1965b) indicated that these groupings did not result from pooling of data from a number of cats. At that time Kiang, Watanabe, Thomas, and Clark (1965b) suggested that there may be four fiber groups, each innervating a different row of hair cells in the organ of Corti. However, they also stated that the data were insufficient at that time to support such a hypothesis. A later study (Kiang et al., 1970) produced the frequency distribution of spontaneous rates presented in Fig. 10-14. Except for the peak formed by fibers with rates below 10 spikes/sec, no other peaks are visible. Examples of data from individual cats in this later study (Fig. 13 in Kiang *et al.*, 1970) also do not appear to be grouped in the manner that individual cat data were in the earlier study (Kiang *et al.*, 1965b).

All sampled cochlear fibers appear to be of a single homogeneous population on the basis of temporal pattern of spontaneous discharge (Kiang *et al.*, 1965b). Their discharge is random and irregular. Although spontaneous rates vary widely, the general shapes of interspike interval (ISI)

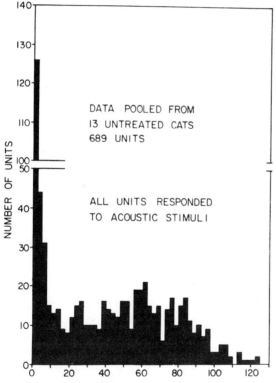

RATE   OF   SPONTANEOUS   ACTIVITY   IN   SPIKES / SEC

Fig. 10-14. Cat. Histogram of the distribution of spontaneous activity rates of 689 cochlear nerve fibers from 13 cats. Bin width is 2.5 spikes/sec. (Kiang *et al.*, 1970) From *Sensorineural Hearing Loss*, CIBA Symposium 1970. Ed. G.E.W. Wolstenholme and J. Knight; London; Churchill.

distributions produced by spontaneous activity are extremely similar from fiber to fiber (Fig. 10-15). All ISI distributions have a modal value between four to seven msec that is followed by an exponential drop in the number of interspike intervals longer than the mode. The ISI distributions of all cochlear fiber spontaneous activity can be described by a Poisson process with a dead-time factor to represent the refractory properties of the fiber.

RESPONSE TO TONAL STIMULI

TUNING CURVES

Each cochlear nerve fiber responds to a limited range of stimulus frequencies (Kiang *et al.*, 1965b). The tuning curve defines the frequencies and the threshold stimulus levels required to elicit a "just detectable" response (Fig. 10-16). The response area of an auditory unit defines all the frequencies and stimulus levels capable of eliciting a change in discharge rate. The frequency to which a unit is most sensitive, the apex of the tuning curve, is called the characteristic (critical or best) frequency (CF).

The characteristic frequency of a cochlear nerve fiber appears to be determined by the locus of innervation of the peripheral processes of the spiral ganglion cell along the longitudinal extent of the cochlea. Fibers with high CF's are located superficially in the nerve trunk, where fibers innervating the basal turn of the cochlea are located (Kiang *et al.*, 1965b). Fibers with lower and middle CF's are located centrally in the nerve trunk, where fibers innervating the apical and middle turns of the cochlea are located. In cats treated with kanamycin, which destroys cochlear receptor cells, fibers unresponsive to acoustic stimuli were encountered where high CF fibers are normally encountered (Kiang *et al.*, 1970). Histological examination of the cochleas of kanamycin-treated cats revealed loss of hair cells extending apically starting from the basal end of the cochlea. Schuknecht and Sutton (1953) demonstrated behaviorally that mechanical injury limited to the basal turn of the cochlea resulted in high-frequency hearing loss in cats.

Normal cochlear fiber tuning curves are roughly U or V shaped, with thresholds increasing monotonically for frequencies above and below the CF. There is a "break" in the low-frequency limb of the tuning curve; i.e., at high stimulus levels the rate of threshold increase decreases from that at lower stimulus levels (Fig. 10-16). The extent of the high frequency limb of the tuning curve appears to be limited, while the low frequency limb broadens considerably with high stimulus levels.

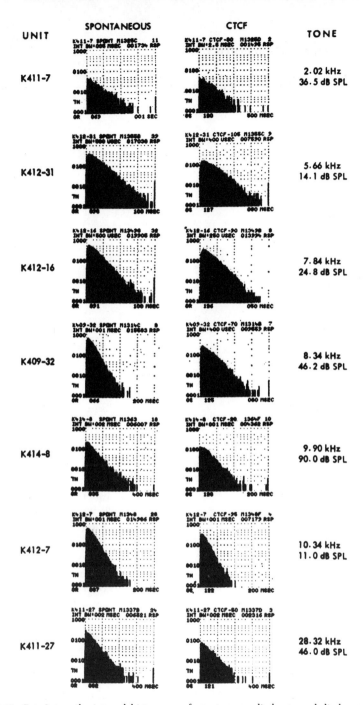

Fig. 10-15. Cat. Interspike interval histograms of spontaneous discharge and discharge to a continuous tone at the characteristic frequency (CTCF) for seven cochlear nerve fibers. (Kiang, 1968) Reproduced with the permission of Dr. Kiang and *Annals of Otology, Rhinology and Laryngology*.

291

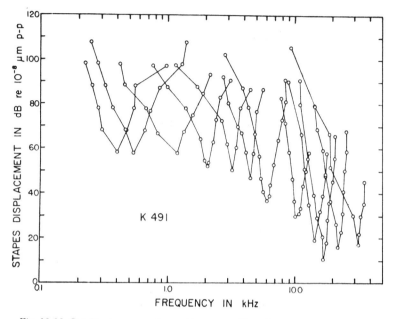

Fig. 10-16. Cat. Tuning curves for cochlear nerve fibers from one cat with stimulus levels expressed in terms of stapes displacement. (Kiang *et al.*, 1970) From *Sensorineural Hearing Loss*, CIBA Symposium 1970. Ed. G. E. W. Wolstenholme and J. Knight; London; Churchill.

Turning curves of cochlear nerve units appear to be similar in shape and differ only with respect to the frequency range covered. Fibers with CF greater than 2.0 kHz appear to be more sharply tuned than low CF fibers, with the degree of sharpness related to CF for fibers with CF above 2.0 kHz. Kiang *et al.*, (1962; 1965b) do not observe a separation of cochlear fibers on the basis of the symmetry of their tuning curves as was suggested by Katsuki and co-workers (1962). In addition, the CF and sharpness of the tuning curve do not appear to be related to a fiber's spontaneous activity rate.

It has been suggested that separate populations of cochlear fibers exist on the basis of threshold difference (Stevens and Davis, 1938). Initially it was reported that units having the same CF may have threshold differences as great as sixty dB (Kiang *et al.*, 1965b). More recently Kiang, Marr, and Demont (1967) report that when CF thresholds are measured with "improved" sound isolation and are expressed in terms of stapes displacement, the spread of CF thresholds of cochlear nerve units with similar CF in individual cats is only 20 dB. The narrow range of thresholds for fibers with similar CF in individual cats suggests that there is a single population of cochlear nerve fibers with respect to CF threshold. However, cochlear nerve fibers producing low spontaneous-discharge rates are reported to have higher thresholds than fibers with high spontaneous rates, with the greatest differences existing for fibers with rates lower than two spikes/sec (Kiang *et al.*, 1965b; 1970).

In kanamycin-treated cats, there are cochlear fibers with low CFs and abnormally shaped tuning curves and extremely high thresholds. The low-frequency limbs of these abnormal tuning curves are similar to the low-frequency limbs of normal tuning curves of fibers with higher CF. The high-frequency limbs of the abnormal tuning curves extend into frequencies that correspond to portions of the cochlea in which damage to outer hair cells is greater than 90 percent and in which inner hair cells appear normal. However, the spontaneous-discharge rates of fibers with abnormal tuning curves do not appear to differ from those of fibers with normal tuning curves.

DISCHARGE PATTERN

All cochlear nerve fibers can be excited by tones of the appropriate frequency or by "white" noise. The response is tonic and the increased activity lasts as long as the duration of the stimulus (Kiang *et al.*, 1965b). Although stimulus-elicited discharge rate decreases gradually even after many minutes of stimulation, the elicited rate never decreases to levels at or below spontaneous rates. With tone- or noise-burst stimuli the discharge is greatest at stimulus onset and gradually decreases to a relatively stable rate of discharge. At the end of the noise burst, there is a sharp decrease in activity to below spontaneous levels followed by a gradual recovery to the previous spontaneous discharge level (Fig. 10-17). At high-stimulus levels the transient increase in discharge becomes prominent as does the transient decrease in activity following the termination of the tone or noise burst. Under the stimulus conditions utilized by Kiang *et al.*, (1965b) spontaneous activity was never observed to be suppressed either at the onset of a tone burst or during the duration of the burst. Also phasic response patterns to onset or offset of the stimulus and after-discharges following tone bursts were never observed.

The general shapes of all cochlear nerve PST histograms generated by tone bursts appear to be similar to that pictured in Fig. 10-17. However, when the discharge pattern produced by tone-burst stimuli is examined in detail for units with low CF (below 4.5 kHz), the discharges are seen to be phase-locked to individual cycles of a low-frequency tone. Low CF units tend to fire during a preferred time within a cycle of the stimulus frequency and not to fire outside this preferred time. The low CF unit usually fires only once every several cycles, but only during a certain phase of the stimulus cycle. At high stimulus levels there sometimes occurs a shift in the phase of the stimulus cycle to which the unit fires, especially when stimulus frequencies are lower than the CF of the unit (Gray, 1966; Kiang *et al.*, 1969). Some fibers with CF greater than 5.0 kHz do display phase-locked discharge to individual cycles of a low-frequency tone, but only at high-stimulus levels.

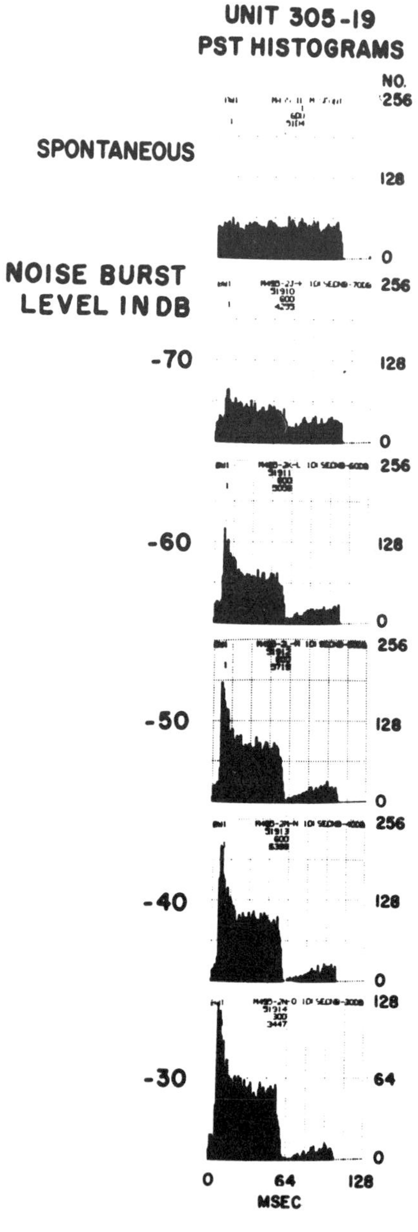

UNIT 305-19
PST HISTOGRAMS

SPONTANEOUS

NOISE BURST
LEVEL IN DB

-70

-60

-50

-40

-30

0   64   128
      MSEC

Fig. 10-17. Cat. Discharge pattern of a cochlear nerve fiber to bursts of noise as a function of stimulus level. Unit CF: 4.49 kHz; total analysis time: 1 minute except at -30 dB at which it is 30 sec; zero time: 2.5 msec prior to onset of electrical input to the earphone. Reprinted from *Discharge Patterns of Single Fibers in the Cat's Auditory Nerve* by N.Y-S. Kiang, T. Watanabe, E.C. Thomas, and L.F. Clark by permission of The M.I.T. Press, Cambridge, Massachusetts. Copyright © 1965 by the Massachusetts Institute of Technology.

The ISI histogram measured for discharge to a continuous CF tone (Fig. 10-15) is very similar to that measured for spontaneous activity for all units except those with low CF (Kiang, 1968). The ISI histograms of continuous CF tone elicited spike trains of all cochlear nerve units have modal values less than 10 msec, followed by a roughly exponential decay of interspike intervals longer than the mode (Gray, 1966). The ISI histograms generated by units with CF below 5.0 kHz to continuous CF tones have the same envelope as high CF units. However, when examined in detail, ISI histograms of low CF units show peaks of activity that are related to the period of the stimulus frequency indicating that the stimulus phase-locked activity observed in PST histograms of low CF fibers is maintained for long periods of time by low CF units.

INTENSITY FUNCTIONS

The rate of discharge of cochlear nerve units changes as a function of stimulus level. The rate of discharge of cochlear fibers to a continuous tone at CF increases as stimulus level increases and reaches a maximal value 20 to fifty dB above threshold. Typically the discharge rate of cochlear nerve fibers to continuous CF tones increases monotonically with stimulus level to some maximal value that does not change with further increases in stimulus level (Kiang, 1968). Other cochlear fibers generate nonmonotonic intensity functions to continuous CF tones in which increases in stimulus level beyond that eliciting the maximal rate produce decreases in discharge rate (Kiang *et al.*, 1965b; 1969). The CF of a fiber does not appear to be related to whether the fiber produces nonmonotonic or monotonic CF intensity functions (Kiang *et al.*, 1969). Nonmonotonic intensity functions can be produced with stimulus tones at, above, or below the fiber's CF, but the nonmonotonic drop in discharge always occurs at the lowest stimulus levels for frequencies below CF. The drop in discharge rate usually occurs at high-stimulus levels, above ninety dB-SPL. The discharge may drop to spontaneous levels, but appears to return to maximum with a further 10-dB increase in stimulus level. High-stimulus levels producing a nonmonotonic drop in discharge also produce large phase shifts in the preferred time of firing of low CF fibers (Gray, 1966; Kiang *et al.*, 1969).

The maximum rate of discharge to continuous CF tones is less than two hundred spikes/sec (Kiang *et al.*, 1965b). However, higher rates (up to one thousand spikes/sec) can be transiently elicited during the onset of intense tones and during electrical stimulation of the cochlea. Electrical stimulation of the cochlea with high shock levels can elicit a maintained one-to-one ratio of spike to shock for rates as high as five hundred spikes/sec for several minutes of stimulation (Moxon and Kiang, 1967). Thus, the maximal rate of acoustically elicited discharge is not limited by the conduction properties of cochlear nerve fibers. The factors determining a fiber's maximal discharge rate to a continuous CF tone also appear to determine its spontaneous activity rate. Fibers with high maximal discharge rates tend to have high spontaneous rates and vice versa. In kanamycin-treated cats, cochlear fibers that are unresponsive to acoustic stimuli rarely exhibit spontaneous discharge but do discharge to electrical stimulation of the cochlea.

CLICK STIMULI

All cochlear nerve fibers respond to click stimuli with a single spike or burst of spikes (Kiang et al., 1965b). The general shape of the PST histograms of unit responses to click stimuli appear to differ for low and high CF units (Fig. 10-18). In general the duration of the entire click-evoked spike train is shorter for units with high CF than for units with low CF (Kiang et al., 1965b). Units with CF below 5.0 kHz produce click PST histograms that can be described as consisting of a number of peaks separated by relatively constant peak intervals. These peak intervals are related to the period of the characteristic frequency of the fiber. This relationship appears to be a linear one with peak interval of the click-generated PST histogram directly proportional to the characteristic period of the unit. Units with CF above 5.0 kHz tend to produce single-peaked PST histograms to repetitive click stimuli, although units with CF between five to eight kHz may often display a second peak at a time interval unrelated to the unit's characteristic period. At high click levels even high CF units show repetitive discharge, but the period of the discharge does not appear to be related to the CF of the units.

The latency of the first spike, as measured with respect to the delivery of an electrical pulse to the ear phone, appears to be related to the CF of the unit responding. For units with CF below 2.5 kHz, latency decreases from approximately 5 msec to 2 msec as CF increases. For units with CF above 2.5 kHz latency is fairly stable at approximately 1.3 to 1.8 msec. The click latency-CF relationship does not appear to result from differences in conduction velocity of units innervating low or high frequency areas of the cochlea; since latency of response to electrical shock applied to the cochlea is approximately 0.5 sec for all fibers sampled (Moxon and Kiang, 1967). Kiang et al. (1965b) suggest that the systematic change in click latency with CF for low CF units probably results because low-frequency sound energy must travel a greater distance than high-frequency energy and appears to do so at a slower rate (Békésy, 1960). Thus, latency of the click response is dependent upon the longitudinal position along the cochlear partition of the terminal part of the peripheral process of the cochlear nerve unit.

Increasing click-stimulus level appears to result in decreases in latency, increases in discharge, and appearance of multiple-peaked PST histograms for high CF units. For low CF units increasing click-level results in an increase in PST histogram peak height and in appearance of new peaks, with

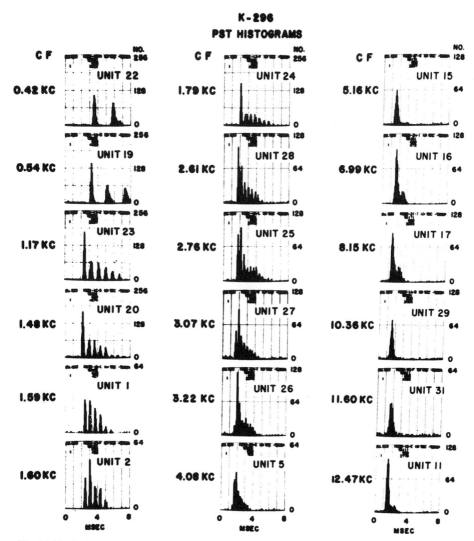

Fig. 10-18. Cat. Post-stimulus time histograms of responses to clicks from eighteen cochlear fibers obtained in a single cat. The CF of each fiber is indicated to the left of each histogram. Reprinted from *Discharge Patterns of Single Fibers in the Cat's Auditory Nerve* by N.Y-S. Kiang, T. Watanabe, E.C. Thomas, and L.F. Clark by permission of the M.I.T. Press, Cambridge, Massachusetts. Copyright © 1965 by the Massachusetts Institute of Technology.

no change in peak latencies. The rate of time-locked discharge of low CF units appears to increase monotonically with stimulus level, with total spike activity (time-locked and spontaneous activity) increasing at a lower rate. Total activity increases at a slower rate because there is a decrease in discharge, below the spontaneous level, between the peaks of the histogram. Kiang et al. (1965b) suggest that the peaks and the dips in the PST histogram result from increased activity to outward motion of the stapes and decrease in activity below spontaneous level with inward motion of the stapes. Reversing the polarity of the click stimulus results in a shift in the preferred times of firing of low CF units by one half the period of the CF, indicating that only one polarity of the mechanical motion stimulates.

MONAURAL COMPLEX STIMULI

The discharge of cochlear nerve fibers to clicks and tone-burst stimuli are affected by the introduction of background noise (Kiang et al., 1965b). The effect is one of reducing the discharge to click- or tone-burst stimuli (Fig. 10-19). Increasing the level of the background noise does not result in increases in activity to background noise that is sufficient to overshadow the click and tone-burst response in PST histograms. Rather the increase in background noise level results in both a reduction in click and tone-burst discharges and an increase in background activity.

The discharges of cochlear nerve fibers to CF tones can be reduced by the simultaneous presentation of a second non-CF tone to the same ear, provided the second tone is of the proper frequency and amplitude (Sachs and Kiang, 1968). Sachs and Kiang (1968) define the inhibitory area of a fiber as the stimulus frequencies and levels required to reduce discharge to continuous CF tone by 20 percent. Each fiber has two inhibitory areas, one above and one below CF, that overlap the excitatory response area of the fiber (Fig. 10-20). The sharpness of tuning of the high- and low-frequency inhibitory areas increase with fiber CF, as does the sharpness of excitatory tuning curves of cochlear fibers. Within the high frequency inhibitory area, there are stimulus frequencies that are capable of reducing discharge to a continuous CF tone at stimulus levels as much as 10 dB below the CF level used. Within the low frequency inhibitory area, the stimulus frequencies must be from 10 to forty dB greater in level than the continuous CF tone to affect a reduction in discharge.

The general time course of monaural two-tone inhibition using a continuous tone at CF and a tone-burst at an inhibitory frequency is illustrated by the PST histograms in Fig. 10-21. Following the onset of the inhibitory tone burst, there is an initial reduction in discharge that may drop to below the level of spontaneous discharge. The discharge gradually returns to a level above the spontaneous rate, but does not reach the level of

UNIT 282-20
PST HISTOGRAMS

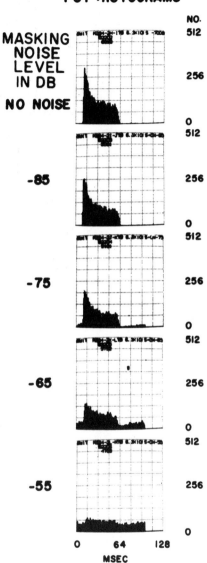

MASKING
NOISE
LEVEL
IN DB

NO NOISE

-85

-75

-65

-55

0   64   128
MSEC

Fig. 10-19. Cat. Post-stimulus time histograms for responses of a cochlear nerve fiber to tone bursts masked by broadband noise as a function of noise level. Zero time of each histogram is five msec before the onset of the tone electric input to the earphone. Reprinted from *Discharge Patterns of Single Fibers in the Cat's Auditory Nerve* by N.Y-S. Kiang, T. Watanabe, E.C. Thomas, and L.F. Clark by permission of The M.I.T. Press, Cambridge, Massachusetts. Copyright © 1965 by the Massachusetts Institute of Technology.

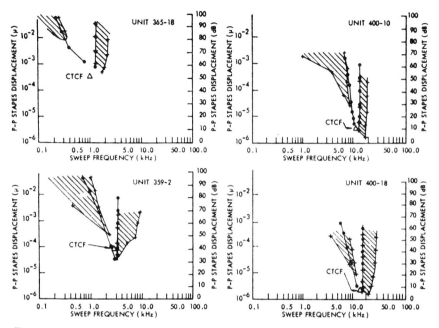

Fig. 10-20. Cat. Excitatory and inhibitory areas for four cochlear nerve units. Excitatory areas represent the frequencies and levels of monaural tones capable of eliciting discharge 20 percent greater than the spontaneous rate. Inhibitory areas represent the frequencies and levels of tone bursts that are capable of reducing by 20 percent the discharge to a continuous CF tone. The inhibitory areas are hatched. The dots represent the boundary of the response area. (Sachs and Kiang, 1968)

discharge elicited by the continuous CF tone alone. The reduction in discharge is maintained for the duration of the inhibitory tone burst and has been observed to last as long as five minutes. Following the offset of the inhibitory tone burst, there is a large transient increase in discharge that gradually decreases back to the level of discharge elicited by the CF tone alone.

The reduction in discharge produced by the inhibitory tone does not appear to be dependent upon brain-stem efferent mechanisms, since it was observed in single fibers of the peripheral stump of a transected cochlear nerve (Kiang et al., 1965b). Sectioning both the crossed and uncrossed olivocochlear bundles also did not affect monaural two-tone inhibition (Kiang, 1968).

According to Sachs and Kiang (1968), the population of cochlear nerve fibers sampled in their study was homogeneous with respect to general features of monaural two tone inhibition. The CF of the fibers sampled ranged from 0.2 to 35.0 kHz and spontaneous discharge rates varied from less than 1 spike/see to over 50 spikes/sec. Discharge of all fibers to a continuous

UNIT 362-9

SPONTANEOUS

TONE BURST
DURATION
IN MSEC.

50

100

400

900

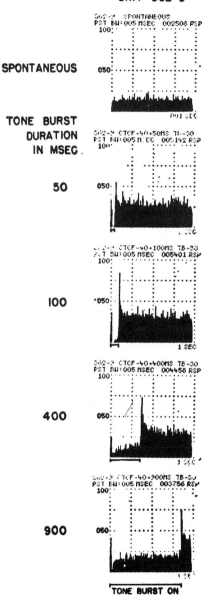

Fig. 10-21. Cat. Post-stimulus time histograms of responses of a single cochlear nerve fiber to tone bursts of various durations presented simultaneously with a continuous tone at fiber CF. Unit CF: 7.83 kHz; 1 min. of data. (Sachs and Kiang, 1968)

CF tone could be reduced by a second tone of proper frequency and amplitude. The general time course of reduction of discharge was similar for all fibers and inhibitory areas differed only with respect to CF, with high CF fibers having more sharply tuned inhibitory areas.

Simultaneous monaural presentation of two tones can also produce an increase in discharge, when the frequencies of the two tones, f1 and f2, where the ratio f2/f1 is less than 2 and greater than 1, produce a combination frequency 2f1-f2 that is approximately equal to the fiber's CF (Goldstein and Kiang, 1968). For fibers with CF greater than 4.0 kHz an increase in discharge rate always occurs when the combination tone 2f1-f2 falls within the fiber's tuning curve, even when f1 and f2 do not elicit discharge when presented alone. For low CF fibers the intensity functions produced by simultaneous presentation of two tones yielding a combination tone equal to the fiber's CF were similar to the intensity functions produced by a single CF tone.

All units with low CF (0.28 to 3.86 kHz) were found to produce spike trains in which discharge could be time-locked to the combination tone 2f1-f2. When the two stimulus tones fall within the tuning curve of a unit, there is synchrony of firing with each of the two tones, f1 and f2, with 2f1-f2 and with 2f2-f1 at slightly higher stimulus levels. When the two stimulus tones, f1 and f2, were selected so that they fall outside the unit's tuning curve (i.e., the unit shows no response to either of the two tones presented alone), discharge synchronized with 2f1-f2 occur, if 2f1-f2 is close to the CF of the unit. The time-locked responses to 2f1-f2 could be canceled by adding a third, externally produced tone equal to 2f1-f2 of the appropriate amplitude and phase. The effect was a reduction in spikes firing in synchrony with the internally produced combination tone, without an overall increase in the discharge of the fiber. Goldstein and Kiang (1968) conclude that the discharges to the combination tone (2f1-f2) are generated by a mechanism located in the inner ear, although they do not attribute the mechanism to any one inner ear process: mechanical, electrical, or chemical.

EFFERENT CONTROL OF COCHLEAR NERVE OUTPUT

Fex (1961) first reported on the effects of electrical stimulation of the crossed olivocochlear bundle (COCB) on single unit activity of cat cochlear nerve fibers. Members of the Eaton-Peabody group (Wiederhold and Kiang, 1970, and Wiederhold, 1970) have also reported on investigations of the effects of electrical stimulation of the COCB on cochlear nerve unit activity. Because the results of the Eaton-Peabody group are comparable to the studies of the cochlear nerve unit activity we have just described, we will concentrate on their results. In the Eaton-Peabody experiments, cats were anesthetized with

Dial-urethane and the tendons of middle ear muscles were severed. The cerebellum was removed to expose the floor of the fourth ventricle for placement of stimulating electrodes in the COCB at the midline. Electrical stimulus levels were kept below levels resulting in stimulation of the facial nerve root that produced facial twitches. The effect of the electrical stimulus upon the fibers of the UOCB could not be assessed in these studies.

Electrical stimulation of the crossed olivocochlear bundle produces a reduction in discharge of all cochlear nerve fibers except those with high CF and extremely low CF (Wiederhold and Kiang, 1970). Stimulation of the COCB reduced spontaneous activity only in fibers that had extremely low thresholds. The spontaneous-activity levels of most cochlear fibers were not affected by COCB stimulation. Stimulation of the COCB at shock rates from fifty to one thousand shocks/sec reduced discharge to CF tones. When the shock rates are below one hundred/sec, the reduction in discharge is synchronized with each shock in the shock train. Above this rate the reduction can no longer "follow" the shock train and the time course of the reduction becomes irregular. At shock rates above one hundred shocks/sec the ISI histograms of the reduced discharge resembles the histograms elicited by a lower level of CF tone presented alone.

The effectiveness and time course of electrical stimulation of the COCB are dependent upon the level of the acoustic stimulus and upon the fiber CF. The COCB effect (reduction in acoustically evoked discharge) is least at acoustic levels eliciting minimal and maximal discharge and is greatest at intermediate levels. At low acoustic levels COCB stimulation results in a small decrease in discharge that appears as a flattening of the acoustic discharge PST histogram. At higher acoustic levels, there is a large, transient decrease in discharge to the onset of the shock train, with gradual recovery of discharge over two to three sec to a rate somewhere between the spontaneous rate and the rate to the CF tone alone (Fig. 10-22). Under certain stimulus conditions the reduction of the acoustically elicited discharge can be maintained with shock trains several minutes long. Offset of the shock train is often followed by a transient increase in discharge above the rate to the CF tone alone, especially if discharge is greatly reduced just before the COCB shocks are terminated. At acoustic levels eliciting maximal discharge when CF tone is presented alone, the reduction in discharge with COCB stimulation is less than at lower acoustic levels.

The time course of the COCB effect differs for low and high CF fibers. High CF fibers take longer to be affected by COCB stimulation and recover faster from COCB stimulation than do low CF fibers. High CF fibers also appear to have a transient period of recovery in discharge after the initial large reduction in discharge with shock rates greater than two hundred shock/sec. This transient recovery period is seen as a peak after the initial drop in the PST histograms of Fig. 10-22.

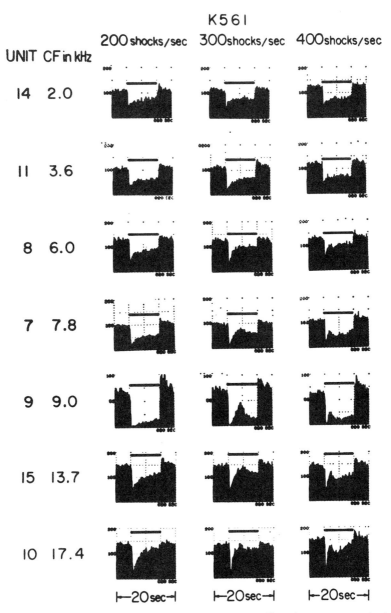

Fig. 10-22. Cat. Post-stimulus time histograms showing effect of varying COCB shock repetition rate on discharge of seven cochlear nerve fibers to continuous tones at CF. (Wiederhold and Kiang, 1970)

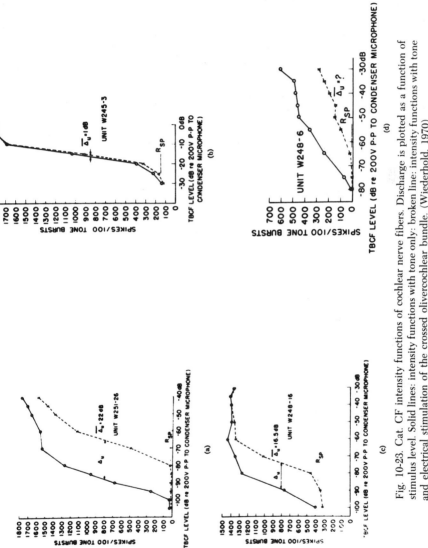

Fig. 10-23. Cat. CF intensity functions of cochlear nerve fibers. Discharge is plotted as a function of stimulus level. Solid lines: intensity functions with tone only; broken line: intensity functions with tone and electrical stimulation of the crossed olivecochlear bundle. (Wiederhold, 1970)

For all cochlear fibers, electrical stimulation of the COCB results in a shift in the intensity function to higher acoustic levels (Wiederhold, 1970). The shifts were constant for most cochlear fibers, so that intensity functions were displaced horizontally to higher levels with no change in the shape of the curves (Fig. 10-23). For a small number of units the shift was not constant, so that the slope of the intensity function was decreased with COCB stimulation (Fig. 10-23, Unit W248-6). For fibers producing horizontal shifts of constant value with COCB stimulation, the electrical stimulation of COCB resulted in CF intensity function shifts ranging from one to twenty-five dB. The effect of COCB stimulation on non-CF intensity functions was much less than for acoustic stimuli of frequency at or near CF. In some fibers no effect is seen if the frequency is far enough from CF.

The magnitude of the shift in CF intensity functions with COCB stimulation does not appear to be related to the spontaneous-activity rate of the fiber or to its threshold to CF tone. The magnitude of the shift is related to CF, with the largest shifts occurring in the frequency range to which cats are most sensitive (Fig. 10-24). The magnitude of the shift increases with CF

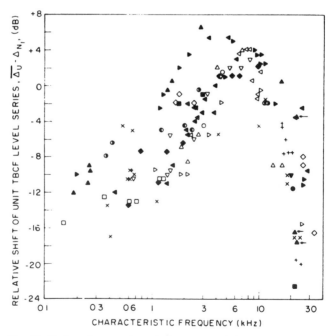

Fig. 10-24. Cat. Scatter plots of the average shift in CF intensity functions with COCB stimulation against cochlear nerve fiber CF (Wiederhold, 1970)

up to six to 10 kHz and does so at a rate of 14 dB/octave for frequencies below six kHz. Above 15 kHz the shift appears to decrease rapidly with increasing CF.

COCHLEAR NUCLEUS COMPLEX

ANATOMY

Within the cranial cavity the eighth cranial nerve root travels a short distance to the brain stem and enters the medulla ventrally. All cochlear nerve fibers appear to terminate within the cochlear nuclear complex (Powell and Cowan, 1962; Osen, 1970b). The cochlear nuclear complex of the cat forms a bulge on the lateral surface of the brain stem that overlies the inferior cerebellar peduncle (Fig. 10-25). A ventral portion of the cochlear nuclear complex, the ventral ganglion of Lorente de Nó, extends from a position near the point where the eighth and seventh nerves enter the brain stem to a more dorsal position near the ventral borders of the inferior and superior cerebellar peduncles (Fig. 10-25). The dorsal portion of the cochlear nucleus, the acoustic tubercle of Lorente de Nó, overlaps part of the caudal surface of the ventral group and extends dorsally over the lateral and dorsal surface of the inferior cerebellar peduncle.

The ventral division of the cochlear nuclear complex is divided into the anteroventral (AVCN) and posteroventral (PVCN) nuclei by the entering fibers of the cochlear nerve root (Fig. 10-26). The cochlear nuclear area located along the course of the entering cochlear root fibers is called the interstitial nucleus (ISN). The dorsal cochlear nucleus has a distinct laminated structure along its dorsolateral surface that caps or encloses a less defined central nuclear area. The ependymal cell layer covers the free surface of the DCN and the molecular and granular (or pyramidal) layers are usually distinguished beneath it. The central nuclear area is defined as the deep portion of the DCN that underlies the molecular and granular cell layers.

Within the area of the interstitial nucleus the cochlear root fibers bifurcate into ascending and descending branches. The ascending branches enter the AVCN and form small parallel bundles that course dorsally and rostrally (Fig. 10-26). The descending branches take a converging course and become packed into dense fascicles that travel dorsally through the PVCN, and turning, travel dorsorostrally into the DCN. According to Lorente de No (1933a), cochlear nerve fibers from the basal turn of the cochlea (high frequencies) bifurcate ventrally and project into ventral areas of the ventral cochlear nuclear group, while fibers from the apical turn (low frequencies) bifurcate and terminate dorsally. However, recent anatomical (Sando, 1965; Van Noort, 1969; Osen, 1970b) and neurophysiological (Rose et al., 1959; Kiang et al., 1965a) studies of the cochlear nuclear complex indicate that the

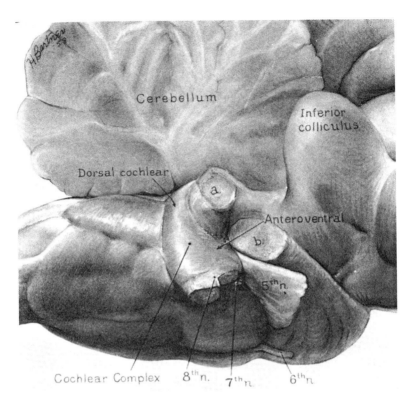

Fig. 10-25. Cat. Upper: Lateral view of the right cochlear nuclear complex of cat after removal of the homolateral cerebellum. The inferior and superior cerebellar peduncles have been cut at a; b is the cut edge of the middle cerebellar peduncle. The eighth cranial nerve has been cut in two steps. The dorsal extension of the cochlear complex is formed exclusively by the dorsal cochlear nucleus. The anterior portion of the complex is formed by the anteroventral nucleus. Right: A closer view of the cochlear nuclear complex indicating the relative positions of the dorsal cochlear nucleus (Dc), the posteroventral cochlear nucleus (Pv), and the anteroventral cochlear nucleus (Av). The interstitial nucleus is located along the course of the entering cochlear nerve root. 1, cochlear nerve fibers innervating the apical portion of the organ of Corti; 2, cochlear nerve fibers innervating the basal portion. Reprinted from Rose, J.E., Galambos, R. and Hughes, J.R., "Microelectrode Studies of the Cochlear Nuclei of the Cat", *Bulletin of the Johns Hopkins Hospital*, Vol. 104, No. 5 (May 1959), p. 214 and 245. © The Johns Hopkins Press.

sequence is the reverse; that is, the fibers from the apical turn bifurcate and terminate ventrolaterally and fibers from the basal turn bifurcate and terminate dorsally in both the ventral and dorsal cochlear nuclei.

CELL TYPES OF THE COCHLEAR NUCLEUS

Lorente de Nó (1933b), using Golgi-stained material, described the cochlear nuclear complex as containing fifty different cell types that are organized into 15 distinct nuclear regions. His descriptions of these cells are very skimpy and none are given for cells located in the anteroventral cochlear nucleus. More recently Osen (1969a, 1969b), using Nissl-stained material, described nine types of cochlear nuclear cells that formed a basis for dividing the cochlear nucleus into nine partially overlapping cell areas. Cochlear nerve terminals associated with these cell types were also described by Osen (1970b) in normal tissue stained with Glees method and in tissues stained with the Nauta method of animals with the entire cochlea destroyed. Because Osen gives detailed descriptions of the cell types, their distribution and the

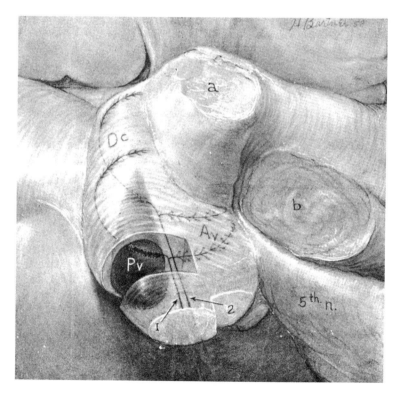

Fig. 10-25 contd.

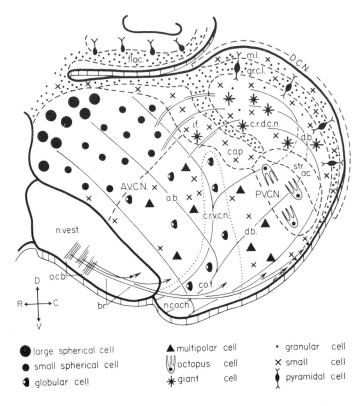

● large spherical cell   ▲ multipolar cell   • granular cell
● small spherical cell   〰 octopus cell   × small cell
◑ globular cell   ✳ giant cell   ⚲ pyramidal cell

Fig. 10-26. Cat. Semidiagrammatic camera lucida drawing of a sagittal section of the cochlear nuclei and adjacent structures. The extent of the dorsal nucleus (DCN) is indicated by the superficial stippled line in the upper right. Dotted line indicates the border of the cochlear nerve root and interstitial nucleus (c.r.v.c.n.) while stippled lines indicate the borders of the granular cell layer (gr.cl.), peripheral cap of small cells (cap), root of acoustic striae (str.ac.), and central regions of the dorsal and ventral nuclei. The distribution of areas of the nine cell types are shown by symbols. Abbreviations: A.V.C.N., anteroventral cochlear nucleus; n. coch., cochlear nerve; n. vest., vestibular nerve; P.V.C.N., posteroventral cochlear nucleus; st. ac. interm., intermediate stria of Held; a.b., ascending branches of the cochlear nerve; d.b., descending branches of the cochlear nerve. Reproduced from K. Osen and K. Roth, "Histochemical localization of cholinesterases in the cochlear nuclei of the cat, with notes on the origin of acetylcholinesterase-positive afferents and the superior olive," *Brain Research*, Vol. 16 (1969), pp 165-185, Figure 1.

cochlear nerve terminals associated with these cell types, we will concentrate upon her description of cochlear nucleus organization.

The rostral half of the anteroventral cochlear nucleus contains large and small spherical type cells. The spherical cells appear round and without visible processes in Nissl-stained sections. One or two opposing processes may be seen in Glees preparations in which parts of the dendrite are stained. The nucleus is centrally located in the cell body and the Nissl substance forms a distinct nuclear cap and a concentric ring of coarse granules. The two types of spherical cells are distinguished on the basis of size. The dorsorostral portion of the AVCN contains large spherical cells exclusively (Fig. 10-26). The small spherical cells and a few small cells are found ventrocaudal to the large spherical cell area (Fig. 10-26). The somas of large and small spherical cells appear to be enveloped by two to four thick fingerlike processes described as typical bulbs of Held. The terminals associated with the large spherical cells are thicker and branch more than those associated with small spherical cells. The preterminal fibers in the large spherical cell area are thicker than those in the small spherical cell area. There also appear to be small bouton-type terminals associated with these cells that degenerate along with the bulbs of Held when the spiral ganglion is destroyed.

The central area of the ventral cochlear nucleus, (the caudal AVCN, ISN and the rostral PVCN) contains several types of cells. The caudal half of the AVCN bordering the interstitial nucleus contains multipolar, globular, and small cells. The multipolar cells have irregularly shaped cell bodies from which two to three cell processes extend. The nucleus is usually located centrally and the Nissl granules, which are evenly dispersed, vary from fine to coarse. Multipolar cells are also found in the rostral part of the PVCN that borders the ISN. The area of the interstitial nucleus contains globular cells exclusively. The globular cells characteristically contain an eccentrically placed nucleus that often appears to bulge from the cell surface. The cell body contains fine, darkly staining Nissl granules diffusely dispersed within the cell body. In some cases, large Nissl granules are observed on the nuclear membrane or at the periphery of the cell. In Glees preparations, heavily branching dendrites are observed to form a dense network near the cell body. Globular cells are also found in the caudal portion of the AVCN along with multipolar and small cells. The area of the PVCN adjacent to the ISN contains both multipolar and small cells. The small cells vary considerably in appearance but are smaller than all other cells except for the granular cells. The nuclei of small cells are usually small and the Nissl granules appear coarse and dark in some, and fine and pale in others. Small cells are found throughout almost the entire extent of the cochlear nuclear complex. At the dorsal margin of the ventral nucleus, the small cells form the "peripheral cap of small cells" that contains small cells exclusively.

In the central area of VCN, containing multipolar, globular, and small cells, small ring-type terminals and irregular bouton-type endings of various shapes and staining properties are observed. The ring-type terminals appear to be related to the cell bodies and dendrites of multipolar cells, while the irregular boutons appear to be associated with the globular cells. The small cells of the peripheral cap of small cells appear to be associated with bouton-type endings that arise from tiny bundles of cochlear nerve fibers coursing up from the underlying portion of the complex. Destruction of the spiral ganglion results in degeneration of these fibers and terminals.

The dorsocaudal portion of the PVCN contains octopus cells exclusively. The octopus cells are characterized by their long dendrites, which are often located on one side of the cell like the arms of an octopus. The octopus cell nucleus is centrally or slightly eccentrically placed, and Nissl granulates are dispersed throughout the cytoplasm of the cell body. The octopus cell is not found in any other area of the cochlear nucleus. The area of the octopus cells contains numerous small ring-shaped boutons that appear to be located on cell body and dendrites. Rasmussen (1967) described the PVCN area as containing large bouton-type endings, two to three microns in diameter, and smaller endings, one micron or less, dispersed between the larger endings.

Both granular- and small-type cells are sparsely scattered within the molecular layer of the DCN. The granular cells are the smallest cells in the cochlear nucleus and contain the smallest nuclei. The cell nucleus is round or oval in shape and is surrounded by very little and lightly staining cytoplasm. Granular cells are found more densely packed in the granular layer of DCN and are also found in the central nucleus of DCN. The granular cells also form a continuous layer that covers the entire free surface of the cochlear nucleus laterally, ventrally, and caudally. Dorsal to the peripheral cap of small cells, granular cells form a granular cell layer that is continuous rostrally with the granular layer of the flocculus. The granular cell layer overlying the peripheral cap of small cells shows very little terminal degeneration with destruction of the spiral ganglion.

The granular or pyramidal layer of the DCN contains granular, small, and pyramidal cells. The pyramidal cells have cell processes that extend from opposite poles of the cell, giving it a bipolar appearance. The cell body contains a nucleus that is centrally or eccentrically placed and medium-sized Nissel granules arranged longitudinally. The pyramidal cells are arranged in an irregular row and often occur in clusters of from three to five cells. Pyramidal cells are found only within the granular layer of DCN. It is not certain whether pyramidal cells are directly innervated by primary afferents.

The central nuclear layer of DCN contains granular, small and, giant cells. The giant cells contain the largest nuclei found in the cochlear nucleus. The cell body is disc shaped and contains coarse Nissl granules. Cell processes radiate in all directions from the cell body. A few giant cells are also found in the region of the peripheral cap of small cells. There appear to be a large number of cochlear nerve terminal fibers and boutons in the small cell area of the central nucleus but very few in the area of the giant cells.

INTRINSIC AND EFFERENT INNERVATION OF THE COCHLEAR NUCLEUS

Following destruction of the spiral ganglion, fewer degenerated fibers are observed in the DCN than in the VCN. Fewer degenerated fibers are observed in the large and small spherical cell areas of AVCN than in other areas of the VCN (Osen, 1970b; Rasmussen, 1967). Almost all fibers in the globular and octopus cell areas are degenerated. Within the DCN the density of degeneration is greatest in the central nuclear area and decreases progressively toward the molecular layer, which contains no signs of degeneration. The granular cell area overlapping the peripheral cap of small cells shows no sign of terminal degeneration.

The neurons of the cochlear nuclear complex give rise to intrinsic axons, which terminate within the complex, and to extrinsic axons, which terminate in other nuclear groups of the brain stem. There are reciprocal connections between the AVCN and the DCN and between the PVCN and the DCN. Reciprocal connections between the AVCN and the PVCN have not been described. Intrinsic fibers interconnecting the DCN and AVCN pass through the peripheral cap of small cells and the overlying granular cell area (Lorente de Nó, 1933b; Osen, 1970b). Intrinsic fibers interconnecting the PVCN and DCN travel along the medial border of the PVCN (Warr, 1969). Fibers from the PVCN have also been described as terminating upon scattered cells located within the acoustic stria (Warr, 1969).

There are four different "efferent" inputs to the cochlear nucleus, which have been described; the olivocochlear bundle, the recurrent bundle of Rasmussen; the recurrent bundle of Held; and the recurrent bundle of Lorente de Nó. The efferent input from the dorsomedial periolivary nucleus via the olivocochlear bundle has been described previously. Collateral fibers of the OCB traverse the glial portion of the vestibular nerve and enter the AVCN (Rasmussen, 1960; 1967). Most of these fibers appear to terminate in the granular cell areas of the cochlear nuclear complex (Rasmussen, 1960; 1967; Osen and Roth, 1969). The fibers of the recurrent bundle of Rasmussen (1960; 1967) arise in the homolateral lateral superior olive, travel in the intermediate acoustic stria, and terminate in the ventral cochlear nucleus. According to Osen and Roth (1969), fibers of this bundle may arise from small cells near the periphery of the lateral superior olive and may terminate as small boutons in the region of the large and small spherical cells of the AVCN. The source of the recurrent bundle of Held has not been fully described. Some of the fibers of this bundle arise from the contralateral ventral nucleus of the lateral lemniscus (Rasmussen, 1960). These fibers travel in the dorsal acoustic stria and terminate in the granular and central nuclear area of the DCN (Held, 1893; Rasmussen, 1960). The fibers of the recurrent bundle of Lorente de No take origin in the inferior colliculus (Rasmussen, 1960; 1967). They descend the brain stem as part of the tectobulbar tract, decussate dorsal to the trapezoid body, and travel in the dorsal acoustic stria to the DCN (Lorente de Nó, 1933b; Rasmussen, 1960; 1967).

NEUROPHYSIOLOGY

The fact that the cochlear nucleus is a complex consisting of many cell types that are associated with different types of cochlear nerve terminals and different efferent inputs suggests that subdivisions of the cochlear nucleus might differ functionally. Because the only systematic neurophysiological studies of the cat cochlear nucleus that relate electrophysiological data with location of units in the cochlear nucleus are those of the Eaton-Peabody group, we will concentrate upon their findings (Kiang and Goldstein, 1962; Kiang, 1965; Kiang, Pfeiffer, Warr and Backus, 1965a; Koerber, Pfeiffer, Warr and Kiang, 1966; Pfeiffer and Kiang, 1965; Pfeiffer, 1966a, b).

The Eaton-Peabody group recorded with indium-filled, platinum-tipped pipettes with which lesions were made either at the recording site or at the end of an electrode track. The locations of these cochlear nuclear units were determined histologically. Other units were located using neurophysiological criteria based upon the tonotopic organization of the cochlear nucleus as described by Rose, Galambos, and Hughes (1959). Cochlear nucleus units were classified as falling into three subdivisions: the anteroventral cochlear nucleus or AVCN, the interstitial and posteroventral cochlear nuclei or ISN and PVCN, and the dorsal cochlear nucleus or DCN. The stimulus conditions utilized in these studies of the cochlear nucleus were similar to those utilized in studying the cochlear nerve, which makes direct quantitative comparisons of results possible.

SPONTANEOUS ACTIVITY

Not all cochlear nucleus units produce spontaneous discharges in the absence of experimenter-produced acoustic stimuli (Pfeiffer and Kiang, 1965). Spontaneous discharge rates vary from 0 to 289 spikes/sec, with 20 percent of the sampled units displaying no spontaneous activity. The majority of units have spontaneous rates above 5 spikes/sec and below 100 spikes/sec. As in the case of cochlear nerve fibers, the rates of spontaneous discharges of cochlear nucleus units do not appear to be related to the CF of the units.

The interspike interval histograms of cochlear nucleus unit spontaneous activity are of at least four types (Pfeiffer and Kiang, 1965). One type of spontaneous-activity ISI histogram is bimodal and reportedly occurs infrequently. The other three are unimodal, but differ with respect to symmetry about the modal interspike interval or with respect to the rate of decay of intervals longer than the mode (Fig. 10-27). The modal interspike interval values of cochlear nucleus units producing unimodal histograms vary from approximately two msec up to over one hundred msec. One group of units produced histograms that were symmetric about the mode and had modes greater than 12 msec. Two other groups produced histograms that were asymmetric about the mode, but differed in the rate of decay of

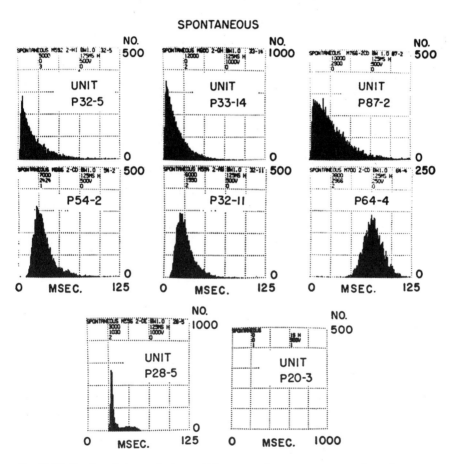

Fig. 10-27. Cat. Sample interspike interval histograms of spontaneous activity for eight units in the cochlear nucleus. These histograms represent a survey of the various shapes of histograms encountered in the cochlear nucleus. The height of each bar in the histogram represents the number of intervals with the time duration indicated by the abscissa. (Pfeiffer and Kiang, 1965)

intervals longer than the mode: One had an exponential rate of decay; the other had nonexponential rates of decay. The temporal pattern of spontaneous discharges is stationary over many hours of recording time and the shape of the ISI histogram of spontaneous activity of any given unit does not vary over time. The shapes of the ISI histograms do not appear to be related to the unit CF or to its spontaneous activity rate.

According to Koerber, Pfeiffer, Warr, and Kiang (1966), the occurrence of bimodal ISI histograms is related to the condition of the cochlea of the animals studied. Only 2 percent of the units sampled from intact animals had bimodal histograms, while 12 percent of the histograms in cats with cochleas destroyed were bimodal. In addition, three of the four intact cats with units generating bimodal histograms were demonstrated to have abnormal cochleas. The spontaneous activity of cochlear nuclear units having short interval modes also appears to be dependant upon the condition of the receptor organ. Destruction of the homolateral cochlea results in the immediately disappearance of all spontaneous activity characterized by short interval mode ISI histograms. The spontaneous activity of units that have long interval modes did not appear to be affected greatly by cochlear destruction.

RESPONSE TO TONAL STIMULI

Units in the different subdivisions of the cochlear nucleus do not appear to differ with respect to the range of frequencies to which they respond, or to shapes of tuning curves, or to characteristic frequencies represented (Kiang et al., 1965a). The tuning curves of cochlear nucleus units vary in shape from a broad and shallow U to a deeper and sharper V (Fig. 10-28). Cochlear nucleus units do appear to have slightly broader tuning curves than do cochlear nerve units (Kiang et al., 1965a).

The tonotopic organization of cochlear nuclear units first described neurophysiologically by Rose, Galambos, and Hughes (1959) has been confirmed by Kiang et al., (1965a). The characteristic frequencies of units in the dorsal, posteroventral, and anteroventral cochlear nuclear subdivisions progress from high to low in a dorsoventral sequence with the boundaries between the subdivisions corresponding to abrupt changes in the orderly sequence of CF. The neurophysiological descriptions of the tonotopic organization of the cochlear nucleus is in agreement with the anatomical description of the pattern of termination of cochlear nerve fibers (Sando, 1965; van Noort, 1969).

The discharge patterns of cochlear nucleus units to tone bursts vary from a phasic, on-type response to a tonic response similar to that elicited from cochlear nerve units (Fig. 10-29). There are four types of cochlear nuclear

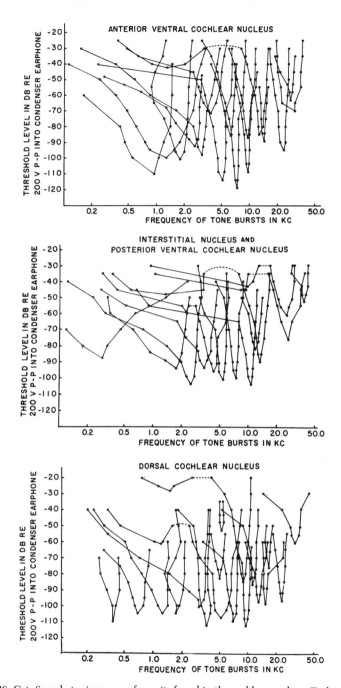

Fig. 10-28. Cat. Sample tuning curves for units found in the cochlear nucleus. Each curve was obtained by varying the level of tone bursts and recording the extremes of frequencies at which discharge was elicited. The tip of the tuning curves designates the threshold and the characteristic frequency (CF) of the unit. (Kiang *et al.*, 1965a) Reproduced with the permission of Dr. Kiang and *Annals of Otology, Rhinology and Laryngology*.

SCHEMATIC REPRESENTATION
OF PST HISTOGRAMS

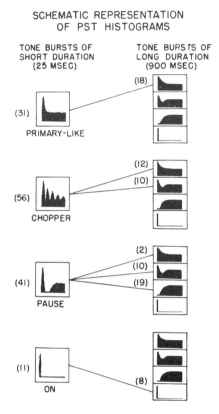

Fig. 10-29. Cat. Summary of cochlear nucleus unit post-stimulus time histogram types elicited by tone bursts with high on-off ratio (900 msec. on, 100 msec. off). Units are initially classified on the basis of shapes of response pattern to tone bursts of short duration (left column). (Pfeiffer, 1966b)

units classified on the basis of the shapes of the PST histograms generated by tone-burst stimuli (Pfeiffer, 1966b). The "primarylike" PST histograms are similar in shape to the PST histograms of tone-burst discharge of cochlear nerve units. The primarylike PST histogram is characterized by an initial high rate of activity that follows stimulus onset and a gradual drop to a steady rate of activity higher than the spontaneous rate. The offset of the tone burst is followed by a brief period of reduction of spontaneous activity from which the unit gradually recovers. The shape of the PST histograms of units with primarylike discharge does not appear to change with increases in stimulus level or with changes in stimulus frequency. While cochlear nerve unit PST histograms become flattened with high tone burst on-off ratios (nine hundred msec. on to one hundred msec off), the PST histograms of primarylike cochlear nucleus units do not change shape with high on-off ratios (Fig. 10-29).

The "chopper"-type PST histogram is characterized by regularly spaced peaks of activity, which are time-locked to the onset of each tone burst. The chopping effect is most prominent at the beginning of the tone burst response and gradually disappears as the tone is left on. The chopper respose pattern is not the result of spikes being phase-locked to the sinusoidal stimuli, as is the case for low CF cochlear units stimulated with low-frequency stimuli. A unit with a chopper-type PST histogram may exhibit a chopper or pause-type PST histogram at stimulus levels twenty-five dB greater than the unit's threshold. In addition, a unit displaying a chopper-type PST histogram with tone burst of low on-off ratio may display a primarylike or pause-type histogram with larger on-off ratio (Fig. 10-29).

The "pause"-type PST histogram is characterized by an initial burst of activity that forms one or two peaks, followed by a short period of depressed activity. This so-called silent period is then followed by a train of spikes that lasts as long as the tone burst. Many units that exhibit pause-type PST histograms change discharge pattern when the on-off ratio is increased (Fig. 10-29). The PST histograms to tone bursts with larger on-off ratios take the form of primary-type, pause-type or build-up type histograms. The build-up type PST histogram displays no initial burst of spikes to stimulus onset and may either exhibit a constant, flat rate of activity with tone on, or may exhibit a gradual increase in discharge to a steady rate that is maintained as long as the tone is on.

The "on"-type PST histogram is characterized by a peak or peaks of activity at the onset of the tone burst with little or no activity following. This is a phasic response that does not appear to change with stimulus level or with increases in on-off ratio of the tone burst. Almost 50 percent of the cochlear nucleus units that do not produce spontaneous discharges respond to a continuous CF tone with a phasic response (Pfeiffer and Kiang, 1965). Pfeiffer (1966b) reports that cochlear nucleus units with low CFs show tendencies toward pause and on-type response patterns, along with phase-locking to the sinusoidal stimulus.

The shape of the ISI histogram generated in response to a continuous CF tone is very similar to that generated by the unit's spontaneous activity, provided the time scale is adjusted for the increased rate of activity (Pfeiffer and Kiang, 1965). For some units the histograms do not change their shape as stimulus level is raised to twenty-five dB above threshold. The similarity in the shapes of the ISI histograms for spontaneous and stimulated activity occurs for all shapes of cochlear nucleus histograms, except for those units with no spontaneous activity. Some units with no spontaneous activity respond with phasic discharge to continuous tones, while others respond with sustained discharge (Pfeiffer and Kiang, 1965).

RESPONSE TO CLICK STIMULI

Cochlear nucleus units respond to click stimuli with a short burst of spikes. While all low CF cochlear nerve units produce multiple-peaked PST histograms to click stimuli, not all low CF cochlear nucleus units appear to do so. There appear to be four different types of low CF units on the basis of the shape of click-produced PST histograms. Some low CF units produce click PST histograms similar to those of cochlear nerve units, with multiple peaks at intervals corresponding to 1/CF (Kiang et al., 1965a). Other low CF units produce click PST histograms with a large single peak followed by smaller peaks that are not as clear as those seen in the click PST histograms of cochlear nerve units. Other low CF units produce click PST histograms with a single narrow peak. For these units high levels of click stimuli may produce multiple-peaked PST histograms, but the intervals between the peaks appear to be unrelated to the CF of the unit. Other low CF units produce broad single-peaked PST histograms.

In general the PST histograms generated by discharges of high CF cochlear nucleus units in response to click stimuli have a single peak that is either narrower or broader than is found in click histograms of high CF cochlear nerve units. Cochlear nerve units with CF greater than 4.0 kHz have a unimodal distribution of latency with a peak at approximately 1.6 msec. The latencies of cochlear nucleus units appear to be bimodally distributed, with one peak at approximately 2.8 msec., and a second peak at approximately 4.6 msec. The broad distribution of the click latencies of cochlear nuclear units suggests that many of the long latency units may not be in direct contact with cochlear nerve fibers.

COCHLEAR NUCLEUS UNIT POPULATION

The discharge characteristics of units in the different cochlear nucleus subdivisions have been summarized in a paper by Kiang, Pfeiffer, Warr, and Backus (1965a). A single type of unit is found excusively within the rostral portion of the AVCN, which probably corresponds to the spherical cell areas of Osen (1969a). The response characteristics of a "typical" rostral AVCN unit is presented in Fig. 10-30. The ISI histograms of spontaneous discharges of AVCN units are unimodal and skewed, with modes less than 12 msec. and decays faster than exponential. PST histograms of these units produced by tone-burst stimuli are of the primary type. The PST histograms produced by click stimuli differ for low and high CF units. Low CF units produce histograms with a large single peak that is followed by smaller multiple peaks whose intervals are related to unit CF. The high CF units produce a single, narrow-peaked histogram with latencies that range from 2.1 to 3.3 msec. The waveform of spikes recorded extracellulary from units in the rostral AVCN

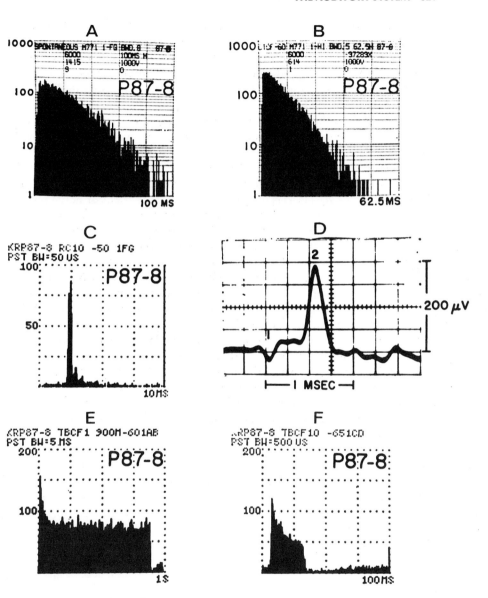

Fig. 10-30. Cat. Discharge characteristics of a single unit located in the anterodorsal portion of the anteroventral cochlear nucleus. A. Interspike interval histogram of spontaneous activity. B. Interspike interval histogram of discharges in response to a continuous tone at the CF (1.9 kHz) of the unit. C. Post-stimulus time histogram of responses to rarefaction clicks. D. Waveform of the spike discharge. E. Post-stimulus time histogram of response to tone bursts (900 msec. on, 100 msec. off) at the CF. F. Post-stimulus time histogram of response to tone bursts (25 msec. on, 75 msec off) at the CF. (Kiang et al., 1965a) Reproduced with the permission of Dr. Kiang and Annals of Otology, Rhinology and Laryngology.

are unique, with a positive deflection occurring 0.5 to 0.7 msec before the onset of the large negative spike (Pfeiffer, 1966a).

Units recorded in the posterior part of the ventral cochlear nucleus — that is, the caudal AVCN, ISN and PVCN — appear to be of three types (Fig. 10-31). The "primarylike" unit has discharge characteristics similar to those of cochlear nerve units. The ISI histograms of spontaneous activity of these units tend to have a short mode (less than 12 msec.) and an exponental decay from the mode. Tone-burst stimuli produce primary-type PST histograms. Primarylike units with low CF produce multiple-peaked PST histograms to click stimuli with peak intervals corresponding to 1/CF. Units with high CF produce click PST histograms that have a single peak with latency less than 3.5 msec. Kiang et al., (1965a) do not believe these are cochlear nerve units because: (1) The type of electrode used does not record from fibers in the cochlear nerve. (2) They can be recorded from over a large distance of electrode movement. (3) These units show injury discharge typical of dying cells. Primarylike units are found only in the ISN and PVCN.

The second type of unit encountered in the posterior VCN group is classified as a "chopper" type on the basis of the shape of the PST histogram produced to tone-burst stimuli (Fig. 10-31). The spontaneous-activity ISI histograms of these units have either short or long modes and decays from the mode that are never faster than exponential. The PST histograms produced by tone bursts exhibit regular peaks that are time-locked to the onset of the stimulus (chopper-type), when the tones are above threshold levels. The click-evoked PST histograms of both low and high CF chopper units have a single peak of short latency, less than 3.5 msec. for units with CF above four khz. The chopper-type units are also found in the DCN, but are mainly in the ISN and PVCN.

The third type of unit in the posterior VCN responds with phasic discharge to tone-burst stimuli and is called an "on" unit (Fig. 10-31). These "on" units have little or no spontaneous activity and do not produce multiple-peaked PST histograms to click stimuli. Most of these units respond phasically to the onset of a continuous tone and do not fire anytime thereafter. Multiple peaks may appear in click-produced PST histograms when high stimulus levels are used. However, the peak intervals are not related to the CF of the unit. On-type units are found most often in the ISN and PVCN and are only rarely encountered in the caudal AVCN and in DCN.

The DCN appears to contain a variety of unit types. However, all DCN units respond to click stimuli with broad single-peaked PST histograms, whose latencies are usually longer than the first peak of the click PST histograms of ventral cochlear nucleus units (Fig. 10-32). The ISI histograms

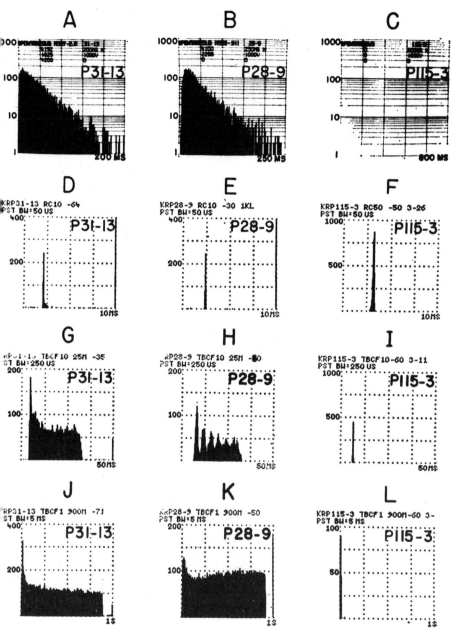

Fig. 10-31. Cat. Discharge patterns for three different units located either in the posteroventral cochlear nucleus or in the interstitial nucleus. A, B, and C. Semi-logarithmic plots of interspike interval histograms of spontaneous activity. D, E, and F. Post-stimulus time histograms of responses to rarefaction clicks. G, H, and I. Post-stimulus time histograms of responses to 25 msec tone bursts at the CF of the units. J, K, and L. Post-stimulus time histograms of responses to 900 msec. tone bursts at the CF of the units. (Kiang et al., 1965a) Reproduced with the permission of Dr. Kiang and Annals of Otology, Rhinology and Laryngology.

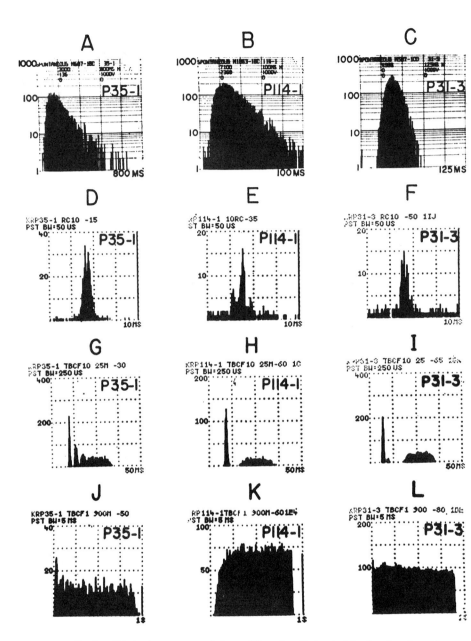

Fig. 10-32. Cat. Discharge patterns of three different units located in the dorsal cochlear nucleus. A, B, and C. Semi-logarithmic plots of interspike interval histograms of spontaneous activity. D, E, and F. Post-stimulus time histograms of responses to rarefaction clicks. G, H, and I. Post-stimulus time histograms of responses to 25 msec tone bursts at the CF of the units. J, K, and L. Post-stimulus time histograms of responses to 900 msec. tone bursts at the CF of the units. (Kiang *et al.*, 1965a) Reproduced with the permission of Dr. Kiang and *Annals of Otology, Rhinology and Laryngology*.

324

of spontaneous activity of DCN units have a variety of shapes. The ISI histogram modes of DCN units are usually longer than those of units in the VCN. The asymmetric ISI histograms never have decays from the mode that are faster than exponential, and they tend to be more symmetrical than those of VCN units. While spontaneous activity characterized by short mode (less than 12 msec.) histograms disappears in the VCN following cochlear destruction, no type of spontaneous activity is eliminated in the DCN. As mentioned previously, very few DCN units respond phasically to tonal stimuli and some display a chopper-type response to tone bursts. Some of those with chopper-type response at moderate levels of tone bursts respond with a pause-type response to higher stimulus levels. Units with a pause-type response to tone-burst stimuli are only found in the DCN.

SUPERIOR OLIVARY COMPLEX

The superior olivary complex receives input from the cells of the cochlear nuclear complex (Fig. 10-33). The superior olivary complex (SOC) consists of two distinctive nuclei and a number of less distinctive surrounding nuclei (Fig. 10-34). The two most prominent superior olivary nuclei are the lateral superior olive (LSO) or S-segment and the medial or accessory superior olive (MSO). The lateral superior olive appears S-shaped in cross section and the medial superior olive crescent-shaped. Surrounding these two nuclei are various trapezoid body nuclei and periolivary nuclei that are named according to their position relative to the lateral and medial superior olives. The medial nucleus of the trapezoid body or the medial trapezoid nucleus (MTB) is located within the fibers of the trapezoid body, medial to the medial superior olive. Located also within the fibers of the trapezoid body, ventral to the medial trapezoid nucleus and ventromedial to the medial superior olive, are the cells of the ventral nucleus of the trapezoid body (VTB), also called the medial or internal preolivary nucleus of Cajal. The lateral nucleus of the trapezoid body (LTB), also called the lateral or external preolivary nucleus, is located within the fibers of the trapezoid body ventral to the lateral superior olive. The posterior periolivary nucleus (PPO) is located caudal to the lateral superior olive and is often continuous with the caudal pole of the lateral trapezoid nucleus. The ventromedial periolivary nucleus (VMPO) is located near the ventrolateral border of the medial superior olive and is surrounded by the medial trapezoid nucleus medially and the ventral trapezoid nucleus ventrally. The ventrolateral periolivary

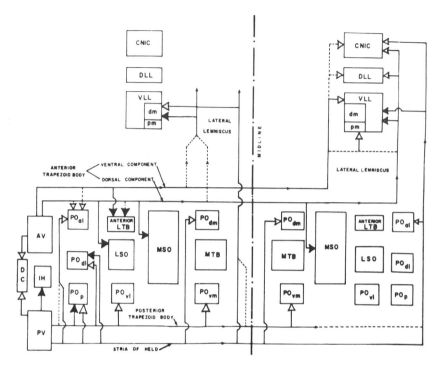

Fig. 10-33. Cat. A schematic representation of the output of the rostral pole of the anteroventral cochlear nucleus (AVCN) and the posteroventral cochlear nucleus (PVCN). The dotted lines indicate minor pathways. The abbreviations are as follows: CNIC: central nucleus of the inferior colliculus; DNLL: dorsal nucleus of the lateral lemniscus; VNLL: ventral nucleus of the lateral lemniscus; VNLLdm: dorsomedial part of the VNLL; VNLLpm: posteromedial part of the VNLL; POal: anterolateral periolivary nucleus; POdm: dorsomedial periolivary nucleus; POdl: dorsolateral periolivary nucleus; POp: posterior periolivary nucleus; POvm: ventromedial periolivary nucleus; LTB: lateral nucleus of the trapezoid body; MTB: medial nucleus of the trapezoid body; MSO: medial superior olivary nucleus; LSO; lateral superior olivary nucleus; AVCN; anteroventral cochlear nucleus; PVCN: posteroventral cochlear nucleus; DCN: dorsal cochlear nucleus; INSH: interstitial nucleus of stria of Held. (Warr, 1969) Courtesy of W. B. Warr, Boston University School of Medicine.

nucleus (VLPO) is a small group of cells located near the ventrolateral border of the lateral superior olive. The dorsomedial periolivary nucleus (DMPO) or retro-olivary nucleus is located dorsal to the medial trapezoid nucleus and the medial superior olive and extends laterally from the dorsal border of the medial trapezoid nucleus to the dorsomedial edge of the lateral superior olive. The dorsolateral periolivary nucleus (DLPO) is located dorsal to the lateral superior olive and extends laterally from the midportion of the lateral superior olive over its dorsolateral edge. The anterolateral periolivary nucleus (ALPO) appears rostral to the lateral superior olive and is continuous with the

dorsal border of the rostral lateral trapezoid nucleus.
More rostrally located nuclei also receive input and send output to the cochlear nuclear complex. The nuclei of the lateral leminscus consist of a ventral and dorsal division. The ventral nucleus of the lateral lemniscus (VLL) is continuous with the rostral pole of the lateral trapezoid nucleus and the anterolateral periolivary nucleus and extends dorsally and rostrally along the lateral lemniscus to the dorsal nucleus of the lateral lemniscus. The dorsal nucleus of the lateral lemniscus (DLL) is located dorsal to the rostral half of the ventral nucleus of the lateral lemniscus.

AXONS OF THE COCHLEAR NUCLEUS

Three fiber groups, the dorsal, intermediate, and ventral acoustic stria, contain fibers traveling to and from the cochlear nuclear complex (Fig. 10-33). The ventral acoustic stria or trapezoid body is the largest of the three. The fibers of the trapezoid body appear along the ventromedial border of the rostral two thirds of the ventral cochlear nucleus. These fibers travel rostrally and medially ventral to the inferior cerebellar peduncle and the spinal trigeminal tract and nucleus. The fibers of the trapezoid body travel through and below the superior olivary complex, forming a wide band of fibers that decussate dorsal to the pyramids. The intermediate acoustic stria appears as a compact bundle of fibers along the lateral border of the posteroventral cochlear nucleus that travels dorsally and is joined by the dorsal acoustic stria at the dorsal margin of the posteroventral cochlear nucleus. The fibers of the two striae continue to ascend between the dorsal cochlear nucleus and lateral surface of the inferior cerebellar peduncle. Upon reaching the dorsal surface of the peduncle, the fibers of the two striae separate. The fibers of the intermediate stria break up into small fascicles that travel ventrally along the medial surface of the peduncle, passing through the vestibular nuclear complex and the spinal trigeminal tract and nucleus. The fibers then take a medial course, passing through the homolateral superior olivary complex. They decussate just dorsal to the trapezoid body and enter the contralateral superior olivary complex and lateral lemniscus. The fibers of the dorsal acoustic stria form a compact bundle that takes a medial course through the vestibular nuclear complex and reticular formation. They cross the midline dorsally as a bundle of scattered fibers ventral to the medial longitudinal fasciculus and tectospinal tract and converge toward the contralateral superior olivary complex.

COCHLEAR NUCLEUS INPUT TO THE SUPERIOR OLIVARY COMPLEX

The axons of the dorsal cochlear nucleus appear to travel in the dorsal acoustic stria to the contralateral superior olivary complex, the nuclei of the lateral lemniscus, and the inferior colliculus (Stotler, 1953; Fernández and Karapas, 1967; van Noort, 1969). According to Fernández and Karapas (1967), a small number of fibers enter the homolateral superior olivary complex. After crossing, some of the fibers enter the dorsomedial and dorsolateral periolivary nuclei and the rostral lateral trapezoid nucleus of the contralateral superior olivary complex. The majority of the dorsal acoustic stria fibers join the contralateral lateral lemniscus on its medial aspect and terminate predominantly in the ventral nucleus of the lateral lemniscus. Some fibers continue into and terminate in the dorsal nucleus of the lateral lemniscus and the inferior colliculus (Fernández and Karapas, 1967; van Noort, 1969).

The cochlear nuclear fibers of the intermediate stria appear to arise from the caudal or octopus area of the posteroventral cochlear nucleus (Lorente de Nó, 1933b; Osen, 1969b; van Noort, 1969). Homolateral to the cells of origin, fibers of the intermediate stria arborize around cells within the posterior, dorsolateral, and anterolateral periolivary nuclei (Warr, 1969). These fibers provide input to only a fraction of the multipolar cells in the posterior periolivary nucleus. The input to the dorsolateral periolivary nucleus is greatest caudally and decreases rostrally. The input to the cells of the anterolateral periolivary nucleus is sparse, as is the input to the homolateral ventral nucleus of the lateral lemniscus. There is also an extremely sparse input to the dorsomedial periolivary nucleus prior to decussation. After decussating the stria penetrates the dorsomedial periolivary nucleus where a few fibers terminate. Rostrally the stria provides moderate input to the anterolateral periolivary nucleus and a large input to the ventral nucleus of the lateral lemniscus. At progressively more rostral levels, the input to the ventral nucleus of the lateral lemniscus decreases. None enter the dorsal nucleus of the lateral lemniscus, and a few enter the posterior inferior colliculus.

Other axons of the posterior two thirds of the posteroventral cochlear nucleus travel rostrally and join the caudal portion of the trapezoid body. According to Warr (1969), the fibers range in size from small to large and are scattered throughout the dorsoventral extent of the caudal trapezoid body. Ipsilateral to their origin, the posteroventral cochlear nuclear trapezoid fibers give off small bundles of fibers that terminate among cells of the posterior, dorsolateral, and ventrolateral periolivary nuclei. There is also a small input to the caudal pole of the ipsilateral ventromedial periolivary nucleus. These posteroventral cochlear nuclear trapezoid fibers represent a major input to the posterior periolivary nucleus, which also receives a smaller input from the posteroventral cochlear nuclear fibers of the intermediate acoustic stria. The posteroventral cochlear nuclear trapezoid fibers to the dorsolateral periolivary nucleus represent a minor input, its major input coming from posteroventral cochlear nuclear fibers in the intermediate acoustic stria. The posteroventral cochlear nuclear fibers in the trapezoid body send only minor inputs to the ventrolateral and ventromedial periolivary nuclei. The remaining fibers cross the midline within the decussation of the caudal one third of the trapezoid body. Most of the crossed fibers appear to terminate caudally within the contralateral ventromedial periolivary nucleus (Warr, 1969).

The rostral two thirds of the anteroventral cochlear nucleus send fibers into the rostral three fourths of the trapezoid body. The fibers from the anteroventral cochlear nucleus appear to separate into two groups: a dorsally located group of fibers twice the diameter and twice the number of a second, more ventrally, located group of fibers. While the dorsally located anteroventral cochlear nuclear fiber group occupies three fourths of the rostrocaudal extent of the trapezoid body, the ventrally located anteroventral cochlear nucleus fiber group occupies only one third of its rostral end. There is some evidence that the ipsilateral distribution of collateral and terminal fibers of the dorsal and ventral fiber groups may differ (Warr, 1966; 1969). The dorsal anteroventral cochlear nuclear fiber component appears to send a major input to the medial and lateral superior olive. The ventral component of the anteroventral cochlear nuclear trapezoid fibers appears to send a major input into the rostral third of the lateral trapezoid nucleas. Fibers from both dorsal and ventral anteroventral cochlear nuclear fiber groups also appear to project a major input to the ipsilateral dorsomedial portion of the ventral nucleus of the lateral lemniscus.

Trapezoid fibers of the dorsal anteroventral cochlear nucleus fiber group decussate in the dorsal part of the trapezoid body and send a major input into the contralateral medial superior olive. Fibers of the ventral anteroventral cochlear nuclear group decussate just dorsal to the pyramidal tract, bypass the superior olivary complex, and join the lateral lemniscus. Fibers from both the dorsal and ventral groups ascend in the lateral lemniscus and project a major input into the ventral nucleus of the lateral lemniscus and minor inputs into the dorsal nucleus of the lateral lemniscus and the inferior colliculus.

According to van Noort (1969), the cells of the central area of the ventral cochlear nucleus give rise to large diameter fibers that travel in the caudal half of the trapezoid body. Within the trapezoid body these fibers are located between the superficially located fine diameter fibers and the dorsally located medium-sized fibers. These large diameter fibers decussate without sending inputs to ipsilaterally located nuclei and terminate principally within the medial trapezoid nucleus. The rostral half of the medial trapezoid nucleus is reported to receive input from the caudal anteroventral cochlear nucleus, and the caudal half, from the rostral posteroventral cochlear nucleus (van Noort, 1969). Cells in the central area of the rat ventral cochlear nucleus, similar to the large globular cells of the cat, appear to give rise to large axons that terminate in the contralateral medial trapezoid nucleus in the form of large calyces of Held (Harrison and Irving, 1965; 1966; Harrison and Feldman, 1970).

Within the superior olivary complex the projections of the posterior two thirds of the posteroventral cochlear nucleus and the anterior two thirds of the anteroventral cochlear nucleus do not overlap (Fig. 10-33). The posteroventral cochlear nucleus projects exclusively to the periolivary nuclei, while the anteroventral cochlear nucleus projects to the medial and lateral superior olivary nuclei and the rostral part of the lateral trapezoid nucleus. The only area of overlap of projections is in the ipsilateral anterolateral periolivary nucleus. Within the nuclei of the lateral lemniscus, there is considerable overlap of projections of the anteroventral and posteroventral cochlear nuclei. Most fibers cross the midline to terminate in the contralateral nuclei of the lateral lemniscus. Major inputs are provided to the principal cell mass of the contralateral ventral nucleus of the lateral lemniscus by both anteroventral and posteroventral nuclei. Minor inputs are provided by these cochlear nuclei to the posteromedial portion of the ventral nucleus of the lateral lemniscus, the dorsal nucleus of the lateral lemniscus, and the inferior colliculus. Ipsilaterally only the dorsomedial portion of the ventral nucleus of the lateral lemniscus receives input from the cochlear nuclei. According to Warr (1969), the principal cell mass of the ventral nucleus of the lateral lemniscus is the only cell group of the nuclei of the lateral lemniscus to receive a massive convergence of heterogeneous inputs.

CELL TYPES OF NUCLEI OF THE SUPERIOR OLIVARY COMPLEX

The medial superior olive (MSO) extends longitudinally from the level of the rostral pole of the facial nucleus up to the level of the trigeminal motor nucleus. It is surrounded by a dense neuropile that separates it from the surrounding SOC nuclei (Fig. 10-34). The MSO is composed of a flat band of spindle-shaped cells arranged in three to four parallel layers (Stotler, 1953). Within the soma of the MSO neurons there are a variably centered nucleus and coarse to fine Nissl granules (Taber, 1961). The cell bodies are elongated with one or more dendrites extending horizontally from each pole of the cell body. These dendrites extend dorsolaterally and ventromedially into the surrounding dense neuropile. According to Osen (1969b), the cells of the MSO receive bilateral input via the trapezoid body from the large spherical cells of AVCN. The afferent preterminals form a bushlike formation around the dendrites and terminate as boutons along dendrites and cell body in an orderly fashion (Stotler, 1953). The majority of the terminals on the right pole of the MSO neuron appear to arise from the right cochlear nucleus and the majority of those on the left pole from the left cochlear nucleus (Stotler,

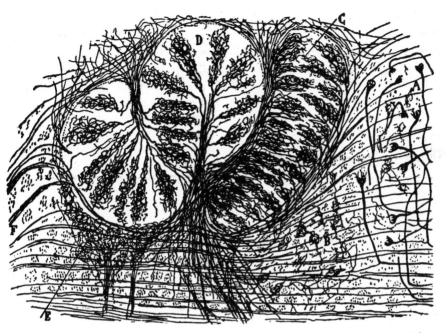

Fig. 10-34. Cat. Nerve arborizations in the superior olivary complex of cat as seen in Golgi-stained cross section of the cat's brain stem. A, medial nucleus of trapezoid body; B, ventral nucleus of trapezoid body; C, medial superior olivary nucleus; D, lateral superior olivary nucleus; E, lateral nucleus of trapezoid body; F, trapezoid body fibers. (Ramón y Cajal, 1909)

1953; Warr, 1966). Ventrolateral areas of the AVCN (low-frequency areas) project to dorsal areas of MSO, while more dorsomedial areas (higher-frequency areas) project ventrally (Warr, 1966).

The lateral superior olive (LSO) first appears caudally just rostral to the caudal pole of the MSO, and extends rostrally to the level of exit of the facial root fibers. The LSO is composed of a plate of cells several layers thick that is folded into an S-shaped configuration. The medial limb or loop of the S-shaped nucleus has a greater rostrocaudal extent than does its lateral limb; the former extending approximately three quarters the length of the MSO, the latter only one-half (Papez, 1930). There appear to be three types of cells within the LSO. The most frequently observed are spindle-shaped cells that appear to be similar in shape to the cells of the MSO (Ramón y Cajal, 1904; Stotler, 1953; Taber, 1961). The cell body of this type of neuron contains an eccentric nucleus and coarse, intensely straining Nissl granules (Taber, 1961). These cells possess large polar dendrites that take a longitudinal course. Intermingled with these spindle-shaped cells are smaller, fusiform cells containing moderately staining cytoplasm (Taber, 1961). Taber (1961) also mentioned observing a small number of "typical motor type neurons."

According to Ramon y Cajal (1904), there are multipolar cells located along the contours of the LSO, which he called the marginal cells. Most of the marginal cells possess dendrites that do not enter the LSO.

The LSO is surrounded by a dense neuropile that appears to arise primarily from medium-sized fibers of the trapezoid body (Ramon y Cajal, 1904). These fibers enter through the hilus and along the convex surface of the LSO. Two or more preterminal fibers form a bushlike formation that surrounds four or more LSO neurons (Ramón y Cajal, 1904). These fibers terminate as boutons along the dendrites and cell body of LSO neurons (Stotler, 1953). The LSO receives input from the homolateral AVCN (Warr, 1966) or, more specifically, according to Osen (1969b), from the small spherical cells of the AVCN. Cells in the ventrolateral area of AVCN (low frequency) project to the lateral limb of the LSO and cells in more dorsomedial areas of AVCN project to more medial areas of LSO (Warr, 1966). A second input from the homolateral MTB has been described by Rasmussen (1967). Because the MTB receives input from the contralateral cochlear nucleus, this second input to LSO represents input from the contralateral ear.

The medial nucleus of the trapezoid body (MTB) extends throughout most of the length of the SOC. The MTB is located medial to the MSO among the fibers of the trapezoid body. Its dorsal and lateral boundaries fuse with the dorsomedial periolivary nucleus (DMPO) and the ventral nucleus of the trapezoid body (VTB). The cells of the MTB have been described in some detail by Morest (1968). The most numerous are the principal neurons that have a spherical or oval cell body containing an eccentric nucleus and fine Nissl substance. Two to four short dendrites extend from the cell body in a horizontal direction. The cell body of the principal neuron makes contact with a single calyx of Held while the dendrites are surrounded by endings of a peri-dendritic plexus. The elongate neuron has an oval cell body a bit smaller than the principal neuron that contains a central nucleus and coarser Nissl substance. Four to five long dendrites extend from the cell body in a dorsoventral direction. Axonal endings on the elongate neurons appear to arise from sparsely branched collaterals of axons passing through the MTB. The third cell type, the stellate neuron, may correspond to the multipolar cells described by Taber (1961). Its cell body is larger than that of the principal neuron and its large dendrites radiate in many directions. Within the cell body the nucleus is centrally placed, and thin Nissl granules appear as darkly stained tigroid substance. A network of fine, short terminals with numerous small boutons envelope the cell body and dendrites of stellate neurons. The cells of the MTB have been reported to receive terminals from the large caliber fibers located between the superficial fine fibers and the deep medium-sized fibers of the trapezoid body (van Noort, 1969). According to van Noort (1969), these fibers arise from the contralateral caudal AVCN and rostral PVCN. Warr (1966; 1969) did not observe cells in MTB receiving terminals from either the rostral AVCN or caudal PVCN.

NEUROPHYSIOLOGY OF THE SUPERIOR OLIVARY COMPLEX

Only those single unit studies of the SOC will be considered in which the location of the units studied were determined histologically. Guinan (1968) recorded from single units in the SOC and NLL and classified them in terms of such response characteristics as waveform of the spike potential, various discharge measures to tone- and noise-burst stimuli, and type of response (excitation or inhibition) elicited by stimulating the ipsilateral and contralateral ear. Over half of the units studied were located in the MTB; the rest were located in the surrounding nuclei. Units generating spike potentials of complex waveform, similar to that generated by units in the AVCN, were located almost exclusively within the MTB where calyces-type endings are also found. Most of the units that discharge only at the off-set of the stimulus were also located in or around the MTB. Units that respond tonically during the stimulus were located throughout the SOC and included all MTB units with complex spike waveform and approximately half the MTB units with simple spike waveform. In general, units excited by stimulation of the ear contralateral to them were located medial to the MSO, while units excited by stimulation of the ipsilateral ear were located lateral to the MSO.

MEDIAL NUCLEUS OF THE TRAPEZOID BODY

Approximately three types of units are found in the MTB. The largest group is composed of MTB units that generate spikes of complex waveform (class 1 units). Class 1 units were found only within the MTB. Because the waveform of the spike potential resembles that of AVCN neurons receiving calyces of Held endings, Guinan suggests that the class 1 units may be the principal neuron of the MTB that Morest (1968) described as receiving calyx-type terminals. Some of these class 1 MTB units appear to be spontaneously active, and all respond with tonic discharge to stimulation of the contralateral ear. Compared with tuning curves of other groups of SOC units, the tuning curves of these MTB units are relatively narrow. In general, class 1 MTB units with high CF are located ventromedially, those with low CF, dorsolaterally. Other types of MTB units do not appear to be organized with respect to CF. The discharge pattern of class 1 MTB units to tone-burst stimuli are of the primary or pause type. Low CF class 1 MTB units produce phase-locked spike discharge to low-frequency stimuli and multiple-peaked click PST histograms whose peak intervals are related to the CF of the unit.

The discharge of class 1 MTB units to a continuous CF tone is irregular and produces a skewed ISI histogram.

A second group of MTB units, class 2, generates spikes of simple waveform and discharges only to the offset of stimulation of the contralateral ear. These units do not appear to be spontaneously active. Most class 2 units respond with a short burst of spikes to stimulus offset, while a few respond with transient increase in discharge that decays slowly to spontaneous levels. Class 2 neurons are also found in the DMPO, where neurons similar to the stellate and elongate neurons of the MTB are located.

A third group of MTB units (class 4) generates spikes of simple waveform and discharges tonically to stimulation of the contralateral ear.. Although most of these units respond only to stimulation of the contralateral ear, a few also respond to stimulation of the ipsilateral ear. Class 4 MTB units made up approximately 29 percent of the total number of SOC units with class 4 response characteristics. Other class 4 units were located in the trapezoid body, VTB, and NLL. Because data were grouped for all class 4 units regardless of histological location, the response characteristics of MTB class 4 units cannot be described separately. Some class 4 units displayed spontaneous activity, while others were silent. Some units were narrowly tuned, while others responded to a relatively broad band of frequencies. The PST histograms produced by tone-burst stimuli varied from the on type, pause type, chopper type, to primary type. Some low CF units produced phase-locked discharge to low-frequency stimuli. The discharge to continuous tones for class 4 units fell into two categories: Most of the units had irregular discharge that produced a skewed ISI histogram, while the others had regular discharge that produced more symmetric ISI histograms.

MEDIAL SUPERIOR OLIVE

Many investigators have presented data from units reported to be localized in or around the MSO, as determined by the gross potential response elicited by click stimuli (Moushegian *et al.*, 1964a, b; Rupert *et al.*, 1965; Hall, 1965; Clark and Dunlap, 1969). The gross potential responses elicited by click, noise-burst, or tone-burst stimuli have been demonstrated to reverse polarity in the region of the MSO cell layer (Galambos *et al.*, 1959; Tsuchitani and Boudreau, 1964). However, the click evoked potential is complex in shape, and often different components of the response reverse polarity at different positions around the MSO cell layer. Therefore the results of studies in which the polarity reversal of the click potential was used to classify units as MSO units without determining histologically if the polarity reversal was actually located within the MSO in the animals from which single unit data were collected will not be reviewed.

According to Guinan, Norris, and Swift (1967) and Guinan (1968), who localized units in the MSO histologically, single units in the MSO of cat are extremely difficult to isolate. These investigators utilized platinum-tipped, metal-filled pipettes, fluid-filled pipettes, and stainless steel microelectrodes. Of the few MSO units Guinan (1968) was successful in isolating, with a 50 percent degree of certainty or greater, there were some units that discharged to stimulation of either ear. Others discharged to stimulation of the ipsilateral ear and were inhibited by stimulation of the contralateral ear at certain stimulus levels and excited at others. A few units were excited only by stimulation of one ear, with stimulation of the opposite ear having no effects. Most of the units encountered in the MSO had CFs below 10.0 kHz (Guinan, 1968).

LATERAL SUPERIOR OLIVE

The LSO appears to be comprised of one type of unit that (1) generates spikes of simple waveform, (2) responds tonically to noise and tonal stimuli, and (3) depending upon unit CF, is only excited by stimulation of the ipsilateral ear, or is excited by stimulation of the ipsilateral ear and inhibited by stimulation of the contralateral ear (Guinan, 1968). Units in the LSO are typically without spontaneous activity: Only 13 percent of the LSO units encountered by Boudreau and Tsuchitani (1970) exhibited discharge in the absence of experimenter-controlled acoustic stimuli. The spontaneous rates are reported to vary from one or two spikes/sec. to much higher rates. Occurrence of spontaneous activity does not appear to be related to unit CF; the CF's of units discharging spontaneously varied from 0.6 to 38.0 kHz. The temporal pattern of spontaneous discharges of LSO units has not been described.

LSO UNIT RESPONSE TO STIMULATION OF THE IPSILATERAL EAR

According to Boudreau and Tsuchitani (1970), LSO units respond either tonically or phasically, with only stimulation of the ipsilateral ear being excitatory. The units discharging in a phasic fashion to onset of the stimulus are described to be injured cells discharging abnormally. The "normal" LSO unit responds to a monaural tone or noise burst with a transient high discharge rate at stimulus onset that drops to a lower rate. Following the initial fairly rapid drop in discharge, the discharge tends to continue to decrease, but at a slower rate, for many minutes of stimulation. When the fine detail of temporal pattern of discharge is examined, the discharges of LSO units with high CF appear to be time-locked to the onset of the stimulus. With short bin times, the discharges of LSO units to tonal stimuli produce chopper-type PST histograms. Low CF units appear to produce discharges that are phase-locked to the individual cycles of the low frequency tonal stimulus.

The monaural tuning curves of LSO units are similar to those of cochlear nerve fibers and cochlear nuclear units. They are U or V shaped, with CF's ranging from below 0.2 kHz to over 40.0 kHz. The units of the LSO are tonotopically organized, with high CF units localized in the ventromedial limb of the S-shaped nucleus and low CF units in the dorsolateral limb (Fig. 10-35). Units with intermediate CF's are localized between, in an orderly and progressive arrangement following the contour of the nucleus (Tsuchitani and Boudreau, 1966). As in the case of the cochlear nerve, threshold differences between LSO units with similar CF's from individual cats are not greater than thirty dB and most often are less than 20 dB (Boudreau and Tsuchitani, 1970).

When LSO tuning curves are normalized by converting stimulus frequency into octave units from CF, the curves of units with CF above about four kHz appear very similar. The average bandwidth of frequencies to which LSO units are responsive at 20 dB above CF threshold is approximately 0.4 octaves for units with CF above three kHz. For units with lower CF, tuning-curve bandwidth decreases from approximately two octaves to 0.4 octave as

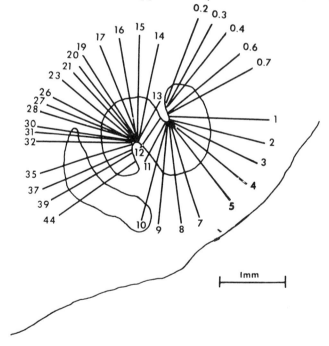

Fig. 10-35. Cat. The tonotopic organization of the cat lateral superior olive. (Tsuchitani and Boudreau, 1966)

CF increases. The slopes of straight lines fitted to the linear portion of the high and low-frequency limbs of the normalized tuning curves also do not appear to differ much for units with CF above four kHz. The mean value of the slopes of the straight lines fitted to the high-frequency limbs is 215 dB/octave. The mean value for the low-frequency limb is 110 dB/octave. As indicated by the bandwidth data, units with lower CF have wider tuning curves and slower rates of change in threshold per octave increase in frequency.

The discharge of LSO units to monaural tonal stimuli increases as the stimulus level is increased up to some maximum discharge rate (Tsuchitani and Boudreau, 1967). Most units generate monotonic intensity functions to two hundred msec duration CF tone bursts (Fig. 10-36). The maximum discharge rates of CF intensity functions range in value from less than 10 spikes/sec. to over six hundred spikes/sec. (Boudreau and Tsuchitani, 1970). The dynamic ranges of the CF intensity functions vary from 15 to fifty dB. Neither maximum rate of discharge nor dynamic range appear to be related to unit CF. Low threshold units tend to have higher maximum rates and greater dynamic ranges than high threshold units.

The intensity functions produced with two hundred msec tone bursts at stimulus frequencies other than CF differ for frequencies above and below CF (Fig. 10-36). With stimulus frequency set near CF, the maximum

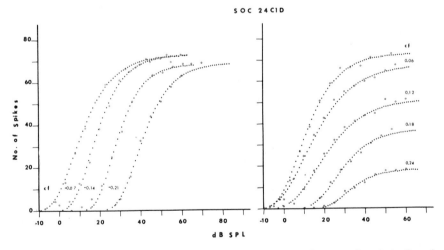

Fig. 10-36. Cat. Intensity functions measured for a lateral superior olive unit when the ipsilateral ear is stimulated with tone bursts at frequency equal to unit CF (cf) or at other frequencies. Stimulus frequency is indicated in terms of octave units from the CF. Tone-burst duration 200 msec. Each CF and non-CF intensity function has been fitted with a Gompertz curve. Right: Intensity functions with stimulus frequency higher than CF. Left: Intensity functions with stimulus frequency lower than CF. (Boudreau and Tsuchitani, 1970)

discharge elicited is near that elicited by the CF tone. As the stimulus frequency is raised, the maximum rate decreases rapidly and appears to do so at similar rates for units with CF greater than four kHz (Tsuchitani and Boudreau, 1967). According to Boudreau and Tsuchitani (1970), the magnitude of the maximum discharge, expressed as percentage of maximum discharge to CF tone, decreases 29 percent per 0.1 octave increase in stimulus frequency. The rate of decrease in maximum rate appears to be lower for units with CF below four kHz (Tsuchitani and Boudreau, 1967). The maximum discharge does not appear to change appreciably for stimulus frequencies below CF, for both low and high CF units. The dynamic ranges of non-CF intensity functions tend to decrease progressively as the stimulus frequency is increased or decreased from CF.

When CF and non-CF intensity functions of units with CF's above 4 kHz are normalized by expressing discharge as percentage of the unit's maximum discharge to CF tone, the functions appear very similar in shape. Boudreau and Tsuchitani (1970) report that these intensity functions could be fitted by the Gompertz function:

$$S = Mg^{h^x}$$

where S is the number of spikes elicited, M is the maximum discharge, h and g are parameters determined from the data, and x is stimulus level in dB above threshold. The median values obtained by fitting 99 CF intensity functions were utilized to describe an "average" intensity function.

LSO UNIT RESPONSE TO BINAURAL TONES

Simultaneous presentation of a tone to the contralateral ear does not affect the discharge of LSO units to tones presented to the ipsilateral ear, if the unit has CF below about 1.0 kHz. The discharge of higher CF units to ipsi-laterally presented stimuli can be inhibited by simultaneous stimulation of the contralateral ear (Galambos *et al.*, 1959; Goldberg *et al.*, 1963; Boudreau and Tsuchitani, 1968; Guinan, 1968). The inhibitory effect is tonic with stimuli two hundred msec in duration.

The discharge elicited by stimulation of the ipsilateral ear with a CF tone can be inhibited only by simultaneous stimulation of the contralateral ear with a tone burst of proper frequency and level or by noise (Boudreau and Tsuchitani, 1968). The inhibitory tuning curve describes the stimulus frequencies and threshold stimulus levels of tones presented to the contra-lateral ear that are capable of inhibiting a single spike discharge elicited by a CF tone presented to the ipsilateral ear (Fig. 10-37). The inhibitory tuning curve of a unit appears to be similar in shape to the excitatory tuning curve, as determined by stimulating the ipsilateral ear alone (Boudreau and Tsuchitani, 1968; 1970). The CF's of the inhibitory and excitatory tuning

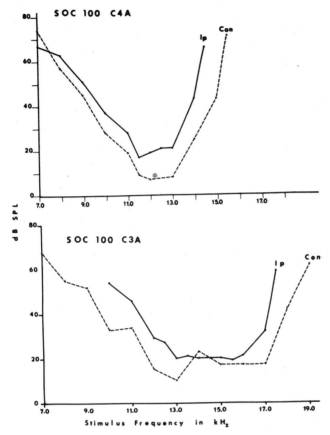

Fig. 10-37. Cat. Ipsilateral excitatory (Ip) and contralateral inhibitory (Con) tuning curves measured for two lateral superior olive units. The inhibitory tuning curves were measured by determining the stimulus levels at which different frequencies presented to the contralateral ear inhibit a one spike discharge elicited by an ipsilateral CF tone. (Boudreau and Tsuchitani, 1970)

curves tend to be similar, and their CF thresholds tend to be equal. The inhibitory tuning curves are slightly wider than the excitatory tuning curves. The average value of the slopes of straight lines fitted to the high-frequency limbs of inhibitory tuning curves is 192 dB/octave, for tuning curves with CF above four kHz. The average value for the low-frequency limb of these high CF tuning curves is ninety-three dB/octave.

The effect of increasing the level of the contralateral tone is to increase the reduction in discharge elicited by stimulating the ipsilateral ear (Tsuchitani and Boudreau, 1969). To study the effects of contralateral CF stimulus level on discharge, a family of binaural intensity functions were generated (Fig.

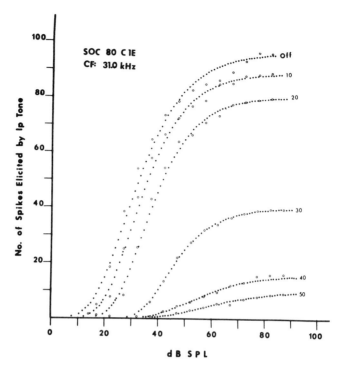

Fig. 10-38. Cat. A family of binaural CF intensity functions for a single lateral superior olive unit. The stimulus level of the contralateral tone was set at the fixed levels indicated on each curve (Off, ten, twenty, etc.) and the stimulus level of the simultaneously presented ipsilateral tone was varied in five dB steps. Each binaural intensity function has been fitted with a Gompertz curve. Stimulus frequency was set to CF of the unit. Tone bursts two hundred msec duration. (Boudreau and Tsuchitani, 1970)

10-38). Each binaural intensity function was generated by setting the contralateral tone at a fixed level and counting discharge as a function of ipsilateral stimulus level increased in five dB steps. Following the acquisition of one binaural intensity function, the stimulus level of the contralateral tone was increased 10 dB and another binaural intensity function was determined. Families of binaural intensity functions were thus generated (Fig. 10-38). As the level of the contralateral tone was increased, maximum discharge to the binaural stimulus decreased progressively. Binaural maximum discharge, expressed as percentage of maximum discharge to a monaural CF tone, decreases linearly at a rate of 2.3 percent per one dB increase in the level of the contralateral tone. The stimulus level of a CF tone delivered to the ipsilateral ear necessary to elicite a five-spike discharge increased linearly as the level of the contralateral tone was increased up to forty-five dB above the contralateral threshold. This binaural five-spike threshold, expressed as dB change from threshold to stimulation of the ipsilateral ear alone, increased at a rate of 0.68 dB per one dB increase in the level of the contralateral tone. Similar results occur when the frequency of the binaural stimulus was set to values other than CF; that is, maximum discharge decreased and five-spike threshold increased as the contralateral stimulus level was increased. Binaural CF and non-CF intensity functions were also fitted with the Gompertz function (Boudreau and Tsuchitani, 1970).

LSO UNIT POPULATION DISCHARGE

Using some of the average unit discharge measures just described, Boudreau and Tsuchitani (1970) have developed a descriptive model of LSO population discharge to monaural and binaural acoustic stimuli. The response properties incorporated into the model unit include tuning curves (threshold functions) as described by average slope values of straight lines fitted to individual tuning curve data, and intensity functions as described by the average intensity function. Also incorporated into the model were (1) the threshold function describing the relationship between the contralateral inhibiting tone level and the ipsilateral threshold shift; (2) the function describing the rate of change in maximum discharge of non-CF intensity functions with increases in stimulus frequency above CF; and (3) the function describing the decrease in maximum discharge as the contralateral stimulus level is increased.

With this model the distribution of population discharge in the LSO under various stimulus conditions was described. The model population consists of cellular elements (model units) that differ only with respect to CF; threshold differences between elements with different CF are ignored. The response of the model population to a monaurally presented 12 kHz tone is illustrated in Fig. 10-39. When the stimulus level is near threshold, the distribution of activity is centered over the elements with CF near 12 kHz. As stimulus level is increased, discharge of elements initially activated increases up to a limiting value. Accompanying this increase in discharge is a recruitment of elements with CF higher and lower than the 12 kHz stimulus frequency. The recruitment is not symmetrical; elements with CF lower than the stimulus tone are recruited at a slower rate than elements with higher CF. Also, the rate of increase in discharge is slower for elements with CF lower than the stimulus tone. Thus, the resulting distribution of activity is asymmetrical, with greater changes occurring for elements with CF greater than the stimulus frequency. As stimulus level is increased, one end of the distribution becomes anchored over low CF elements, while the spread of activity over the high CF elements continues. Stimulus level increases result in an increase

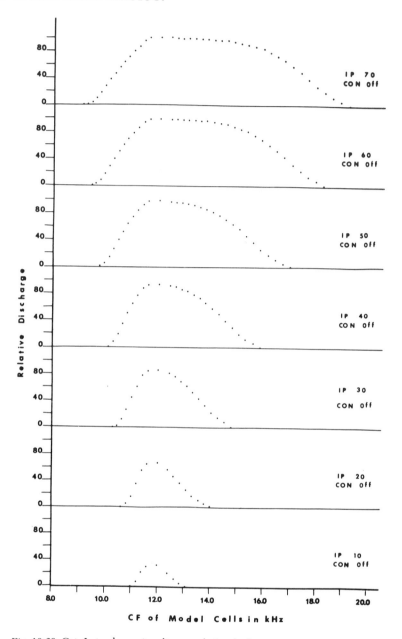

Fig. 10-39. Cat. Lateral superior olive population discharge to a monaural ipsilateral twelve kHz tone as a function of stimulus level. Elements of the model olive are represented by their CF. Discharge level of elements with different CFs predicted by a descriptive model. Stimulus level in decibels above threshold of elements with CF equal to twelve kHz. (Boudreau and Tsuchitani, 1970)

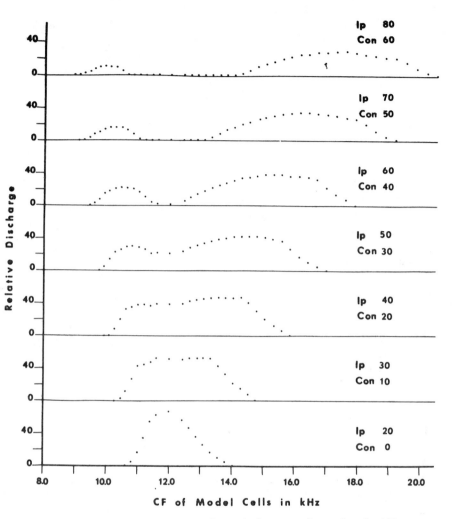

Fig. 10-40. Cat. Lateral superior olive population discharge to a binaural twelve kHz tone as a function of binaural stimulus level. Elements of the model LSO population are represented by their CF. Stimulus level in decibels above threshold of elements with CF equal to twelve kHz. At all stimulus levels, there is an interaural intensity difference of twenty dB. (Boudreau and Tsuchitani, 1970)

in the range of CF's of elements discharging maximally, so that at high stimulus levels the model LSO population appears to be broadly tuned.

Under conditions simulating binaural stimulation with tones of equal frequency but different magnitudes, the distribution of activity across the model LSO population is quite different from that under monaural stimulus conditions. The distribution of activity across the model LSO population generated by a binaural tone 12 kHz in frequency, with the ipsilateral level always 20 dB greater than the contralateral level, is presented in Fig. 10-40. The distribution of activity with binaural stimulation resembles that of monaural stimulation only at low binaural stimulus levels. As the binaural stimulus level is increased, elements with CF equal to the stimulus frequency begin to decrease discharge, while elements with CF further from the stimulus frequency become activated by the binaural tone. As the binaural stimulus level is increased to higher levels, the discharge of elements with CF similar to the stimulus frequency reaches zero and the area of decreased activity spreads to elements with CF near the stimulus frequency. The resulting distribution of activity is bimodal, with a narrow peak of activity corresponding to elements with CF below the stimulus frequency and a broad peak of activity corresponding to elements with CF greater than the stimulus frequency. Still further increases in the binaural stimulus level results in a continued spread of decreased activity, with the two peaks of activity moving farther and farther apart.

The distribution of monaurally evoked activity illustrated in Fig. 10-39 would probably not occur unless the cat were functionally deaf in one ear. Interaural intensity differences depend upon the orientation of the head and ears of the cat with respect to the sound source and the frequency of the sound source (Wiener et al., 1965). With the pinna in its normal position, interaural intensity differences as great as 20 dB can occur (Fig. 10-6).

SUMMARY

The structure and function of the cat's auditory system is better understood than any of the other sensory systems covered in this book. Carefully controlled experimental and stimulus conditions have provided quantitative data that are reliable and representative of the preparations utilized. Psychophysical studies have provided information concerning the capabilities of the cat and human auditory systems. The transform characteristics of the outer and middle ear of the cat have been quantitatively described and modeled (Wiener et al., 1965; Guinan and Peake, 1967). Although Békésy's studies of cochlear partition motion to high-intensity, low-frequency sinusoidal stimuli provide quantitative measures of some cochlear mechanics, the transfer function of the inner ear is not known (Békésy, 1960). At the present time it is not known what aspects of mechanical motion of the various structures in the inner ear are directly relevant to the transfer of sound energy from the middle ear to the sensory receptor cells. Even less is known about the transform characteristics of the cat auditory receptor cell. A major source of difficulties is that the techniques for recording from receptor cells in a normally functioning organ of Corti are not developed to a satisfactory state. Thus, at present the function of the inner ear can only be studied in combination with that of the cochlear nerve fibers; that is, in terms of an input signal as specified by stapes motion (the middle ear output) and an output recorded from the cochlear nerve.

Neuroanatomical studies have provided a structural basis for identifying and classifying neuron types within neural structures. They have also provided the "wiring diagram" of the system, indicating the structure of the interconnections of neurons within the auditory system. Differences in the morphology of neurons within a neural structure and in the interconnections made by neurons should serve as a warning to neurophysiologists that possible functional differences may also exist. Thus, the studies of Spoendlin (1966) on the afferent innervation of the cat organ of Corti indicate that Kiang and his associates are missing a segment of the population of cochlear nerve fibers, possibly due to recording electrode bias. Anatomical studies of the cochlear nuclear complex and superior olivary complex indicate that these neural structures are complexes of subnuclei that differ with respect to the types and arrangements of terminal endings and cells. Although the functional significance of these differences is not known, no systematic study of these structures can afford to ignore the existence of these differences. Unless care is taken to determine systematically the response characteristics of neurons sampled, these structures will appear to consist of heterogeneous populations that cannot be characterized in terms of the response measures taken. An investigator may be forced to report that there exist more types of units in these structures than can possibly be classified and that every cell is different. When the responses are studied systematically and when locations of the neurons studied are determined histologically or electrophysiologically, functional and anatomical data can be correlated and neurons classified, as in the case of the studies of Kiang and associates on the cochlear nuclear complex and of Tsuchitani and Boudreau, and Guinan on the superior olivary complex.

Recent advances in stimulus control, recording techniques, and data processing of single unit spike discharges have enabled the quantitative description of single unit responses. The discharges of single units in the cat cochlear nerve to simple auditory stimuli (tone bursts or clicks) and to more complex stimuli (two tones or tone and electrical stimulation of the efferent olivocochlear bundle) have been described quantitatively by Kiang and his associates. The response characteristics of the sampled cochlear nerve fibers indicate that the population of fibers sampled is homogeneous with differences in response pattern related to the characteristic frequency of the fiber. Thus, if the characteristic frequency of the fiber is known, one can predict certain aspects of the discharge of the fiber to tonal or click stimuli. Similarly, the statistical characteristics of spontaneous activity of cochlear nerve fibers indicate that the population of nerve fibers sampled is homogeneous. In contrast, single unit studies of the cochlear nuclear complex by

Kiang and associates indicate that the cochlear nuclear complex consists of a population of heterogeneous units with respect to spontaneous-activity patterns and response characteristics to click and tonal stimuli. The differences in the response characteristics of cochlear nerve fibers and cochlear nuclear units indicate that recoding of stimulus information occurs at the level of the cochlear nucleus. The heterogeneity of the response characteristics of cochlear nucleus units indicate that this recoding takes various forms. The cochlear nuclear complex appears to consist of a number of different functional types or sets of neurons, each of which transforms the incoming cochlear nerve fiber inputs in a different manner. The cochlear nuclear complex is the first station where sensory information carried by the cochlear nerve is recoded, probably with different properties of the auditory stimulus represented by the outputs of different types of cochlear nuclear units.

Because the afferent connections of the cochlear nuclear complex with the superior olivary complex have been described in some detail, the input to neurons in the superior olivary complex that arise from the cochlear nucleus can be specified. The neurons of the medial nucleus of the trapezoid body (MTB) receive input from the central area of the contralateral ventral cochlear nucleus. MTB units that Guinan (1968) calls class 1 units respond similarly to the "primarylike" units of the ventral cochlear nucleus. However, it is not known if the primarylike units of the central area of the ventral cochlear nucleus terminate upon these class 1 MTB cells. Guinan believes that because the class 1 MTB units produce spikes with waveforms similar to cochlear nucleus neurons receiving calyces of Held, class 1 cells are the primary neurons of the MTB that Morest (1968) described as receiving calyx-type endings. Neurons of the lateral superior olive receive ipsilateral inputs from the anteroventral cochlear nucleus (AVCN) and contralateral inputs most likely from the homolateral medial trapezoid nucleus. The response characteristics of AVCN neurons differ from those of neurons in other divisions of the cochlear nuclear complex and from those of the neurons in the MTB. The neurons of the AVCN and MTB do appear to be similar in the type of ending found in these nuclei (end bulbs or calyces of Held), and in the waveform of the spike potential generated (Guinan, 1968). The response characteristics of lateral superior olivary (LSO) neurons differ from those of both AVCN and MTB neurons. The tone-burst produced spike trains of AVCN neurons generate primarylike PST histograms, those of class 1 MTB units generate primarylike and pause-type PST histograms, while LSO units produce chopper-type PST histograms to monaurally presented tones. Simultaneous activation of the "contralateral" MTB input to the LSO with tones of appropriate frequency and amplitude can completely inhibit the discharge elicited by stimulating the ipsilateral AVCN inputs to LSO for LSO units with CF above 1.0 kHz. Perhaps because the AVCN input is excitatory and the MTB input inhibitory, very few units of the LSO display spontaneous activity. Neurophysiological data indicate that low CF LSO units do not receive an inhibitory contralateral input. Detailed anatomical studies of the MTB input to the LSO have not been described for the cat.

The value of the systems analysis approach to sensory systems and the value of knowledge of the neuroanatomical structure of sensory systems are most obvious in the study of the auditory system. The systems analysis approach was used in investigating and describing the transform characteristics of the receptor organ. Although the transfer functions of the inner ear and auditory receptor cells are not known, the transfer function (stimulus-response characteristics) of the peripheral sensory component, consisting of the inner ear, receptor cell, and cochlear nerve fiber, has been investigated. Because the response characteristics of cochlear nerve fibers can be quantitatively described, the input to the cochlear nuclear units can be specified for certain stimulus conditions. Because the response characteristics of certain cochlear nucleus units can be specified and because the connections of these units with units in the superior olivary complex have been described, the transfer functions of neurons in the superior olivary complex can be and have been investigated. Because little is known about the response characteristics of superior olivary complex neurons and about the afferent connections of higher-order auditory neurons, the inputs to higher-order neurons cannot be specified and the transfer functions of these neurons cannot be investigated directly.

11
THE VISUAL SYSTEM

Visible objects within the cat's environment consist of radiant sources and reflecting surfaces that emit or reflect light. Light, which effectively stimulates visual receptors, is a form of electromagnetic radiation of which the visible spectrum forms a very narrow band (390 to 760 millimicrons). Light may be emitted from a source, such as the sun or an incandescent light bulb, or reflected off surfaces. Objects are perceived when they emit or reflect light that differs in level or wavelength (for some animals) from the immediate surround. The level of light emitted from a radiant source is measured in photometric units of luminous intensity (lumens). The amount of light falling upon a surface (surface illumination) is expressed in units of illuminance (lumen/sq. m or in millilamberts/sq. m—mL/sq. m). The amount of light reflected from an illuminated surface is expressed in units of luminance (candles/sq. m—cd/sq. m). The amount of light illuminating the retina is measured in units of trolands (td). The wavelengths of visible light extend from above that of ultraviolet to below infrared radiation. The subjective color of an object is determined by the wavelengths of light that it reflects. Not all animals appear to be capable of appreciating differences in the wavelengths of light reflected by an object; that is, not all animals can perceive color differences (Walls, 1942).

The eye is an optical device that functions to gather and organize light energy such that an image is produced upon the photoreceptive surface of an organism. The mammalian eye is a versatile instrument that functions under a wide range of illumination levels. It can focus upon near and far objects and extracts various attributes from the light world such as object form, distance, movement, and in some cases, color. The type of eye an animal possesses is most closely related to its activity pattern, for different optical and receptor properties are required for visual perception under low and high illumination levels. The structure of the eye of nocturnal animals is quite distinct from that of diurnal animals, regardless of the family or genus of the animals.

The cat is an arhythmic animal, being active either during the day or night. As a carnivore, a cat must adapt his activity pattern to those of the species upon which it preys. In hunting at night, the cat uses his large cornea and pupil and a highly reflective tapetum within the eye to make maximum use of the light available at low illumination levels. However, the cat can also function effectively under high illumination conditions because his eye has developed other features that restrict retinal illumination and prevent overstimulation of the eye. As in most predatory animals, the eyes of the cat are positioned frontally, giving it a large binocular field and providing depth perception cues.

Because we cannot communicate verbally with cats, we do not know how the visual world appears to the cat. However, behavioral studies can provide clues to some of the aspects of the visual world the cat can perceive. Behavioral studies indicate that cats can make brightness discriminations (Mead, 1942; Thorn, 1970), can perceive stationary and moving objects (Kennedy and Smith, 1935; Smith, 1936), can discriminate between different patterns (Voneida and Robinson, 1970), and probably can make wavelength discriminations (Mello and Peterson, 1964; Sechzer and Brown, 1964).

ANATOMY OF THE EYE

The structure of the eye of the cat is similar to that of most mammals. The eyeball or globe of the eye is spherical in shape and is located within the bony orbit surrounded by connective tissue and orbital fat. The ocular muscles, which control the position and movement of the eyes, attach to the outer wall of the globe. The exposed portion of the eye is covered by the conjunctiva, a delicate mucous membrane that passes under the inner surfaces of the eyelids. The surface of the conjunctiva is kept lubricated and clean by the secretions of the lacrimal gland.

In addition to the upper and lower eyelids, the cat (unlike the human) possesses a prominent third eyelid, the nictitating membrane (Fig. 11-1). The nictitating membrane appears to function to protect the eye from irritating agents, for it will protrude rapidly and cover the eye when the cornea is mechanically stimulated (Rosenblueth and Bard, 1932). The nictitating membrane is capable of extending at least two thirds the distance across the cornea of the eye. Normally, this membrane is reflected back into the inner margin of the eye when the eye is opened. When the eye is closed, the retractor bulbi, an extraocular muscle not evident in man, withdraws the globe into the orbit and causes the nictitating membrane to be pushed forward over the eye.

The wall of the globe is composed of three concentric coats or tunics, which enclose the transparent media of the eye. The outer or fibrous tunic consists of the cornea and sclera (Fig. 11-2). The sclera is a thick connective tissue membrane, white in color, which forms the posterior 70 percent of the outer tunic. The sclera helps maintain the shape of the globe, serves to protect the structures within, and acts as a place of attachment for the ocular

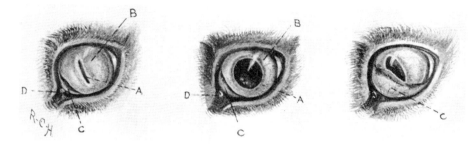

Fig. 11-1. Cat. Drawings of the eye of the cat indicating pupil size and shape and position of nictitating membrane: A, pupil; B, iris; C, nictitating membrane. (Simpson, 1903)

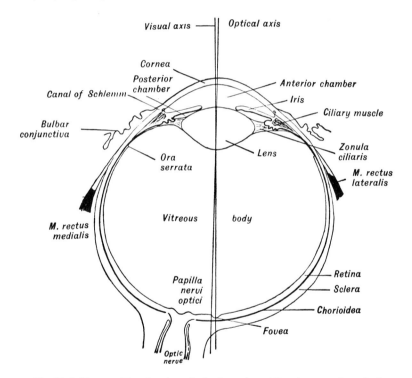

Fig. 11-2. Human. Line drawing of a horizontal meridional section through the human eye. Reproduced by permission from Bloom, W. and Fawcett, D.W. (1968) A *Textbook of Histology*, Ninth Edition, W.B. Saunders Co., Philadelphia, Pa.

muscles. At the posterior pole of the globe, the sclera is reduced to a thin membrane, the lamina cribrosa, containing perforations permitting the passage of bundles of nerve fibers and retinal blood vessels.

The cornea, the avascular and transparent portion of the fibrous tunic, forms the anterior 30 percent of this tunic (Fig. 11-4). The cornea is the first refracting medium interposed between the external light source and the internally located photoreceptors. The percentage area of the globe surface occupied by the cat cornea is almost twice the percentage area occupied by the human cornea (compare Figs. 11-2 and 11-4). The large area of the cornea, along with a large pupil diameter, is typical of nocturnal and arhythmic animals (such as the cat), and permits the entry of the maximum amount of light into the eye.

The middle or vascular layer of the globe consists of the choroid, the ciliary body, and iris. The choroid is the largest segment of the vascular layer and covers most of the inner surface of the sclera. It is a thin, soft, and richly vascularized membrane, which is darkly pigmented. Through its rich vascular supply it provides nutrients to the inner ocular tissue and, with its pigmented cells, serves as a dark, light-absorbing lining.

Anteriorly the choroid merges with the ciliary body, a thickening of the vascular tunic surrounding the outer perimeter of the lens. The ciliary body consists of three parts: the obiculus ciliaris, the ciliary processes, and the ciliary muscles. The obiculus ciliaris joins the choroid and is considered a direct continuation of the choroid. The ciliary processes appear as radiating ridges, seventy-six in number, on the inner aspect of the ciliary body. These processes extend out toward the equator of the crystalline lens. The ciliary muscles are located near the base of the ciliary processes. Attached to the ciliary processes are the suspensary ligaments or the zonule, which appears to attach the ciliary processes to the lens. The ciliary body functions to control the position and shape of the lens through the tension exerted on the lens capsule by the ciliary muscles, the ciliary processes, and the zonule.

The iris, the most anterior part of the vascular layer, extends over the anterior surface of the lens. The iris is a thin, pigmented annular-shaped structure with an opening in its center, the pupil. The iris contains two sets of smooth muscles that control the size of the pupil aperture. The fibers of the sphincter muscle are vertically oriented and are located near the pupillary margin. Constriction of the sphincter muscle decreases the horizontal diameter of the pupil. the vertical meridian being relatively immobile. The fibers of the dilator muscle are prominent in all parts of the iris except along the vertical meridian. In the cat the pupil is round in shape when dilated and forms a vertical slit when contracted (Fig. 11-1).

The pupil of the cat is highly mobile, adjusting its size to control the amount of light entering the eye and also to control depth of focus of the eye.

The maximally dilated pupil attains a diameter of 14 to 16 mm (Thieulin, 1927), while the maximally constricted pupil can close entirely at its center, leaving a pair of terminal pinholes at either end of the vertical slit (Walls, 1942). In mammals the fully closable slit pupil occurs only in prosimians, most small species of Felidae, seals, and dormice (Walls, 1942). The large species of Felidae and some of the smaller species possess pupils that are round when dilated and when fully contracted. The slit pupil appears to be an adaptation for arhythmic activity pattern that permits maximal light entry at low light levels and prevents excessive stimulation at high light levels. Cats appear also to utilize pupil aperture size to aid in focusing on objects at different distances. Under a constant ambient illumination level, the pupil aperture size can be seen to adjust rapidly as the cat views different objects in the environment.

The third or innermost coat of the eye is the nervous tunic or retina. The photoreceptive retina, or retina proper, covers the choroid and extends anteriorly to just behind the ciliary body, where it ends abruptly at the ora serrata. The outermost layer of the retina, which lines the choroid, is a layer of epithelium that is pigmented in most areas. The nonphotosensitive portion of the retina, consisting of a double layer of epithelium, continues forward to cover the inner surface of the ciliary body and iris.

There are regional differences in the superficial appearance of the cat retina or fundus (Fig. 11-3). The upper half of the fundus, excluding the far periphery, contains a triangular area of high reflectivity. In this area the tapetum lucidum is found between the epithelial layer of the retina and the choroid. The epithelium covering the tapetum is completely devoid of pigment, allowing light to pass freely to and from the tapetum. The tapetum acts as a mirror reflecting light back through the retina, thus utilizing the light twice. The presence of this mirror in the cat's eye accounts for the eyeshine observed when light is directed into the cat's eyes at night. The epithelial layer of the lower and extreme periphery of the retina where the tapetum is absent contains a dark brown pigment.

The optic disc or optic nerve head lies near the center of the posterior pole of the eye, just at or above the inferior border of the tapetum (Fig. 11-3). It is approximately 0.93 mm in diameter and is marked by a shallow depression. The optic disc is the area of the retina at which retinal processes exit the globe to form the optic nerve externally. This area also marks the point of entry and exit of the retinal vessels, which appear to arise from the margin of the disc.

The cat does not possess a macular (yellow-colored) area or a fovea (depression in the retina). There appears to be a specialized area known as the area centralis, which, according to Bishop *et al.*, (1962), is coincident with the visual pole (the point at which the visual image is brought into focus). Under ophthalmoscopic examination, this area appears free of visible blood

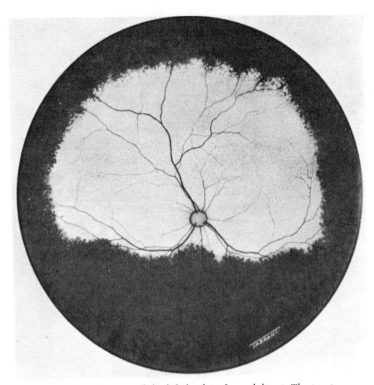

Fig. 11-3. Cat. Painting of the left fundus of an adult cat. The tapetum, which appears light in color, forms a triangular area in the superior half of the fundus. Blood vessels can be seen radiating from the optic disc, a dark circular area in the tapetum. The blood vessels can be seen taking an arcuate course above and below the area centralis, which is located temporal to the optic disc. (Henkind, 1966)

vessels and has a greenish hue as compared to the golden color of the tapetum. Bishop *et al.* (1962) state that blood vessels can be seen sweeping laterally in an arcuate course above and below this area (Fig. 11-3). The area centralis lies in the superior temporal area of the retina, approximately 20 to twenty-five degrees above a horizontal axis drawn through the center of the optic disc (Henkind, 1966). The center of the area centralis is approximately 3.42 mm away from the center of the optic disc (Bishop *et al.*, 1962).

The interior of the globe is filled with the transparent media of the eye (Fig. 11-4). The crystalline lens is located behind the iris and in front of a gelatinous mass called the "vitreous humor." The crystalline lens is a transparent biconvex structure contained within an elastic lens capsule. It is suspended in the eye by the zonule fibers of the ciliary body that are attached to the lens capsule. The anterior chamber of the eye, located between the cornea and the iris and anterior surface of the lens, is filled with the watery

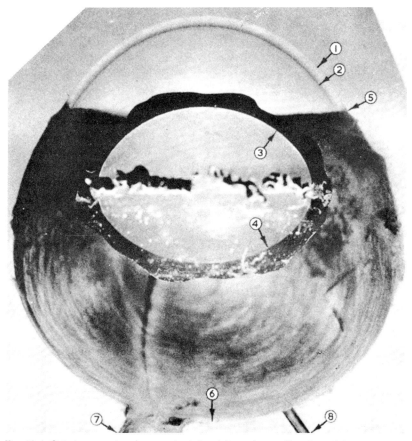

Fig. 11-4. Cat. A composite photograph of the globe and crystalline lens of the cat eye: 1-2, cornea; 3-4, crystalline lens; 5, corneo-scleral junction; 6, posterior surface of the sclera; 7, optic nerve. (Vakkur and Bishop, 1963)

aqueous humor. The posterior chamber, a ring-shaped space located between the posterior surface of the iris and lens and the anterior surface of the vitreous, is also filled with aqueous humor. Posterior to the lens is the vitreal cavity, which is filled by the third and most voluminous transparent body, the gelatinous vitreous humor.

IMAGE FORMATION

The image-forming mechanism of the eye is similar to that of a camera. The cornea and crystalline lens form the lens of the camera; the pupil and iris, the aperture and diaphragm respectively of the camera; the ciliary body, the lens-focusing mechanism; and the retina, the photographic plate. The curved transparent surface of the cornea is the first interface of refracting media light encounters in its course to the retina. Light is most strongly refracted upon entering the eye. Light rays refracted by the cornea are further refracted by the crystalline lens. The cornea and crystalline lens produce a single, inverted image on the retina that is smaller than the object viewed.

Because the image-forming mechanisms of the eye of the cat have been adapted for maximum performance under low level light conditions, the dioptics of the cat eye differ somewhat from that of man (compare Fig. 11-2, schematic of the human eye, and Fig. 11-4, the cat eye). The large corneal surface (30 percent of the total outer surface) along with the large size of the pupil, allow a greater amount of light to enter the eye. However, the large diameter of the cat cornea makes it a weaker refracting medium. The lens is enlarged both to compensate for the loss in refracting power of the cornea and to accommodate the wide beam of light entering the eye (Fig. 11-4). Since the lens is enlarged, its center is shifted back from the cornea. The resulting image, formed by an enlarged, more powerful lens situated far back from the cornea, is 5.2 times brighter but 0.74 times smaller than the image formed on the human retina (Vakkur and Bishop, 1963). The physical characteristics of the cat's eye have been studied by Bishop and co-workers who developed a model schematic eye for the cat (Bishop et al., 1962; Vakkur et al., 1963; Vakkur and Bishop, 1963).

Like a camera, the eye has the capability of altering its refracting powers through the process of accommodation. In accommodation the dioptics of the lens are modified by alteration of the shape and position of the lens via the action of the ciliary body. Theoretically, in man when the eye is at rest, images of objects from infinity to approximately six meters away can be clearly focused on the retina by the cornea and unaccommodated lens. The process of accommodation comes into play in focusing on objects closer than six meters away.

The mechanics of lens accommodation are not fully understood, and there are conflicting theories as to the mechanical actions involved. It has been suggested that, in the eye at rest, the suspensary ligaments are under tension and exert a radial pull on the elastic lens capsule, causing it to flatten the crystalline lens. In accommodation the ciliary muscles contract and, acting as a sphinctor, pull the ciliary processes anteriorly and inward, toward the crystalline lens, thus reducing the tension on the suspensary ligaments. The reduction of this tension on the lens capsule results in an increase in lens curvature and a shift in the position of its anterior surface. The lens thus becomes more refractive and can focus clear images of near objects on the retina. In a 12-year-old boy the accommodative process permits the eye to focus a clear image of an object from six meters to seven cm away (amplitude of accommodation of 14 diopters).

The lens' accommodative process has not been studied in the cat and may differ from that in the primate (Vakkur and Bishop, 1963). It has been suggested that the development of a thick crystalline lens in the cat may result in reduced range of accommodation to approximately four diopters, compared to 14 diopters for a young human (Hartridge and Yamada, 1922; Vakkur and Bishop, 1963).

ANATOMY OF THE RETINA

Although the cat is one of the more frequently used subjects in neurophysiological studies of the visual system, not much is known of the neuroanatomy of the cat retina. The retinal neural elements have been studied using light microscopic observations of whole flat-mount retinas and thinly sectioned retinas stained with silver or methylene blue. Few electron microscopic studies have been made of the cells and synapses of the cat retina as compared with the guinea pig and frog retinas.

The retinal layer of the eye is derived from neural tissue, having developed from an outpocketing of the frontal end of the embryonic neural tube. The retina is a unique receptor surface, in that it contains at least four structurally distinct neurons in addition to the receptor cells. These neural elements include two vertically oriented neurons, the bipolar and ganglion cells, and two horizontally oriented neurons, the horizontal and amacrine cells. In the cat, as in most mammals, ten distinct retinal layers can be distinguished (Fig. 11-5). The retinal epithelium, forming the outermost layer immediately joining the choroid, is a single layer of cuboidal cells that usually contains a dark brown pigment. Protoplasmic expansions of these epithelial cells extend into and pass between processes of the photoreceptors lying within the next layer of the retina. The bacillary or receptor layer lies immediately adjacent to, and is partially enveloped by, the retinal epithelium. This layer is composed of the rodlike or conelike inner and outer segments of the photoreceptor cells. The outer limiting membrane appears as a sharp line separating the bacillary layer from the layers within. This layer is formed by the outer elements of the supporting neuroglial radial fibers of Muller. The outer nuclear layer is composed of the cell bodies of the photoreceptors. The outer plexiform layer, adjoining the outer nuclear layer, represents the area of termination of the photoreceptors, bipolar and horizontal cells. The inner nuclear layer contains the cell bodies of the horizontal, bipolar and amacrine cells and of the supporting Muller cells. Within the inner plexiform layer the processes of the bipolar, amacrine, and ganglion cells appear to terminate. The ganglion cell layer consists of the cell bodies of the ganglion cells. The ninth layer, the optic-nerve layer, consists primarily of the unmyelinated axons of ganglion cells in their course to the optic disc, where they leave the eye to form the optic nerve. The innermost layer, bounding the retina from

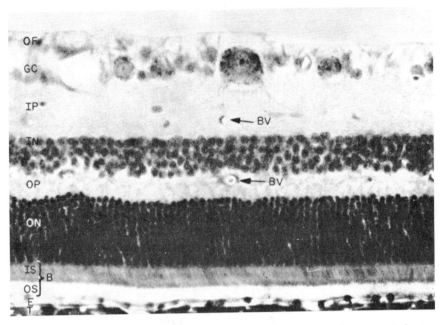

Fig. 11-5. Cat. Horizontal section of the cat's retina some distance from the area centralis: T, tapetum; E, retinal epithelium; B, bacillary layer; OS, outer segment of receptor cells; IS, inner segment of receptor cells; ON, outer nuclear layer; OP, outer plexiform layer; IN, inner nuclear layer; IP, inner plexiform layer; GC, ganglion cell layer; OF, optic fiber layer. (Donovan, 1966)

the vitreous, is called the inner limiting membrane. It consists of the flattened inner ends of Mullers radial fibers, which appear to be joined to one another.

The visual receptor cell is located in the outermost layers of the retina, separated from the choroid coat by the retinal epithelium. The visual receptor can be divided into five or six parts (Fig. 11-6). The outermost portion, the outer segment, is a laminated structure, which under the electron microscope has the characteristic appearance of a pile of double-walled discs, which may or may not be continuous with the cell membrane. The outer segment is connected to the inner segment by nine eccentrically placed cilia (Tokuyasu and Yamada, 1959; Sjöstrand, 1959). The outer and inner segment of the receptor cell is located within the bacillary layer of the retina. A slender outer fiber may connect the inner segment to the cell body, if the cell body is displaced from it. The cell body contains the nucleus of the cell and surrounding cytoplasm. A slender inner fiber arises from the cell body, and passes through the outer nuclear layer into the outer plexiform layer, where it ends as a receptor terminal.

The retina of the cat apparently contains two types of receptor cells; rods and cones (Fig. 11-6). The original classification of photoreceptor cells into

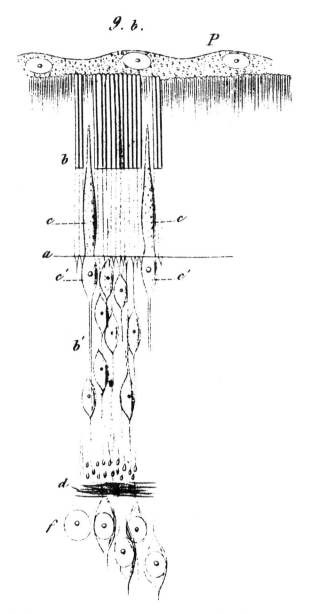

Fig. 11-6. Cat. Schematic drawing of a horizontal section through the cat's retina: a, outer limiting membrane; b, outer segments of receptor cells; c, inner segments of cone cells; c', cell body of cone cells; b', inner fiber of receptor cell; d, outer plexiform layer; f, inner nuclear layer. (Schultze, 1866)

rods and cones was based upon the differences in the shape of the outer and inner segments of the receptors (Schultze, 1866). Menner (1929), who classified cells as rods or cones on the basis of the appearance of the receptor cell body, reported that he did not observe cone-type receptors in the cat retina. The description to follow of the rods and cones of cat retina is based upon the observations of Schultze (1866), Chivetz (1889; 1891), and Ramón y Cajal (1960).

The rod receptor has a slender, cylindrical outer segment which is approximately one to 1.5 microns in diameter and 15 to 20 microns in length. The inner segment of the rod is of the same diameter as the outer segment or a bit thinner and a bit shorter. The rod shape of the inner and outer segments are characteristic of rod receptor cells. The cell body of the rod receptor is approximately the same size as that of the cone receptor (six to seven microns in diameter). However, within the rod cell body the nucleus is much smaller than that of the cone and is surrounded by a greater amount of cytoplasm. The inner rod fiber that connects the cell body to the receptor terminal is much thinner (1 micron or less) than the inner cone fiber. The inner rod fiber terminates in a small pear-shaped end bulb called the "rod spherule."

The cone outer segment is conical or cylindrical in shape and often is shorter than the rod outer segment. The cone inner segment is as long as the rod inner segment, but is four to five microns wide and has a characteristic spindle shape. The cell body of the cone cell contains a larger nucleus and less surrounding cytoplasm than the rod cell body. The inner cone fiber is two to five microns thick and terminates as an enlarged triangular ending called the "cone pedicle."

Very little is known about the distribution of the receptors in the cat retina. Zurn (1902) reports that there is a ratio of twenty-five cones to two hundred rods in the cat's retina. Chievitz (1889), who counted the number of nuclei within the nuclear layers of different areas of the retina, noted a decrease in density of receptor nuclei in the area centralis. Chievetz attributed the decrease of receptor nuclei within the middle of the area centralis to the increase in cone density in this area. He reasoned that, because the inner segments of cones have greater diameter and take up a greater area than those of the rods, an increase in cone density would result in an overall decrease in number of receptor cell nuclei per unit area examined.

Although the classification of visual receptors into rod and cone types was first based upon the appearance of the inner and outer segment of the receptor, Schultze (1866) noted that the shape of these segments varied with the position of the receptor cell in the retina. Chievetz (1891) reported that in the cat's retina the inner segment diameter of cone receptors in the area centralis decreased to two to three microns, compared to inner segment diameters of four to five microns for cones located peripheral to area centralis. Rodlike receptors in the extreme periphery of the cat retina had inner segments with diameters between two to three microns as compared to that of one to 1.5 microns for rod cells located more centrally. Electron-microscopic studies of primate retinas indicate that the fine structure of the outer segments of both centrally and peripherally located cones is distinct from that of the outer segments of rods (Dowling, 1965; Missoten, 1965).

The horizontal cell of the cat's retina is a neuron that may or may not possess an axonal process (Fig. 11-7). The cell bodies of horizontal cells are from six to 20 microns in diameter and lie within the inner nuclear layer, at or near its junction with the outer plexiform layer. These cells give rise to from three to 11 protoplasmic processes that enter and bifurcate further within the external plexiform layer.

Ramón y Cajal (1933) described two main types of horizontal cells in mammalian retinas, small or external horizontal cells and large or internal horizontal cells. The external horizontal cells are flattened and stellate, located immediately near the outer plexiform layer. Numerous processes extend from the cell body and form a thick plexus near the receptor terminals. The internal horizontal cells are located within the inner nuclear layer internal to the outer cells. These inner horizontal cells give rise to thick, short fingerlike ascending processes that terminate nearby. Ramón y Cajal reported that some horizontal cells possess a fine axon that travels horizontally within the outer plexiform layer.

There is considerable disagreement over the number of horizontal cell types and the lamination of horizontal cells in the cat's retina. The most

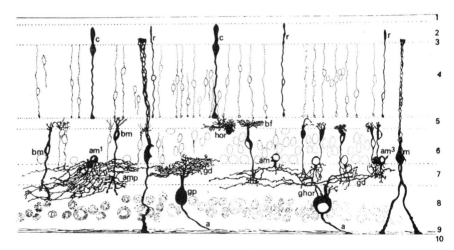

Fig. 11-7. Cat. Schematic drawing of neurons in the retina of a fifteen-day-old kitten, stained with Golgi method: r, rod receptors; c, cones; hor, body of horizontal cell; bm, mop bipolar cell; bf, flat bipolar cell; am1-am3, amacrine cells; gp, bushy ganglion cell; ghor, broad range ganglion cell; m, Mullers supporting cell; a, axon. (Shkolnik-Yarros, 1971)

commonly observed horizontal cell, the outer horizontal cell of Cajal, has a small flattened cell body that lies in the junction of the outer plexiform and inner nuclear layer. It gives rise to thick or medium-sized flattened processes, which spread horizontally and cover an area up to three hundred to five hundred microns in diameter. There is agreement that in the cat this type of cell has no identifiable axon (Gallego, 1965; Dowling *et al.*, 1966; Leichester and Stone, 1967; Honrubia and Elliott, 1969) and that each of its processes appears to be morphologically identical (Dowling *et al.*, 1966).

A second type of horizontal cell, the inner horizontal cell, is found within the inner nuclear layer (Ramón y Cajal, 1960; Dowling *et al.*, 1966; Shkolnik-Yarros, 1971). Dowling *et al.* (1966) describe an inner horizontal cell with a round cell body and thin processes that cover an area one hundred to two hundred microns in diameter. Some of these small cells give rise to a thin process similar to an axon. Other types of horizontal cells, having features intermediate to the first two types, have also been observed (Dowling *et al.*, 1966; Shkolnik-Yarros, 1971).

The highest density of horizontal cells per unit area is within the area centralis where these cells appear to be smaller than in the periphery (Uyama, 1934; Honrubia and Elliot, 1969).

The bipolar cells form a vertical path connecting the inner and outer plexiform layers. The cell bodies of the bipolar cells are located within the inner nuclear layer, internal to the horizontal cells (Fig. 11-8). The ascending portion of some bipolar cells are formed by a single ascending dendrite that branches and terminates in the outer plexiform layer (Ramón y Cajal, 1960; Brown and Major, 1966). When the cell body of the bipolar cell is located close to the outer plexiform layer, the ascending portion of the cell is formed by several dendritic processes that travel to, branch, and terminate in the outer plexiform layer (Brown and Major, 1966). The descending axonal portion of the cell extends into, bifuncates, and terminates within the inner plexiform or gangalion cell layers.

Ramón y Cajal (1960) described two distinct types of bipolar cells in the developing kitten eye. The cone or flat bipolar cell is short and has an oblong cell body. The branched ascending terminals of the flat bipolars pass parallel to the receptor terminals and form a flattened tuft that extends horizontally within the outer plexiform layer. Those flat bipolars with cell bodies located well within the inner nuclear layer send a single axon process to the inner plexiform layer where they form extensive arborizations. Those flat bipolars with cell bodies located close to the inner plexiform layer give rise to a number of axonal processes that branch extensively within the inner plexiform layer. The axonal terminal branches of flat bipolars are found within all levels of the inner plexiform layer (Ramón y Cajal, 1960) and in the middle zones of that layer (Brown and Major, 1966).

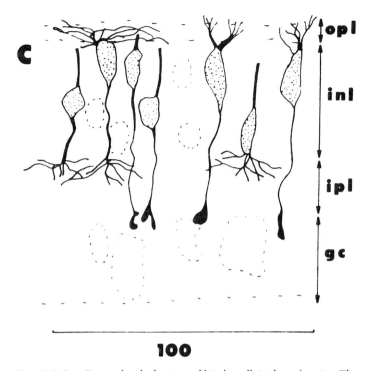

Fig. 11-8. Cat. Camera lucida drawings of bipolar cells in the cat's retina. The axons of the mop bipolar cells end in the region of the cell bodies of ganglion cells. The axons of the flat bipolars branch well within the inner plexiform layer. Scale: 100 microns. Opl, outer plexiform layer; inl, inner nuclear layer; ipl, inner plexiform layer; gc, ganglion cell layer. Reprinted by permission from Brown, J.E. and Major, D. (1966) *Exp. Neurol.* 15: 70-78.

The second type of bipolar cell observed by Ramón y Cajal (1960), the rod or mop bipolar, has a more voluminous cell body and thicker processes. The ascending dendritic portion consists of two or more thick processes that branch and pass vertically as fine ascending tufts into the receptor terminal area of the outer plexiform layer. The descending axonal process travels through the entire inner plexiform layer, and forms one to three branches that terminate as large end bulbs either on the body of a ganglion cell or on the origin of the dendrites of a ganglion cell (Brown and Major, 1966; Shkolnik-Yarros, 1971).

A third type of bipolar cell, the midget bipolar, has been described in primate retinas (Polyak, 1941; Boycott and Dowling, 1969). This type of bipolar cell has not been observed in the cat's retina.

The distributions of the flat and mop bipolar cells have not been described for the cat's retina.

The outer plexiform layer contains the receptor terminals, and processes and terminals of the horizontal and bipolar neurons. According to Dowling and Boycott (1966), the rod spherule and cone pedicle can be distinguished by their size and number of synaptic invaginations. Although the detailed description of receptor terminals given by Dowling and Boycott (1966) is based upon monkey retina, they state that the receptor terminals of cats and rabbits are similar to those of the monkey. The larger (cone) terminals have numerous invaginations, while the small (rod) terminals may have only one. In general, four to seven processes are found in a rod synaptic invagination and three processes in a cone synaptic invagination. Within a synaptic invagination, two deeply placed, laterally located processes are positioned on either side of one to three centrally placed processes that lie more superficially (Fig. 11-10). The two laterally placed processes have been identified as horizontal cell processes and the centrally placed processes as bipolar cell processes. In addition to the invaginated synapses, a superficial, flat contact has been observed on the surface of the receptor terminal. In the primate and frog, the processes forming these superficial contacts have been traced to the flat bipolars and the invaginated centrally located terminals to mop and midget bipolars.

Boycott and Dowling (1969) report that in the primate eye mop bipolars terminate on rods exclusively and the flat and midget bipolars terminate only upon cones. The mop bipolars terminate on from one to several adjacent rod spherules, the midget bipolars on a single cone pedicle, and the flat bipolars on a group of cones. Whether this scheme applies to the cat's retina is not known. The horizontal cell processes of the cat retina have been reported to contact the dendrites and soma of bipolar cells as well as other horizontal cell processes (Dowling et al., 1966).

The amacrine cells are similar to the horizontal cells in that they do not appear to possess an axonal process. The cell bodies of the amacrine cells are located in the inner zone of the inner nuclear layer, adjacent to the inner plexiform layer (Fig. 11-7). The processes of the amacrine cells pass into the inner plexiform layer to end in horizontal nets. Ramón y Cajal (1933) described two main categories of amacrine cells in the mammalian retina on the basis of the position of the branching of their processes within the inner plexiform layer. The processes of the diffuse amacrine cells branch at all levels of the inner plexiform layer. The processes of stratified amacrine cells branch within and are confined within a single horizontal statum of the inner plexiform layer, which Ramón y Cajal divided into four to five stratums. Ramón y Cajal reports observing fusiform- or bipolar-type amacrine cells in retinas of mouse embryos.

Examples of Ramón y Cajal's two main types of amacrine cells and a third, fusiform-type cell have been observed in the cat's retina. Shkolnik-Yarros (1971) reports that the diffuse amacrine cells, which have extremely dense processes that occupy the entire width of the inner plexiform layer, predominate in Golgi-treated retinas of cats and kittens. This type of amacrine cell is reported to give rise to up to 120 processes which cover a span of 600 microns or more. Two types of stratified amacrine cells, both with cell body diameters ranging from 8 to 20 microns, have been observed in the cat's retina. One type, which appears in silver-stained tissue, gives rise to from 3 to 5 thick processes that branch at a level either above or below the ganglion cell dendrites (Gallego, 1965; Leichester and Stone, 1967). The second type, observed only in mythelene blue-stained retinas, gives rise to 4 or 5 short processes that branch to form a single layer in the region of the ganglion cell dendrites (Gallego, 1965; Leichester and Stone, 1967). Fusiform-type amacrine cells with large globular cell bodies have been observed in the middle third of the inner nuclear layer (Leichester and Stone, 1967). The processes of these cells spread vertically toward the inner and outer plexiform layers (Leichester and Stone, 1967; Shkolnik-Yarros, 1971).

The ganglion cells have interested most retinal neuroanatomists because they give rise to the axons of the optic nerve and appear to be the most easily isolated of the spike generators within the cat's retina (Bishop et al., 1962; Gallego, 1965; Stone, 1965; Brown and Major, 1966; Leichester and Stone, 1967; Honrubia and Elliott, 1969; Shkolnik-Yarros, 1971). The cell body of the ganglion cell lies within the ganglion cell layer. Its dendritic processes extend into the inner plexiform layer, and its unmyelinated axons form the optic fiber layer of the retina. Ramón y Cajal (1933) observed only multipolar ganglion cells in mammalian retinas and described two main types of ganglion cells on the basis of the level of branching of their dendrites within the inner plexiform layer. The diffuse ganglion cells possess from three to five main dendrites that ramify loosely and terminate without stratification in almost the entire thickness of the inner plexiform layer. According to Ramón y Cajal, the stratified ganglion cells send their main dendritic processes to one of the five zones of the inner plexiform layer where they branch and terminate. Polyak (1941) observed a third type of ganglion cell, the midget ganglion cell, in the primate retina. These cells are characterized by a single dendrite that enters the inner plexiform layer and forms a few short branches.

Many types of multipolar ganglion cells have been observed in the cat and kitten retina (Fig. 11-7). Although Brown and Major (1966) and Leichester and Stone (1967) report that they did not observe diffuse-type cells in either silver or methylene blue-stained retinas, Shkolnik-Yarros (1971) reports observing diffuse ganglion cells whose dendrites branched and spread throughout the width of the inner plexiform layer. The stratified multipolar ganglion cells appear to be of five types as classified on appearance and horizontal extent of their dendritic ramifications (Shkolnik-Yarros, 1971). There are two types of ganglion cells whose dendritic spread is of moderate size (60 to 200 microns) and whose dendritic arborizations have a bushlike appearance. The bushy, densely branched cells have small- to medium-sized cell bodies (12 to 27 microns) and dendrites that branch extensively. The dendritic processes form a dense bush most often in the upper part of the inner plexiform layer near the cell bodies of the amacrine cells or less often in the lower part of this layer. The sparsely branched ganglion cells have small cell bodies (16-20 microns) and dendrites that branch less extensively. The sparse dendritic bush of these cells is also located in either the upper or lower levels of the inner plexiform layer. In addition, there are three types of ganglion cells with large horizontal dendritic spreads (120-750 microns). The large broad range cells have medium to large diameter cell bodies (18 to 70 microns) and dendrites that branch in the innermost aspect of the inner plexiform layer, near and sometimes within the ganglion cell layer. The small broad range cells have miniature to small diameter cell bodies (7 to 13 microns and 16 to 20 microns) and dendrites that ramify in the middle or outermost aspect of the inner plexiform layer. From the description given by Shkolnik-Yarros (1971), it is difficult to determine the difference between small-sized, small broad-range cells, and the bushy, sparsely branched cells. A third type of horizontal broad-range cell is the unilateral broad-range cell. This type of cell has a medium-diameter cell body (10 to 25 microns) and long dendrites that extend eccentrically from one side of the cell body. Retinal ganglion cells having asymmetrical dendritic fields have also been observed by Gallego (1965) and Honrubia and Elliott (1970). The dendrites of the unilateral broad range cells branch in either the inner or outer zones of the inner plexiform layer. Central-type ganglion cells with small cell body and very narrow dendritic spread also occur frequently in the area centralis of cat retina.

Leichester and Stone (1967) describe only two types of multipolar ganglion cells on the basis of the level of dendritic branching in the inner plexiform layer. The deep multidendritic cells were the most commonly observed cell type. The dendrites of these cells arborize in the upper zone of the inner plexiform layer, close to the bipolar cell layer. The deep multidendritic cells probably correspond to the bushy branched and broad-range small and unilateral cells that branch in the upper part of the inner plexiform layer. The shallow multidendritic cells of Leichester and Stone (1967) have dendrites that branch in the middle third of the thickness of the inner plexiform layer. Some of the shallow cells may correspond to the bushy branched cells whose dendrites branch in the middle third of the thickness of the inner plexiform layer. Leichester and Stone do not report observing multipolar ganglion cells that branch in the lower zone of the inner plexiform layer near the ganglion cell layer. Shkolnik-Yarros (1971) reports observing dendritic arborizations of many busy branched cells, all large broad-range cells, and some unilateral cells within the lower zone of the inner plexiform layer.

Leichester and Stone (1967) report observing single dendrite ganglion cells that are similar to the midget ganglion cells of the primate retina described by Polyak (1941). This type of ganglion cell is observed only in methylene-blue preparations and not in silver-stained material. These cells have small diameter cell bodies (11-21 microns) and a single dendrite that branches in the upper half of the inner plexiform layer. One type of single dendritic cell forms a loosely branched arborization; a second type, a very dense arborization. Both types have dendritic spans that range from 18 to 135 microns in diameter in the periphery of the retina and 15 microns and less in the area centralis.

The distribution of the different ganglion-cell types across the retinal surface has not been investigated. The ganglion cell bodies of area centralis form a partial double layer and those of the peripheral areas form a partial single layer. Stone (1965) has studied the density and distribution of ganglion cells in flat-mount sections of methylene blue-stained retinas. Stone reports that as cell density decreases, cell body size increases so that areas of high density contain small cells predominantly, whereas areas of low density contain larger cells (Fig. 11-9). Within the area centralis the ganglion cells are smaller and most densely concentrated (Fig. 11-9). Eighty-five percent of the ganglion cells in the area centralis have cell body diameters less than 16 microns, and cell density there is approximately four thousand per square mm. Cell density decreases and cell body size increases as the sample area is selected from more peripheral retinal areas. According to Stone (1965) the distribution of cell size at any given area of the retina is always unimodal, with the modal size determined by the relative position of that area with respect to area centralis. Stone (1965) estimates the total number of ganglion cells in the cat's retina to be approximately ninety thousand.

Dowling and Boycott (1966) and Boycott and Dowling (1969), by reconstructing serial sections and by correlating light and electron microscopic observations of silver-stained retinas, have described the synaptic organization of the inner plexiform layer of the human and monkey retina (Fig. 11-10). The most commonly observed synaptic arrangements were the dyad (a bipolar terminal in contact with an amacrine terminal and a ganglion cell terminal) and contacts between amacrine and bipolar cell terminals. Also observed were contacts between two amacrine terminals and between amacrine and ganglion cell terminals. Very few contacts were seen between bipolar terminals and amacrine soma and between bipolar terminals and ganglion cell soma.

Within the optic nerve fiber layer, the axons of the ganglion cells located temporal, superior, and inferior to the area centralis take an arcuate course around the central area, while those of the nasal retina take a fairly straight course to the optic disc. The axons are unmyelinated internal to and within

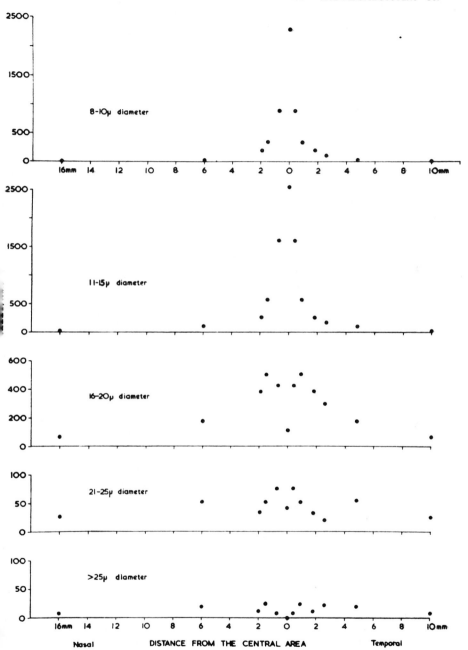

Fig. 11-9. Cat. Density of ganglion cells in terms of cell size. Vertical axis represents density and horizontal axis represents distance in mm from area centralis. (Stone, 1965)

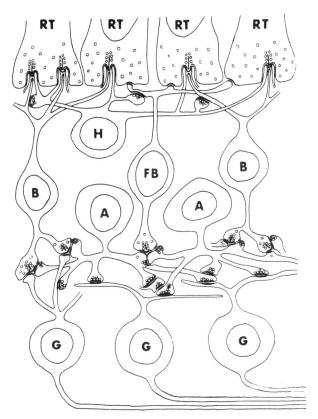

Fig. 11-10. Vertebrate. A schematic drawing of the arrangements of synaptic contacts found in vertebrate retinas. In the outer plexiform layer, terminal processes of the bipolar cells (B) and horizontal cells (H) penetrate into invaginations in the receptor terminals (RT). The terminals of flat bipolar cells (FB) make superficial contacts on the bases of some receptor terminals. In the inner plexiform layer, two basic synaptic contacts appear to occur. Bipolar terminals may contact one ganglion cell (G) dendrite and one amacrine cell (A) process or bipolar terminals may contact two amacrine processes. Amacrine cell processes contact both bipolar and ganglion terminals. (Dowling, 1970)

the lamina cribrosa of the sclera. Externally, the axons are gradually myelinated (Blunt *et al.*, 1965) and one mm from the lamina cribrosa all axons of the optic nerve appear to be myelinated (Bruesch and Arey, 1942). Bruesch and Arey (1942) report that comparison of myelin-stained and axon-cylinder stained fiber counts indicate that the optic nerve of cats does not contain unmyelinated fibers. Within the optic nerve those fibers originating from the nasal retinal quadrant are located in the medial half of the nerve, the temporal quadrant in the lateral half, from superior quadrant in dorsal half and from inferior quadrant in ventral half (Overbasch, 1927).

Donovan (1967), using the light microscope, counted the number of myelinated nerve fibers with diameters greater than 1 micron in cat optic nerves. A total of 85,926 fibers was counted in one nerve and the outside diameter of each fiber was measured. The fiber-diameter frequency histogram (Fig. 11-11) appears to be unimodal and skewed with a peak at 2.5 microns and a maximum diameter value of 10.5 microns. Donovan (1967) suggests that the discrepancies between the results of her study and those of other investigators who describe multiple-peaked distributions of fiber diameter (Bishop et al., 1953; Bishop and Clare, 1955; Chang, 1956; van Crevel and Verbarrt, 1963) result from sampling errors because they took measures from small segments of the nerve or tract. There are more fibers located in peripheral areas as compared to central areas of the nerve, and fibers in the periphery tend to be smaller. In addition, the distribution of fibers in one sector of a cross section of the optic nerve differs significantly from other sectors of the nerve. Thus, a sample taken from selected areas of the nerve would not be representative of the entire nerve since the fibers within the nerve are not homogeneous in distribution or size.

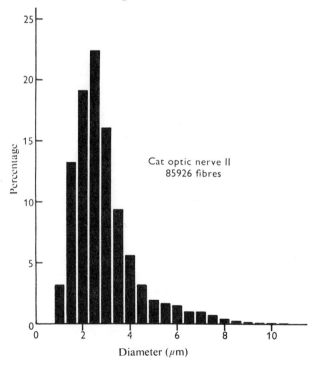

Fig. 11-11. Cat. Fiber-size frequency distribution of myelinated nerve fibers in a cat optic nerve. Reproduced by permission from Donovan, A. (1967) *Journal of Anatomy* 101; 1-11.

The optic nerve enters the cranium of the skull through the optic foramen. Prior to entering the brain, over half of the fibers of the optic nerve cross in the optic chiasm to join the contralateral optic tract. All fibers that arise from ganglion cells located in the retina nasal to a vertical line drawn through the central area decussate in the optic chiasm (Stone, 1966). Seventy-five percent of axons arising from ganglion cells located temporal to the vertical line do not cross. Approximately 50 percent of the fibers arising from ganglion cells within the vertical median strip decussate. Of the crossing vertical strip axons, 60 percent arise from the nasal half of the strip and 40 percent from the temporal half of the strip.

The crossed and uncrossed fibers join to form the optic tract, which enters the brain stem at diencephalic levels. Within the diencephalon the optic tract branches and forms the dorsal and ventral rami of the optic tract. Many of the fibers terminate within the lateral geniculate body of the diencephalon. Other fibers or collaterals travel to the midbrain to terminate in the superior colliculus, pretectal area, and in the nuclei of the accessory optic tract.

NEUROPHYSIOLOGY

There has been a great deal of research on retinal slow potentials; however, in keeping with the general plan of this book, only spike potential data will be reviewed. The bipolar neuron is considered, in the classical sense, the first-order afferent of the visual system. As traditionally viewed, the bipolar neuron receives input from the receptor and sends its output to the ganglion cell, which, in turn, sends its output to the CNS.

Spikes may be recorded from different retinal cell layers. Brown and Wiesel (1959) have reported recording spike discharges when their recording electrode was in the inner nuclear or ganglion cell layer according to depth measures and slow potential maps of the retinal layers. Brown and Tasaki (1961) report recording spike activity when their electrode tip was in either the inner nuclear or ganglion cell layer as determined by histological conformation of electrolytic marks made with the recording tip in position. Werblin and Dowling (1969) have recorded slow and spike potentials from cells in the mudpuppy (Neturus maculosus) retina with intracellularly placed micropipettes. Niagara blue stain was injected into the neurons with the recording pipettes and cell type was determined histologically. According to Werblin and Dowling (1969), both amacrine and ganglion cells produce spike potentials in the mudpuppy retina. In spite of these reports, all investigators recording from electrodes inserted into the cat retina report that they are recording either from the unmyelinated axons of ganglion cells or from their cell bodies. None of the investigators reviewed in this chapter reports histological conformation of the location of recording electrodes in the retina. Therefore, the data of these investigators will be referred to as having originated from retinal units. Data obtained while recording from fibers in the optic nerve, optic chiasm, or optic tract will be referred to as optic-fiber data.

Because there is some evidence that anesthetic doses of barbiturates depress spontaneous activity and alter stimulus-elicited discharge patterns of retinal units and optic fibers (Brown and Rojas, 1965 in the rat; Barlow *et al.*, 1964 in the rabbit; Schmidt and Creutzfeldt, 1968 in cat), most of the investigators reviewed utilized decerebrate, lightly anesthetized, or locally-anesthetized preparations. In the decerebrate preparations the brain was either transected at midbrain or high pontine, pretrigeminal levels. Most lightly anesthetized preparations were given sufficient doses of 60 to 70 percent nitrous oxide (Rodieck and Stone, 1965; Rodieck, 1967a, b; Barlow and Levick, 1969; Sakmann and Creutzfeldt, 1969) or urethane (Cleland and Enroth-Cugell, 1968) to prevent organized movement to noxious stimuli, but insufficient to prevent uncoordinated withdrawal of limbs to noxious stimuli. Of the investigators utilizing lightly anesthetized preparations, only Sakmann and Creutzfeldt (1969) report applying local anesthetics to open wounds and pressure points. In the locally anesthetized animals, long-lasting analgesics were applied to open wounds and pressure points (Herz *et al.*, 1964; Fuster *et al.*, 1965; Spinelli, 1967). With all three types of preparations, paralyzing agents (gallamine thriethiodide and/or d-tubocurarrine) were used to immobilize the animal. It must be noted that to avoid barbiturate effects, these investigators have utilized multiple drug conditions, all of which have central effects.

CONDUCTION VELOCITY

Although the fiber diameter distribution of the optic nerve appears to be unimodal (Fig. 11-11), optic-fiber conduction-velocity distributions have been described to be multimodal. Lennox (1958) electrically stimulated the optic nerve and measured latencies of single unit potentials with micropipettes, recording from the ipsilateral optic tract of cats deeply anesthetized with chloralose-urethane. She reports that conduction velocity estimates from 75 units indicated four populations of uncrossed fibers: one conducting at 16 meters per second (2 to 3 microns); one at 37 meters/second (6 microns); one at 52 meters/second (8 to 9 microns); and one at 66 meters/second (10 to 12 microns). Lennox reports that fast-conducting fibers were encountered more frequently deep within the optic tract. In actual fiber-diameter measurements, the 2 to 3 micron fibers represent 80 percent of the total fiber-diameter population. Lennox attributes the paucity of 2 to 3 micron-fiber diameter estimates to the difficulties involved in recording from small diameter fibers.

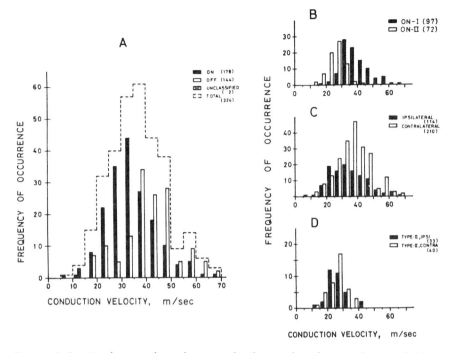

Fig. 11-12. Cat. Conduction-velocity frequency distribution of antidromic spikes recorded in optic chiasm: A. Comparison between excitatory (on-center) and inhibitory (off-center) and unclassified fibers. B. Comparison between phasic excitatory (on-I) and tonic excitatory (on-II) fiber conduction velocities. C. Comparison between uncrossed and crossed fibers. D. Comparison between uncrossed tonic excitatory fibers and crossed tonic excitatory fibers. (Fukada, 1971)

Fukada *et al.* (1966) recorded antidromic responses with tungsten or stainless-steel microelectrodes inserted into the optic disc of the retina. Electrical stimulating electrodes were inserted into both optic tracts so that latencies of uncrossed and crossed fibers could be measured. They report that for both fiber groups, crossed and uncrossed, the distributions of conduction-velocity estimates were bimodal. The distribution measured by stimulating uncrossed fibers (60/201) had peaks at 16 and 34 meters/second, with a greater number within the slow conducting group. The conduction-velocity distribution for the crossed fibers (141/201) had peaks at 14 and 30 meters/second, with a greater number of fibers in the fast conduction group. Fukada *et al.* found very few fibers with conduction velocities above 40 meters/second as compared to the results of Lennox. This discrepancy may be due to the differences in the type and placement of recording electrodes: Lennox recorded orthodromic spikes with pipettes from single fibers in the optic tract that are believed to be myelinated, while Fukada *et al.* recorded antidromic spikes with metal electrodes from single fibers in the optic disc that have been described as unmyelinated.

In a later study by Fukada (1971), antidromic responses were recorded from optic fibers in the optic chiasm with tungsten and micropipette electrodes. The fibers were stimulated electrically with an electrode placed in the optic tract near the lateral geniculate body. The conduction velocities of a total of 324 fibers were measured, with 114 uncrossed fibers and 210 crossed fibers. Conduction velocities ranged from less than 10 m/sec. to nearly 70 m/sec. and formed a unimodal distribution with peak at 35-40 m/sec. (Fig. 11-12). The distributions of conduction velocities of crossed and uncrossed fibers overlap, the crossed fibers having a slightly faster modal conduction velocity (Fig. 11-12). The difference in the distributions of Fukada et al. (1966) and Fukada (1971) probably reflects the differences in the fibers sampled; Fukada et al. (1966) measured conduction velocities of unmyelinated optic nerve fibers in the optic disc, while Fukada (1971) measured conduction velocities of myelinated fibers in the optic chiasm.

As in earlier studies, very few slow-conducting, small-diameter fibers were encountered by Fukada (1971) in the optic chiasm. The majority of the uncrossed fibers had conduction velocities that indicate their fiber diameters range from greater than three microns to less than nine microns. The grouping of conduction velocities of uncrossed fibers observed by Lennox (1958) is not apparent in the distribution of conduction velocities in Fig. 11-12C. Fukada (1971) also determined the location of the visual receptive field of each unit, using a light stimulus of small diameter. Both slow and fast conduction velocities are represented by units with receptive fields in the region of the area centralis.

RECEPTIVE FIELD CONFIGURATION

Many attempts have been made to determine the types of retinal units or optic fibers in the cat's peripheral visual system on the basis of receptive field configuration. Under certain stimulus conditions, the receptive fields of retinal units and optic fibers are complex. Under conditions of light adaptation, a visual receptive field consists of two or three areas that when stimulated elicit a response characterized by excitation (increased discharge), inhibition (decreased discharge), or a more complex discharge pattern. An area within the field is defined in terms of the type of response elicited when it is illuminated; i.e., illumination of an excitatory area elicits an excitatory response. The receptive field configuration is defined in terms of the relative positions of these areas to one another. A concentric type receptive field is organized with a central area that when illuminated elicits one response and a surrounding area that when stimulated elicits the opposite response. A simple type receptive field consists of an area that when stimulated results in one type of response. An asymmetric type receptive field consists of two areas that border one another, without one surrounding the other completely. Because receptive field configuration of retinal units and optic fibers is described in terms of the response elicited from areas within the field, a brief description will be given of the types of responses elicited. It should be noted that most investigators mapping retinal receptive fields classify responses as excitatory or inhibitory on the basis of audio- or oscilloscope-monitored spike trains.

The discharge elicited from retinal units and optic fibers to increased illumination are of three basic types: excitatory, inhibitory, and complex. The excitatory response (Fig. 11-13A at log 1 $=-2$) is characterized by increased discharge to increases in retinal illumination and a brief period of suppression to decreased retinal illumination. The inhibitory response (Fig. 11-13B at log 1 = 1) is characterized by decreased discharge to increases in retinal illumination and a brief period of increased discharge to termination of decreased retinal illumination. The complex response (Fig. 11-13B at log 1 = -1) usually consists of increased discharge to both increase and decrease in illumination. Audiomonitoring of discharge often results in failure of detection of complex responses (Rodieck and Stone, 1965). If spontaneous or maintained activity rates are low, inhibition of discharge will also be difficult to detect with audio and oscilloscopic monitoring.

Vision researchers call units that respond with increased discharge to increased illumination "on-units" and units that discharge to decreased illumination "off-units." We will be using the terms excitatory and inhibitory in preference to the terms on and off. The excitatory response of retinal units and optic fibers is usually tonic (i.e., maintained for the duration of the stimulus) (Donner and Willmer, 1950; Kuffler, 1953; Rodieck and Stone, 1965; Cleland and Enroth-Cugell, 1968; Creutzfeldt et al., 1970). The discharge pattern of most inhibitory type units appears to be similar to that of units in other sensory systems whose discharge is inhibited by stimulation of the receptor organ. When the stimulus that reduces or inhibits discharge is removed, there is usually a phasic increase in discharge that may be interpreted as a release from inhibition. Thus, the "off discharge" of most retinal units may be similar to the after-discharge that occurs in auditory units after removal of an inhibitory stimulus (Sachs and Kiang, 1968; Boudreau and Tsuchitani, 1968). We will be using the term after discharge to designate the phasic increase in discharge that occurs following a stimulus.

RECEPTIVE FIELDS UNDER CONDITIONS OF DARK ADAPTATION

When small spots of light are used to explore the dark adapted retina, two types of units are encountered (Barlow et al., 1957). The excitatory type unit

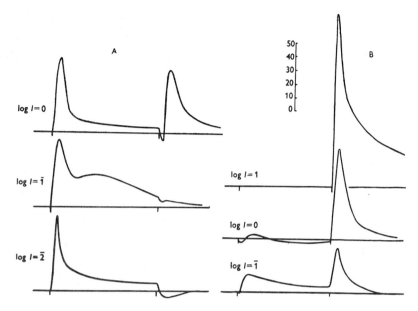

Fig. 11-13. Cat. A. PST histogram of discharge of a retinal unit that changes from an excitatory type to a complex type as the intensity of whole retinal illumination is raised. B. PST histogram of discharge of a retinal unit that changes from a complex type to an inhibitory type as the intensity of whole retinal illumination is raised. Ordinates: impulses/sec. Abscissas: time, with stimulus duration indicated by small vertical markers. (Donner and Willmer, 1950)

responds with increase in discharge to increases in illumination level. The inhibitory type unit responds with inhibition of dark discharge to increases in illumination and with a phasic increase in discharge to decreases in illumination. The receptive fields of dark adapted units appear to be of two types (Barlow et al., 1957; Rodieck and Stone, 1965). The excitatory units have receptive fields in which stimulation of any point in the field results in increased discharge. Increase in illumination of any point within the inhibitory unit receptive field results in decrease in dark discharge, while decrease in illumination results in increase in discharge. Thus, in the dark adapted retina the excitatory type unit has a simple excitatory receptive field and the inhibitory unit, a simple inhibitory receptive field.

The thresholds of dark adapted units to small spots of light are affected by the duration of the stimulus and the area-size of the exploring spot (Barlow et al., 1957). Thresholds to stimuli of long duration (380 msec) are lower than those of short duration (70 msec) and threshold decreases as the area-size of the exploring spot increases. The area-size of the unit's receptive field determines the boundaries beyond which threshold does not increase with further increases in area-size of the stimulus. Increasing the area-size of the exploring spot a few mm beyond the area of the receptive field does not appear to alter threshold or discharge pattern of dark adapted units provided the spot illumination is kept at moderate levels. Whole retinal illumination, especially at high levels, results in alteration of retinal unit discharge pattern.

Granit (1944) reports observing two types of retinal units in the dark adapted eye when it is stimulated with whole retinal illumination. The majority of the units sampled respond with increased discharge to both the onset and cessation of illumination. Although Granit (1944) and others call this the "on-off response," we will be using the term complex response. Granit noted that the magnitude of the excitatory discharge and inhibitory after-discharge of these complex response units was dependent upon stimulus intensity and was affected by light adaptation. Other units respond with an excitatory type response to whole retinal illumination; that is, with increased discharge to increased illumination. Donner and Willmer (1950) noted that the discharge pattern of excitatory type units observed by Granit (1944) could be altered into a complex or inhibitory pattern by increasing whole retinal illumination level two or more log units above the retinal unit's threshold (Fig. 11-13). Similarly, the discharge of complex response type units could be changed to the inhibitory pattern by increasing illumination level. Thus, while studies using small spot stimuli projected on the dark adapted retina indicate that all retinal units are either excited or inhibited by light, studies using whole retinal illumination of dark adapted units indicate retinal units are both excited and inhibited by light. That the latter is the case is illustrated by studies using light adapted retinas.

RECEPTIVE FIELDS UNDER CONDITIONS OF LIGHT ADAPTATION

Using a small spot of light as the exploratory stimulus, Kuffler (1953) reports that on the basis of receptive field organization there are two types of units in the retina of light adapted cats. The typical light adapted unit has a receptive field that is concentrically arranged, with increased illumination of the central area eliciting one type of response and increased illumination of the surround area eliciting the opposite response (Fig. 11-14). The excitatory center type unit has a receptive field with a central area that when illuminated increases discharge and a surround area that when illuminated decreases maintained or background discharge and when un-illuminated results in after-discharge. The inhibitory center unit has a receptive field of opposite configuration; illumination of the center area results in inhibition, while illumination of the surround results in excitation. The center and surround areas appear to be mutually antagonistic so that the excitatory response can be inhibited by simultaneous illumination of inhibitory areas or vice versa.

The response elicited by stimulating the central area of a light adapted receptive field is the same as that elicited by stimulating any area of the dark

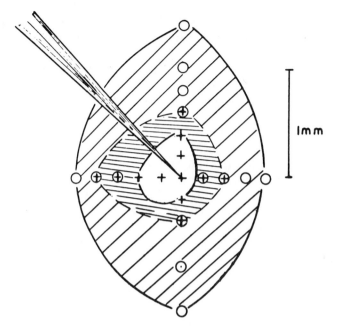

Fig. 11-14. Cat. Concentric-type receptive field under conditions of
light adaptation: Stimulation of the central area with a small light spot
elicited an excitatory response, while in the diagonally hatched
surrounding area, inhibition was elicited. Stimulation of the in-
termediary, horizontally hatched, zone elicited complex discharge.
(Kuffler, 1953)

adapted field. That is, the dark adapted excitatory unit has a light adapted
receptive field that consists of an excitatory center and an inhibitory
surround. For brevity's sake we will call light adapted excitatory center units
"excitatory units"; and light adapted inhibitory center units, "inhibitory
units." The total area of the dark adapted receptive field is larger than the
central area of the light adapted field. However, the area of the dark adapted
field is smaller than the total area (central plus surround) of the light adapted
field (Barlow, 1957; Rodieck and Stone, 1965). The surround area is not
apparent in the dark adapted retina if stimuli of moderate intensity and of
area-size a few mm greater than the receptive field are directed onto the
field. However, increasing stimulus area-size to whole retinal illumination
appears to elicit the surround response, and increasing the level of
illumination appears to increase the surround response.

The most commonly observed light adapted receptive field is the
concentric or center-surround type first described by Kuffler (1953) for the
cat's retina. Units with this type of receptive field are found both in and
around the area centralis and in peripheral areas of the retina (Wiesel, 1960;
Rodieck and Stone, 1965; Fukada, 1971). Units with large receptive fields

tend to have an intermediate annular-shaped area between the center and surround that when stimulated results in complex excitatory inhibitory responses (Kuffler, 1953; Rodieck and Stone, 1965). According to Rodieck and Stone (1965), a few units have receptive fields with an intermediate area of insensitivity between the center and surround areas.

The central area of concentric fields has been described to be roughly circular in shape, with the surround area asymmetrically situated about it (Rodieck and Stone, 1965). The diameter of the central area in terms of angle subtended at the cat's eye has been estimated to range from 0.5 degrees (0.125 mm) to 8 degrees (2 mm) (Wiesel, 1960; Rodieck and Stone, 1965). It has been reported that units located in or near the area centralis tend to have smaller central areas (Wiesel, 1960; Rodieck and Stone, 1965; Winters and Walters, 1970). According to Stone and Fabian (1966) the central areas of units believed to be located in the area centralis ranged in diameter from 0.5 to 1.5 degrees. Wiesel (1960), using the area-threshold method (a circular spot of light of increasing diameter), estimates total receptive field diameters to range from 6 degrees (1.5 mm) to 12 degrees (3 mm). Wiesel (1960) further reports that there appears to be no systematic relationship between the size of total receptive field of units with small central areas and those with large central areas, and that some units with small central areas have large antagonistic surround areas.

Although units with concentric type receptive fields are the most commonly observed in light adapted retinas, Kuffler (1953) states that not all the units he observed were of the concentric type pictured in Fig. 11-14. Rodieck (1967b) has described two units in the periphery of the retina that responded only to contrast stimuli (a light spot in a dark background, or vice versa) and only with inhibition of maintained discharge. Increases in discharge could not be elicited with contrast stimuli, flashing light, or moving lights. This type of unit was probably first observed in the cat by Brown and Wiesel (1958).

Although the majority of retinal units observed to be located within area centralis have concentric-type receptive fields, units with three other types of fields have been observed in area centralis (Stone and Fabian, 1966). The center type unit is similar to dark adapted retinal units in that only one type of discharge, excitatory or inhibitory, could be elicited from any part of the unit's receptive field. However, although no surround response could be elicited by a small spot of light, diffuse retinal illumination produced a "much weaker" response, suggesting a surround effect. The receptive fields of the center type units are the smallest found, with diameters ranging from twenty-two to thirty minutes of angle subtended at the cat's eye. The second type of unit is similar to the center type in that only one type of discharge could be elicited by stimulating any area of the receptive field. However, the response of this type of unit is complex with phasic increase in discharge to onset and cessation of the light and inhibition of discharge while the light is maintained on. The receptive fields of these "on-off" units have diameters ranging from 0.5 to 1.5 degrees. Fukada (1971) reports observing one fiber in the optic chiasm with similar discharge and receptive field configuration. Units having similar characteristics occur more commonly in the frog (Hartline, 1938), pigeon (Maturana and Frenk, 1963), and rabbit (Barlow *et al.*, 1964). The third type of unit observed in area centralis by Stone and Fabian (1966) had a receptive field with an irregular concentric type configuration. These units were characterized by their weak and oscillatory discharge to spot stimuli and are called "diffuse" type units because they have the largest receptive fields observed, fifteen degrees in diameter.

Quantitative descriptions of cat retinal unit or optic fiber receptive field configurations are extremely rare. Usually estimates are given of the diameter of the central area of receptive fields. Only one group of investigators, Cleland and Enroth-Cugell (1968), have made quantitative maps of the threshold distribution of optic fiber receptive fields. However, they limited their investigation to the central areas of excitatory units only. They have plotted the stimulus level required to elicit a threshold response as a function of position in the retina and called the curve a "sensitivity profile" (Fig. 11-15). The sensitivity profiles appear U or V shaped with a peak or plateau of high sensitivity from 0.1 to 2.5 degrees in diameter. This part of the curve is known as the "area of uniform center." For over half of the optic fibers sampled the uniform centers are elliptical, rather than circular in shape. On either side of the uniform center threshold increases exponentially. Examination of the time course of discharge elicited by threshold stimuli at positions where the threshold drop did not follow an exponential course (i.e., Fig. 11-15B) demonstrated that the response elicited was of complex form indicating the surround effect was being elicited. The total central area was defined as the size of the field where threshold had increased by 98 percent. The total central area ranged in diameter from a minimum of 1.1 degrees to a maximum of 8.4 degrees.

FACTORS INFLUENCING RECEPTIVE FIELD CONFIGURATION

The recording electrode is an important factor in determining the minimum physical size of the retinal units or optic fibers sampled. The sampling bias of the recording electrodes may greatly influence the types of units encountered if response type and receptive field configuration are related to unit size. Rushton (1949; 1950) noted that his twenty-five micron tip platinum electrodes probably recorded selectively from the soma of large diameter (thirty-five to fifty microns) ganglion cells. Kuffler (1953) also reports that he believed his platinum electrodes (10 to 15 micron tip diameter) recorded only from retinal units with receptive field central areas of diameters 0.5 mm (two

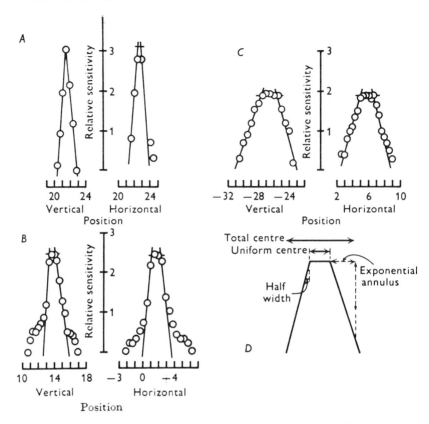

Fig. 11-15. Cat. Sensitivity profiles of three optic fibers: Plots of the stimulus level, re 3.3 log td, required to elicit a threshold excitatory response as a function of position of the exploratory spot. The profiles labled vertical were determined by positioning the exploratory spot along the vertical axis passing through the area of minimum threshold. Those labled horizontal were measured along a horizontal axis through the point of symmetry of the vertical sensitivity profile. (Cleland and Enroth-Cugell, 1968)

degrees) or more. In the same study, micropipettes with tip diameters less than 0.5 micron were capable of recording from retinal units having central area diameters as small as the diameter of the exploring spot used, i.e., 0.5 degrees.

Tungsten microelectrodes appear to be capable of recording from units with even smaller receptive field central areas. Stone and Fabian (1966) recording from retinal units believed to be located in the area centralis report observing a unit with receptive field central area 22 minutes in diameter. Cleland and Enroth-Cugell (1968), recording with tungsten microelectrodes inserted into the optic tract, report observing units with receptive field central areas ranging from 1.1 degrees to 8.4 degrees in diameter. Fukada

(1971), who recorded from tungsten electrodes and micropipettes inserted into the optic chiasm, reports that the central areas of receptive fields had diameters between 0.5 and 8.5 degrees, with the majority within a range of 1.5 to 5 degrees. Conduction-velocity estimates by Fukada (1971) indicate that the majority of these fibers had diameters greater than 3 microns. Thus, Fukada (1971) and perhaps Cleland and Enroth-Cugell (1968) probably sampled fibers that make up only 20 percent of the total population of the optic nerve, since 80 percent of the total population of optic fibers have diameters less than 3 microns.

Kuffler in 1953 reported that, in the cat, discharge pattern, and thus, receptive field configuration of retinal units are highly dependent upon a number of stimulus conditions. Therefore one would expect that in examining receptive field configuration considerable care would be taken to standardize or specify the stimulus conditions under which receptive fields are investigated. Unfortunately, stimulus conditions differ from one investigator to another and different photometric units are used to report stimulus intensity either in terms of luminance or illuminance. Often insufficient data are given to permit comparison of stimulus conditions. To quote one group of investigators in the area, ". . . . . it is often quite difficult to integrate results of different workers ...." since "..... sufficient information is rarely available for translation of one set of results into terms of another investigator's results" (Cleland and Enroth-Cugell, 1968).

Investigators utilize different stimulus configurations to map receptive fields. In some studies the stimulus configuration consists of two light sources that are directed toward the cat's eye: one a small exploratory test spot; the second, a surrounding background light. In other studies a translucent screen may be interjected between the light source and cat. Another stimulus configuration often utilized is a white screen of uniform luminance that serves as the background upon which a small exploratory light is projected. In other studies the background may be a screen (white, black, or gray) and the exploratory spot a black or white disc with illumination of both background and exploratory spot arising from the same or from different sources. In most cases the light source of the exploratory spot is flashed on and off, at different rates for different investigators. However, there are investigators who use exploratory spots of modulated intensity. The background, or in this case, the area surrounding the exploratory spot is illuminated at one level, B. The exploratory light level is modulated, either sinusoidally or rectangularly, from a maximum level H to minimum level L. The period of increased illumination or "stimulus on" condition is that time during which the modulated spot light is at level H and the background or "stimulus off" condition is the time during which the modulated spot light is at level L. In most cases level L is never as low as level B and therefore the background illumination levels of the exploratory spot area is at level L or level L plus B, if they overlap, and the surrounding area is at level B.

Kuffler (1953) reports that factors such as level of background illumination, area-size of the exploratory spot, and the intensity of the exploratory spot all affect discharge pattern, and therefore affect the size and configuration of the receptive field. The effect of background illumination on receptive field configuration is the most obvious as reported in preceeding sections on receptive fields. Only simple excitatory or inhibitory receptive fields are observed in dark adapted retinas, when small exploratory spot stimuli are used. Under conditions of moderate background illumination, concentric-type receptive fields are most commonly observed. According to Barlow and Levick (1969), the effectiveness of the surround area increases with background illumination level. The lowest background illumination at which it is possible to elicit the surround response of excitatory center units is reported to be 10^{-3} cd/m². The surround response of inhibitory center units appears to be elicited at even lower background levels. In addition, Sakmann and Creutzfeldt (1969) report that the threshold of the central area to a small spot of light increases with increases in background illumination.

According to Kuffler (1953), increasing background illumination to "high" levels results in a decrease in receptive field size and a decrease in the surround effect. With high background levels of illumination, the discharge pattern normally elicited from the surround cannot be elicited with small spot stimuli. Increasing the area-size of the spot stimulus to cover both the center and surround areas appears to result in a weak surround response in some units (Kuffler, 1953). It is possible that the center-field type units observed by Stone and Fabian (1966) in the area centralis are concentric-field type units with such low thresholds that the background illumination level used might have been great enough to suppress the surround effect. Although Stone and Fabian (1966) report background illumination could be varied from complete darkness to 5 cd/m², no mention is made as to whether background illumination was, in fact, varied to determine its effect. Stone and Fabian argue that since concentric-type fields were observed with identical background illumination levels, background level was not a factor influencing receptive field organization. However, since they did not demonstrate that the thresholds of center type and concentric type units are equal, it may be that the levels of background illumination that produced surround effects in concentric-type units were capable of suppressing them in center-type units. It was also reported by Stone and Fabian (1966) that center-type units did show indications of surround effects when the stimulus was diffuse retinal illumination. Fukada (1971) also reports observing optic fibers with center-type receptive fields that when stimulated with diffuse light showed signs of surround effects. Fukada superimposed upon a background luminance of 1.5 cd/m² an exploratory spot of light whose intensity was modulated rectangularly. The minimum value of the modulated light was 216 cd/m². Therefore the "background" illumination of the retinal area under the exploratory spot was the sum of the 1.5 cd/m² background and the 216 cd/m² of the modulated light.

The area-size of the exploratory spot determines the stimulus level required to elicit a threshold response, and may also affect discharge pattern (Kuffler, 1953). In both the dark and light adapted retinas, the effect of increasing area-size of the exploratory spot centered on the central area of a unit's receptive field was the reduction of the intensity required to elicit a threshold response (Barlow *et al.*, 1957). Increasing the area-size a few mm beyond the boundaries of the central area results in no change in threshold for dark adapted units and in a slight increase in threshold for light adapted units, according to some (Barlow *et al.*, 1957; Wiesel, 1960) and in no change, according to others (Cleland and Enroth-Cugell, 1968; Winters and Walters, 1970).

Increasing the area-size of an exploratory spot beyond the boundaries of the central area may result in alteration of the discharge pattern elicited. Whole retinal illumination of dark adapted retinas produces excitatory, inhibitory, or complex type responses, depending upon the level of stimulus used (Donner and Willmer, 1950). A large spot of light at stimulus levels several times a light adapted retinal unit's threshold to a small spot of light centered on the central area of the field may elicit a complex response or the surround response (Kuffler, 1953). Thus, if an investigator attempts to map receptive fields with an exploratory spot that is larger than the smallest receptive field, and if the stimulus level is much greater than the center area threshold, he may well elicit a complex or surround response from a concentric field type unit and classify it as a center-type unit or "on-off" type unit.

The sensitivity of a unit's receptive field in the light adapted retina is not uniform over the entire area of the unit's receptive field (Kuffler, 1953). Within the central area of the receptive field, sensitivity has been reported to be maximal at the approximate geometric center and to decrease steadily from the center. The surround area close to the central area may in some cases be as sensitive as the center or may be quite insensitive (Rodieck and Stone, 1965). Within the surround area the area of greatest sensitivity may be located to one side of the central area or may be symmetrically located about the central area.

Because the sensitivity or threshold of a unit is not uniform throughout the entire extent of the receptive field, the stimulus level of the exploring spot must be increased to activate retinal units when the spot is directed onto more peripheral areas of the retinal field. According to Kuffler (1953), stimulus levels one hundred to one thousand times the retinal unit's threshold to stimulation of the central area are required to determine the entire extent of receptive fields. Fukada (1971) reports that decreasing the stimulus level of an exploring spot resulted in decreases in the estimates of size of the central optic-fiber receptive fields. Thus, mapping retinal unit receptive fields with an exploring spot of fixed intensity will result in a partial estimate of field size, if the stimulus is of moderate level. Such may be the case for the few retinal units that Rodieck and Stone (1965) observed as having intermediate areas of insensitivity between the center and surround. Use of exploring spots of fixed, high-stimulus level leads to further complications.

Kuffler (1953) reports that increasing the intensity of the exploratory spot of light to high levels influences discharge pattern of light adapted units. The effect of increasing, by several log units, the intensity of a spot of light, smaller than the central area and positioned on the center of the central area, is pictured in Fig. 11-16. Increasing the level of the exploratory spot two log units above the unit's threshold appears to produce the surround response and, at higher levels, often results in a decrease in overall discharge rate (Stone and Fabian, 1968; Cleland and Enroth-Cugell, 1968; Winters and Walters, 1970). If high-level exploratory spots are used to map an excitatory center receptive field, the most sensitive area of the receptive field, which responds with increased discharge to low light levels, may respond with a complex or inhibitory response and be classified as a complex or inhibitory area. Since it is not known if the most sensitive area of all retinal unit and optic-fiber receptive fields have the same absolute threshold, one cannot argue that the light intensity used is not great enough to alter discharge of the real area of maximum sensitivity. This can only be determined by comparing the stimulus level used with measures of the threshold level required to elicit some minimum response of each area sampled within the receptive field.

DISCHARGE PATTERN

SPONTANEOUS ACTIVITY AND MAINTAINED DISCHARGE TO DIFFUSE RETINAL ILLUMINATION

Retinal units and optic fibers are spontaneously active under conditions of dark adaptation (thirty to ninety minutes in complete darkness). They also maintain tonic activity under conditions of light adaptation, which is often referred to as maintained activity as opposed to spontaneous activity. The dark adapted spontaneous activity is referred to as the dark discharge. The dark discharge does not appear to occur in all retinal cells and mean rates range from 0 to 85 spikes/second (Rodieck, 1967a).

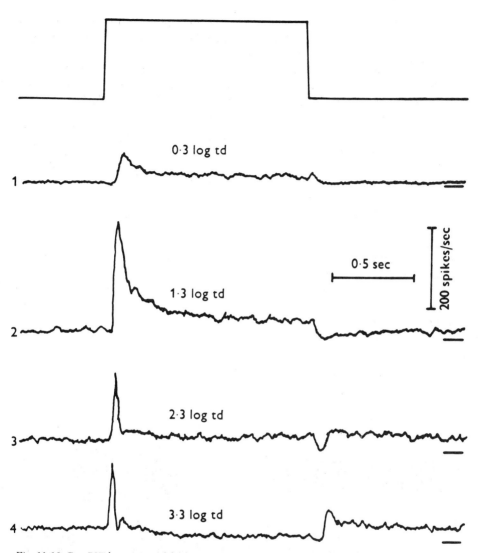

Fig. 11-16. Cat. PST histograms of discharge to small exploratory light centered upon the central area of optic fiber receptive field of light adapted eye. (Cleland and Enroth-Cugell, 1968)

Rodieck and Smith (1966) report observing slow rhythmic fluctuations (two per minute to two per hour) in dark discharge and in maintained discharge (Fig. 11-17). These fluctuations occur as sudden shifts in rate, with the discharge maintained at the new rate for several minutes before it drops abruptly back to the previous level of discharge. These slow rhythms were observed more often in animals anesthetized with nitrous oxide than in animals with midbrain lesions. They were observed to occur in both excitatory and inhibitory units but only under conditions of dark adaptation and at "low" levels of whole retinal illumination (below 4 to 7 x 10^{-2} cd/m²). Slow rhythmic changes in rate were not observed at higher levels of illumination (Rodieck and Smith, 1966) or when the illumination of the receptive field center was maintained at a level different from that of the surround (Rodieck, 1967a). Sectioning of the optic tract did not alter the slow rhythm and the rhythm did not appear to be related to respiration or blood pressure. Barlow and Levick (1969) report observing similar fluctuations in rates in preparations they felt were in good physical condition, but only over a limited range of whole retinal illumination and not at higher or lower levels. The fluctuations occurred around level 10^{-3} cd/m² and not during dark adaptation.

Barlow and Levick (1969) and Cleland and Enroth-Cugell (1970) report that rhythmic fluctuations in dark and maintained discharge were related to the poor physical condition of the preparation. Barlow and Levick report that most cases of rhythmic fluctuations were related to deteriorating conditions of the eye, excessive anesthesia or d-tubocurarine, respiratory obstruction, or general deterioration of the preparation. Barlow and Levick further suggest that instability of mean rate might result from "a wide variety of nonspecific noxious influences." Such noxious influences might occur more frequently in unanesthetized or lightly anesthetized preparations. Whatever the cause, many investigators report the omission of dark or maintained activity data

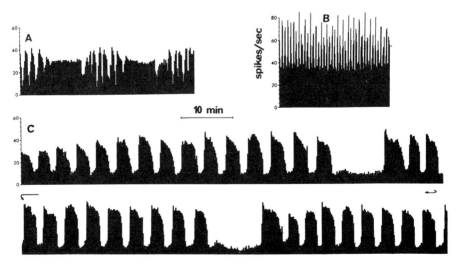

Fig. 11-17. Cat. Mean discharge rate of three unstimulated retinal units during extended periods in the dark. (Rodieck, 1967a)

because of wide fluctuations in discharge rate (Kuffler *et al.*, 1957; Ogawa *et al.*, 1966; Sakmann and Creutzfeldt, 1969).

It has been reported that excitatory unit maintained discharge rate increases monotonically as the luminance of a diffuse source is increased from complete darkness to approximately 10^{-3} cd/m² (Barlow and Levick, 1969; Sakmann and Creutzfeldt, 1969). Increasing the level of luminance to 1 cd/m² either resulted in a decrease in mean rate or in no change in mean rate of maintained activity (Sakmann and Creutzfeldt, 1969). According to Barlow and Levick (1969), increasing the luminance level up to 10^3 cd/m² resulted in further increases in mean rate of excitatory units. Inhibitory units are reported to respond to increases in luminance levels of a diffuse source with decreases in maintained discharge rate (Barlow and Levick, 1969). The decrease in discharge appears to level off at about 10^{-1} cd/m. Sakmann and Creutzfeldt (1969) calculated mean rates of excitatory unit discharge, using the total number of spikes elicited during the fifth minute after raising luminance. Barlow and Levick (1969) did not appear to use any systematic method for determining mean rate. In both studies spike trains with nonstationary mean-discharge rates were eliminated.

There have been many attempts to characterize the statistical properties of dark and maintained activity discharge patterns. However, Rodieck (1967a) reports that in most cases retinal unit spike trains from decerebrate cats in the absence of slow rhythm changes in rate had nonstationary statistical properties and that discharge pattern would change suddenly without much change in mean rate. He did not believe the nonstationarity was due to cell injury because he observed it in fibers as well as cells, and because it occurred without change in the shape of the recorded spike potentials. In Fig. 11-18 are examples of ISI histograms generated by retinal cells in darkness or under diffuse illumination of 4-7 cd/cm² (Rodieck, 1967a). Each histogram contains data that were checked for stationarity. Histograms A and B are from the same cell recorded at different times under the condition of complete darkness. Histograms C and D are from another unit, C in the light and D in the dark. Histograms E and F were both generated by the same unit at different times in light. Rodieck concludes because of nonstationarity, "Thus one cannot, in general, classify retinal ganglion cells into types on the basis of their maintained firing patterns." (1967a, pg. 1052). It is possible, however, that cells might be classified on the basis of the degree and type of nonstationarity shown.

The problem of nonstationarity has been mentioned by others studying dark or maintained discharge. Some investigators mention it in passing (Hughes and Maffei, 1965; Barlow and Levick, 1969) or cite it as a factor for rejecting certain records from analysis (Fuster *et al.*, 1965; Rodieck, 1967a). Many investigators reject all spike trains with widely fluctuating mean discharge rates but do not bother to check the stationarity of the ISI

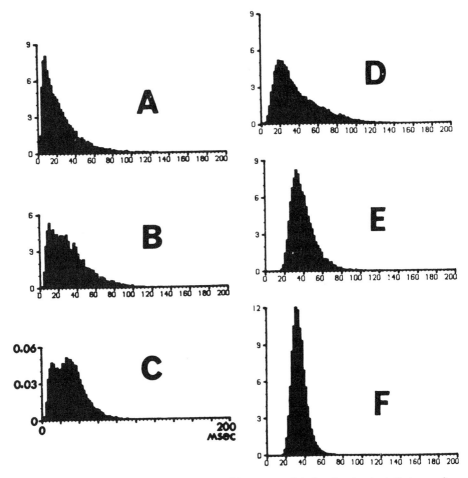

Fig. 11-18. Cat. Normalized interspike interval histograms of dark and maintained discharge of three retinal units. Histograms A and B were produced by the dark discharge of the same unit recorded at different times. Histogram C and D were recorded from another unit, C generated by maintained discharge to light and D by dark discharge. Histograms E and F were produced by the maintained discharge of another unit at different times in light. (Rodieck, 1967a)

histograms (Kuffler *et al.*, 1957; Ogawa *et al.*, 1966; Sakmann and Creutzfeldt, 1969). Fuster *et al.*, (1965) mention rejecting spike trains with nonstationary discharge patterns but do not mention the incidence of occurrence of nonstationarity, or note it as a serious drawback to classifying retinal cells on the basis of ISI distributions of dark and maintained activity. In any case nonstationarity of dark and maintained discharge appears to be a problem with which investigators utilizing paralyzed, unanesthetized, decerebrate, or lightly anesthetized cats must contend.

Nonstationarity of spike trains may account for the variety of results obtained by investigators attempting to classify retinal units or optic fibers on the basis of ISI distributions of dark or maintained discharge. ISI distributions of dark and maintained discharge are reported to range from unimodal to multimodal type distributions (Ogawa et al., 1966; Heiss and Bornschein, 1966; Rodieck, 1967a). Although multimodal distributions have been attributed to barbiturate effects (Ogawa et al., 1966; Rodieck, 1967a; Schmidt and Creutzfieldt, 1968), Heiss and Bornschein (1966) report observing them in unanesthetized, paralyzed preparations. Rodieck (1967a) reports that retinal units in cats anesthetized with nitrous oxide also had a tendency to fire rhythmically with bursts of about three spikes/sec. Some investigators report that the ISI histograms of dark discharge can be described as a Poisson process, with a mode at 12 msec followed by an exponential drop in numbers of longer interspike intervals (Herz et al., 1964; Fuster et al., 1965). Kuffler et al. (1957) state that exponential distributions did not fit any of their ISI histograms. Others report that many of their ISI histograms of dark and maintained discharge could be fitted by a gamma distribution, but that this distribution did not fit in all cases (Kuffler et al., 1957; Barlow and Levick, 1969).

DISCHARGE TO SMALL SPOTS OF LIGHT

The time course of discharge of excitatory retinal units and optic fibers to small spots of light centered on the central area of the receptive field has been examined by several investigators (Rodieck and Stone, 1965; Stone and Fabian, 1968; Cleland and Enroth-Cugell, 1968; Winters and Walters, 1970; Fukada, 1971). Most investigators report that the typical excitatory response consists of an initial burst of high frequency discharge that decays rapidly to a maintained rate that is usually higher than that to background illumination alone. When the spot luminance is decreased, discharge drops to below the level to background illumination alone (the background discharge level), then gradually recovers back to the background discharge level. According to Fukada (1971), there are two types of excitatory optic fibers on the basis of the time course of the discharge elicited by increased illumination of the excitatory central area. The tonic excitatory type fiber (Type II-On in Fig. 11-19) responds with a maintained discharge that is higher in rate than the background discharge level for the duration of increased illumination. The phasic excitatory type fiber (Type I-On in Fig. 11-19) responds with a transient increase in discharge that drops to background discharge levels in one to two seconds following the onset of increased illumination.

The time course of inhibition of maintained discharge to increased illumination of the central area of inhibitory units has not been described for

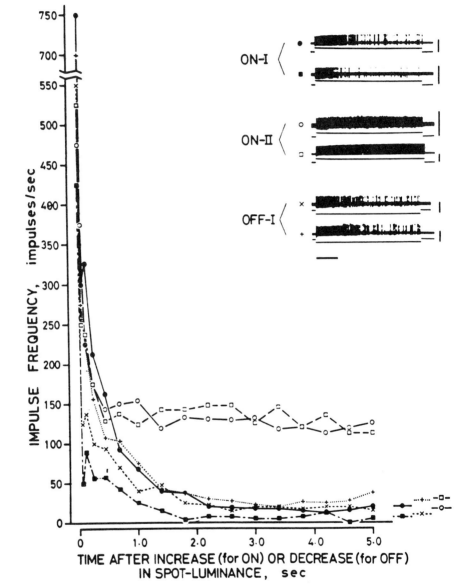

Fig. 11-19. Cat. PST histograms of different types of optic fibers to increased and decreased illumination of receptive field central area: Open circles and open squares represent discharge of fibers classified as tonic excitatory. Solid circles and solid squares represent discharge of fibers classified as phasic excitatory. Plus and X represent after discharge of fibers classified as phasic inhibitory. Background activity levels are represented to the right of the histograms. (Fukada, 1971)

the cat's peripheral visual system. The time course of the discharge to reduced illumination of the central area of inhibitory units has been described (Rodieck and Stone, 1965; Winter and Walters, 1970; Fukada, 1971). Although Rodieck and Stone (1965) report that the time course of the inhibitory after discharge is similar to that of excitatory discharge—i.e., tonically maintained for the duration of reduced illumination—others (Winter and Walters, 1970; Fukada, 1971) report that in most cases the after-discharge is transient and decays rapidly to background discharge levels. Saito, Shimahara, and Fukada (1970) and Fukada (1971) report observing two types of inhibitory optic fibers on the basis of the time course of discharge to a black disc on a white or gray background; that is, to a reduction in spot illumination to below background levels. The phasic inhibitory type optic fiber (type I-off in Fib. 11-19) is the most commonly observed inhibitory fiber. The phasic inhibitory fibers respond with a transient increase in discharge to reduction of illumination of the exploratory spot to background illumination level and below. The tonic inhibitory unit responds differently to the two stimulus conditions. It produces a transient after-discharge to reduction of illumination of the exploratory spot to background illumination level and produces discharge that is maintained for the duration of reduced spot illumination, if its level is reduced to below background levels. The maintained discharge of tonic inhibitory units to "dark" spots does not appear to be an after-discharge or rebound discharge, but appears to be an excitatory response to the stimulus configuration of a "dark" spot centered in a "light" surround.

According to Fukada (1971), the phasically discharging fibers decussate more often (162 crossed to 78 uncrossed) than do tonically discharging fibers (40 crossed to 33 uncrossed). The phasic fibers also appear to have higher conduction velocities and therefore larger axon diameters (Fig. 11-12B). The average conduction velocity was 39.1 m/sec for phasic excitatory fibers and 40.9 m/sec for phasic inhibitory fibers, as compared to 26.1 m/sec for tonic excitatory fibers. The phasic fibers also appear to have larger receptive field central areas. The average size of the receptive field centers was 3.7 degrees for phasic excitatory fibers and was 3.8 degrees for phasic inhibitory fibers, as compared to 2.6 degrees for tonic excitatory fibers.

Phasic and tonic fibers appear to respond differently to conditions of diffuse retinal illumination. Most phasic fibers respond with phasic discharge to onset and cessation of diffuse illumination, although some phasic fibers responded to the diffuse light with discharge characteristic of the central response. Tonic fibers were described to respond "poorly" to diffuse illumination and many tonic fibers responded with decreases in maintained discharge.

The effect of the stimulus level of a small exploratory spot on optic-fiber discharge rate under conditions of light adaptation has been examined (Creutzfeldt *et al.*, 1970; Winter and Walters, 1970). Winters and Walters (1970) report that increasing the intensity of an exploratory spot (0.1 to 7 degrees in diameter and centered upon the most sensitive portion of the central area) up to 2.2 log units above a fiber's threshold resulted in a monotonic increase in discharge rate of the initial high frequency burst of excitatory units, of their maintained activity and of the after-discharge of inhibitory units. At higher intensity levels the discharge rate of all three decreased with increased intensity, presumably because surround effects were elicited (Fig. 11-16).

Creutzfeldt *et al.* (1970) measured discharge rate of excitatory cells as a function of stimulus intensity, position of the stimulus within the receptive field central area, and of area-size of the stimulus. Discharge rate of the first fifty msec of the elicited response of optic fibers was observed to increase monotonically as stimulus level was increased up to two log units above threshold. Moving the position of the stimulus to more peripheral areas of the receptive field center produced a decrease in the slope of the intensity function, i.e., the discharge rate-log intensity plot. The slope of the intensity function varied little within 0.5 to one degree of the most sensitive area, decreased to 60 percent at 1.2 degrees and to below 30 percent at two degrees stimulus eccentricity for half the fibers studied. For the other half the slope decreased to below 60 percent at one degree and to below 30 percent at two degrees stimulus eccentricity. Increasing the area-size of a stimulus centered on the most sensitive portion of the receptive field central area lowered the stimulus level required to elicit a threshold response and increased the slope of the intensity function by a factor of 1.8 when area-size was increased by a factor of one hundred (5 minutes to 50 minutes of angle subtended at the cat's eye). These investigators did not appear to use stimulus levels greater than 2 log units above a fiber's threshold to the stimulus, and therefore do not report observing nonmonotonic intensity functions or complex discharge patterns.

SUMMARY

In our attempt to characterize the constituents of the population of retinal units and optic fibers, we have limited our review of the neurophysiology of the cat's peripheral visual system to studies utilizing relatively simple stimulating conditions. We had hoped to determine if the population is homogeneous or heterogeneous with respect to receptive field configuration and discharge pattern under conditions of dark and light adaptation with whole retinal and central area illumination. However, the results are not too clear because the stimulating conditions used often confounded the results obtained.

From the studies utilizing "simple" stimulus conditions, it would appear that two types of units are most frequently encountered in the retina and optic nerve, chiasm, and tract. These are the excitatory and inhibitory units, characterized on the basis of their response to stimulation of the central area of their receptive fields. These units appear to have concentric or asymmetrical receptive fields consisting of a "central" area that when stimulated elicits one response and a "surround" area that when stimulated elicits the antagonistic response. The surround area is not apparent under conditions of dark adaptation, and appears at low levels of light adaptation. Other types of units classified on the basis of their receptive field configuration may exist. However, the receptive fields of these units should be mapped with a threshold method using an extremely small spot of light of fixed area-size, under conditions of dark adaptation and at various levels of bckground illumination to determine if the stimulating conditions, rather than the unit's true receptive field configuration, are producing the unit type observed.

It is not clear if there are different types of units on the basis of the statistical properties of their discharge to complete darkness or to maintained levels of whole retinal illumination. It has been suggested that the discharge is nonstationary and therefore cannot be characterized by statistical measures (Rodieck, 1967a).

There appear to be four types of optic fibers when grouped on the basis of receptive field configuration and discharge pattern to illumination of the central area of the receptive field. The excitatory center fibers are of two types on the basis of time course of discharge to increases in retinal illumination: One discharges phasically; the other, tonically. The inhibitory center fibers are also of two types on the basis of the time course of discharges to reduction of illumination to levels below surround illumination: One discharges phasically; the other, tonically. These response types were observed only under conditions of light adaptation using high contrast stimuli. It is not known if these fibers respond similarly under conditions of dark adaptation or low level light adaptation or with low contrast stimuli.

There are numerous papers on the response of the cat's retinal units and optic fibers to complex stimulus conditions such as multiple spot stimuli, flickering stimuli, moving stimuli, stimuli with sinusoidally varied intensity, colored lights, etc. However, the data provided by studies using complex stimulus conditions do not further elucidate the types of neurons existing in the peripheral visual system of the cat.

Observing and describing the neuroanatomy and neurophysiology of the retina presents a task of almost bewildering complexity. Whereas most of the peripheral sensory systems described in this book usually consist of a sensory receptor element and a single neural element, the retina consists of two distinct receptor elements and a multitude of neural elements. Unlike most other sensory systems, the extraction of a pulse-coded message apparently can only be performed relatively late in the neural chain. The farther away from the transduction process the measurements are taken, the more difficult it is to determine the nature of the input signal to the neural elements under study. The recordings from the retina take place at a level that probably corresponds to the cochlear nucleus output in the auditory system: The neural population is composed of multiple subpopulations and the degree of abstraction of information is magnitudes greater than that found in the usual "first pulse afferent" in any other sensory system. We are not certain that, without knowledge of the input, structures of the degree of complexity of the retina are readily amenable to presently available techniques of analysis and conceptual understanding, at least to the degree of satisfaction possible in most other sensory systems.

12

CHEMICAL SENSORY SYSTEMS

The chemical senses take on a wide variety of appearances, depending upon receptor organ structure and their specific tasks of chemical measurement and analysis. The complexity of the sensory system is a reflection of the difficulty of the measurement problem: The olfactory system that is responsible for measuring and identifying an almost infinite number of airborne substances has tens of millions of primary nerve cells and fibers, whereas the chemoreceptive fibers bilaterally innervating the taste buds of the fungiform papillae of the tongue probably number between fifteen hundred and eighteen hundred. There are more olfactory fibers than there are fibers in the peripheral nerves of all other sensory systems combined. Probably all moist external surfaces are equipped with one or more chemical senses. The cornea, for instance, is innervated with chemoresponsive fibers as well as those serving other modalities (Dawson, 1962). The oral cavities are innervated by four separate cranial nerves (facial, glossopharyngeal, trigeminal, and vagus), which supply chemoreceptors in the tongue and elsewhere. Three separate nerves (olfactory, vomeronasal, and trigeminal) innervate the nasal cavities and form sensory systems responsive to airborne chemicals. Chemical sensory systems are probably located in other parts of the respiratory and digestive tracts. The digestive tract is in essence a chemical processing plant within which various substances are broken into their constituent parts through mechanical and chemical digestive activities. Undoubtedly these chemical processing procedures are monitored at every stage.

Anyone who has observed cats in their day-to-day activities realizes the importance odors play in a cat's life. Other cats are recognized primarily by odor rather than sight. A newcomer to a group frequently must be sniffed about the mouth and anus before everybody can relax. Food is identified first by sniffing and then, odor proving acceptable, by a flick of the tongue, which is richly supplied with chemoreceptors. There are also species specific cat-produced odors that are capable of completely dominating a cat's behavior. Toms mark with an odorous spray. The odor of a female cat in estrus can put a normally placid tom into a two to four day frenzy.

The chemical senses are not limited to external surfaces in contact with the outer world. The central nervous system monitors the chemical constituency or functioning of many internal organs. The chemistry of the blood is analyzed within complex organs that continuously sample the arterial blood stream. Chemoresponsive fibers have been recorded from in sensory nerves from the liver (Niijima, 1969) and other organs. No doubt many un-discovered chemoreceptive systems exist, since the study of visceral sensory systems is in its infancy (Iggo, 1966b).

In this chapter the anatomy of the chemoreceptor systems of the cat's oral and nasal cavities is reviewed. Adequate neurophysiology only exists for the chemoreceptors of the fungiform papillae of the tongue, however. The anatomy and neurophysiology of the cat's carotid body is also reviewed in this chapter.

CHEMICAL SENSES OF THE NOSE

The nose of the cat has an outer part, the nostrils, and an inner part known as the nasal cavities. The nasal cavities are separated into two halves by a bony division known as the "nasal septum." These two cavities are filled with a complex series of baffles formed by fine bones known as turbinals or conchae (Fig. 12-1). These thin bones run parallel with the air stream and break the nasal cavities into a many-surface organ. The honey-combed inner structure of the nasal cavities is best appreciated by viewing a transverse section through the nose (Fig. 12-2). The turbinals in the anterior and ventral parts of the nasal cavities are known as "maxilloturbinals." They are covered with respiratory mucous epithelium that contains many cilia. The maxilloturbinals function in air-conditioning by heating, moisturizing, and cleaning the air (Negus, 1958). The turbinals of the upper parts of the nasal cavities are known as the ethmoturbinals. According to Jayne (1898), there are seven lateral ethmoidal scrolls and one medial septal scroll. They are lined with both respiratory and olfactory epithelium. Several types of glands bathe the nasal mucosa (Bang and Bang, 1959). During normal respiration, the inspired air stream is directed through the maxilloturbinals and down into the trachea. A sniff is required to direct the air stream into the ethmoturbinals. According to Dawes (1952), the swell body located in the anterior parts of the nasal cavities near the ventral portion of the septum may also be utilized to direct the incoming air into the ethmoturbinals. The swell body is a highly vascularized structure that enlarges with an increase in blood supply (Schmidt, 1957; Negus, 1958).

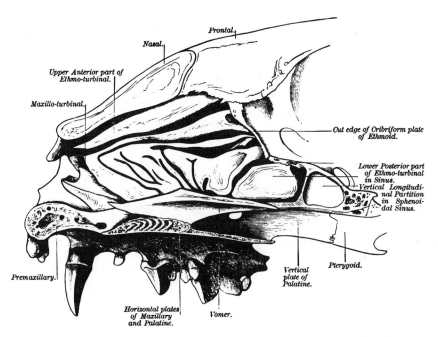

Fig. 12-1. Cat. Bony turbinals of the nasal cavity. The olfactory mucosa is located on the ethmoturbinals. (Jayne, 1898)

According to Read (1908), olfactory epithelium covers about half of the surface of the ethmoturbinals and is restricted to the dorsal and posterior parts of these structures. Olfactory epithelium also lines the dorsal parts of the septum. The olfactory epithelium thus extends over a considerable area. Lauruschkus (1942) estimates that the olfactory epithelium of the cat covers an area of 32 to 37 cm sq. Negus (1958) estimates the area to be 20.8 cm sq, an area larger than that found in either the rabbit or the human.

The olfactory epithelium is bathed by mucous produced by Bowman's glands (Moulton and Beidler, 1967). The olfactory epithelium (or olfactory mucosa, as it is frequently referred to) can be differentiated from the surrounding respiratory epithelium by the absence of respiratory cilia and by its slightly yellow color (Read, 1908). The complexity of the olfactory mucosa is most appreciated microscopically. Transverse sections through the olfactory mucosa reveal that there are several layers of cells in this epithelium. Basically, three different cell types have been identified in mammalian olfactory mucosa (Schultze, 1856): olfactory sensory nerve cells, supporting or sustentacular cells, and small stellate basal cells. These three cell types can be seen in diagrammatic representation in Fig. 12-3. Stellate or basal cells lie near the bottom of the olfactory epithelium, between the bases of the

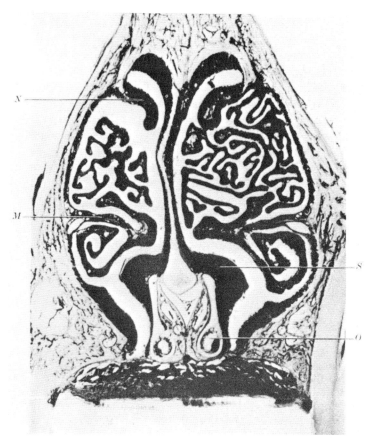

Fig. 12-2. Cat. Cross section through the nasal cavities: M, maxilloturbinals; N, ethmoturbinals; O, vomeronasal organ; S, swell body of the septum. (Schmidt, 1957)

supporting cells. Sustentacular or supporting cells occupy the superficial layers of the olfactory epithelium (Fig. 12-3). The cytoplasm of these cells encircles the olfactory sensory cells and forms different types of contacts with them (Moulton and Beidler, 1967). Andres (1969) has distinguished two different types of sustentacular cells in the cat on the basis of their appearance in electron microscopy (Fig. 12-4). Sustentacular cells extend microvilli into the ventral layers of the overlying mucous. The olfactory cells are evenly distributed between the supporting cells. Their nuclei occupy a zone between the nuclei of the supporting cells and the connective tissue underlying the olfactory epithelium. The apical portion of the olfactory cell extends as a cylindrical process from the nucleus to the surface of the

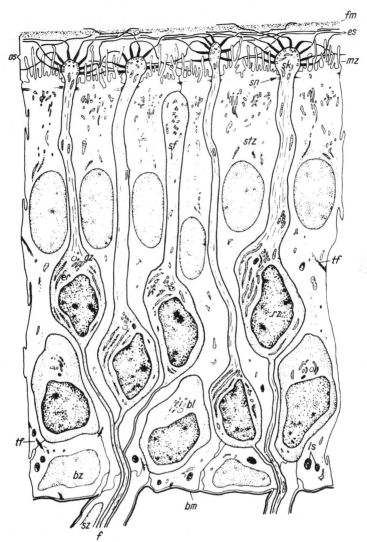

Fig. 12-3. Mammal. Schematic of the cell types found in the olfactory mucosa: Olfactory cells, rz; basal cells, bz; supporting cells, stz. (Andres, 1966a)

epithelium. The proximal end tapers into a thin, smooth filament, an olfactory nerve fiber. In addition to the sustentacular and olfactory cells, Andres (1969), distinguishes another cell type, which—like the olfactory cell—has its cell body located in the deeper layers of the olfactory mucosa and—like the olfactory cell—extends a thin distal process into the mucous layer, where it ends in straight stiff microvilli (Fig. 12-4). This new receptor

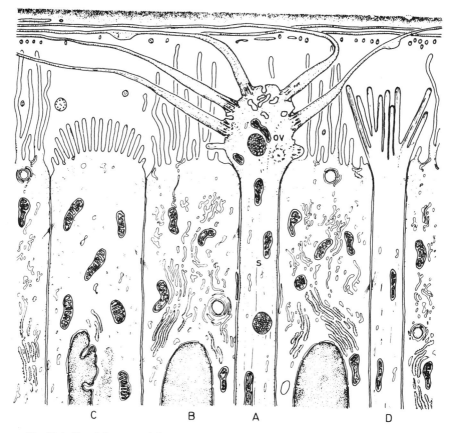

Fig. 12-4. Cat. Schematic of the superficial extensions of the cells in the olfactory mucosa: A, peripheral end of an olfactory sensory cell; B and C, two different types of supporting cells; D, new type of sensory cell. (Andres, 1969)

type is apparently quite rare and is found mainly in the parts of the olfactory mucosa adjoining the respiratory epithelium. On the basal part of this sensory cell a nerve fiber synapses.

The more commonly observed olfactory cell is like no other sensory neuron. It is both a receptor and a first-order neuron. Essentially, it is a bipolar neuron with a cell body in the deeper layers of the olfactory epithelium. From the cell body extends a long thin dendritic process up through the epithelium to the upper parts of the mucous layer, where it forms a knob from which extend a number of long (up to eighty microns) cilia. From the other end of the cell body emerges a thin unmyelinated axon that synapses in the olfactory bulb. Thus, the olfactory cell is in contact with both the outside world and the central nervous system. These olfactory cells can be seen schematically in Fig. 12-3 or in detail of their distal extensions

(Fig. 12-4). Olfactory cells are present in large numbers in the olfactory epithelium. Allison and Warwick (1949) estimate that in the rabbit there are about one hundred twenty thousand cells/mm² or 50 to 100 million in the olfactory epithelium on one side. Muller (1955) estimates there to be from 124 million to 224 million olfactory cells in the different breeds of dog. Mammalian olfactory cells have not been divided into morphologically distinct cell types, (Allison, 1953; Moulton and Beidler, 1967). Andres (1969) reports that cat olfactory cells are constantly degenerating and being reformed.

There is a one-to-one relationship between the number of olfactory receptors and the number of primary olfactory nerve fibers (Gasser, 1956; Clark, 1957). The unmyelinated axons of the olfactory cells range in size from 0.1 to 0.5 microns and conduct impulses at a rate of about 0.2 meters/sec. (Gasser, 1956; deLorenzo, 1957). After leaving the olfactory mucosa, the fibers group together in bundles enveloped by a single Schwann cell. The fiber bundles course through small holes in the cribiform bone and synapse in the glomeruli of the olfactory bulb with the dendrites of the mitral cells (Allison, 1953).

Spike potentials have been recorded from the olfactory receptor layer of the frog (Gesteland et al., 1963, 1965; O'Connell and Mozell, 1969) and vultures (Shibuya and Tucker, 1967). The unit potentials have been reported to be of long duration and to occur at low rates. Spontaneous activity is common.

THE VOMERONASAL SYSTEM

The vomeronasal organ of the cat is a tubular organ bilaterally situated in the anteroventral part of the nasal cavities near the septum (Fig. 12-2). The vomeronasal organ is enclosed in a cartilage capsule and is patent at the caudal end. The anterior part of this tubular organ opens into the nasopalatine duct and thus has access to both the oral and nasal cavities (Negus, 1956, 1958). The organ is lined with columnar ciliated epithelium on its lateral wall and with a thicker epithelium similar in construction to olfactory epithelium on its medial wall. According to Read (1908), the sensory cells of the vomeronasal organ are similar in shape to those found in the olfactory epithelium. Like the olfactory sensory cells, they have long thin dendritic processes extending into the mucous layer, where they form knobs (Fig. 12-5). From the proximal end of the cell bodies, unmyelinated axons arise. These axons travel to the accessory olfactory bulb, where they synapse in glomeruli with cells similar to the mitral cells of the main olfactory bulb (Allison, 1953; Ramón y Cajal, 1902).

Tucker (1963) has recorded from small bundles of axons innervating the vomeronasal organ in the rabbit. The electrical activity in these bundles fluctuated according to several variables, of which changes in the chemical composition of the air entering the nasal cavities seemed the least important. Chemoreceptive discharges were obtained in the rabbit by infiltrating aqueous solutions of odorants into the organ. In the gopher tortoise on the other hand, fibers from the vomeronasal organ responded to a wide range of airborne chemicals (Tucker, 1963).

TRIGEMINAL NASAL CHEMORECEPTORS

In addition to the specialized nerves of the olfactory and vomeronasal mucosa, the nasal cavities are innervated by fibers from other origins. The nervus terminalis innervates various areas within the nasal cavities (Larsell, 1914; McCotter, 1913). Fibers from or passing through the sphenopalatine ganglion innervate extensive areas within the nasal cavities (Read, 1908). These fibers are mostly efferent fibers of autonomic origin but may also contain sensory fibers from the geniculate ganglion of the facial nerve (Larsell and Fenten, 1928; Rhinehart, 1918; Boudreau et al., 1971). In addition to these nerves, the nasal epithelium is innervated extensively by sensory fibers apparently from the trigeminal ganglion via the ophthalmic and maxillary divisions of the trigeminal nerve (Read, 1908). These fibers apparently terminate in the olfactory and respiratory mucosa (Lenhossék, 1894).

Electrical recordings from trigeminal nerve bundles in the rabbit (Beidler, 1960; Tucker, 1963) indicate that this system is responsive to many of the same chemical stimuli that activate primary olfactory fibers.

ORAL CHEMORECEPTORS

Like the nose of the cat, the oral cavity of the cat is endowed with a number of chemically responsive sensory systems, although the medium of delivery is saliva instead of air. Chemoreceptive fibers from the trigeminal ganglion apparently innervate the oral cavity as well as the nasal cavities but the physiology of the oral systems has not been studied at all. In addition, the vagus nerve apparently supplies the taste buds in the epiglottis and larynx of the cat (Tuckerman, 1892; Oppel, 1900).

Fig. 12-5. Cat. A. Vomeronasal organ in an embryo kitten. Section of the cephalic region of the organ, the cartilagenous capsule entirely enclosing it. Two sensory cells are shown in the upper part of the lining of the epithelium. B,C. Sensory cells of the vomeronasal organ, with varicose axons. The cell with the largest axon was drawn from a different region of the same organ (enclosing lines indicate the thickness of the epithelium). D. Section through the middle of the vomeronasal organ; cartilaginous capsule not entire. Note the difference in thickenss of the median and lateral epithelium; an olfactory cell is shown in the epithelium of the median wall. (Read, 1908)

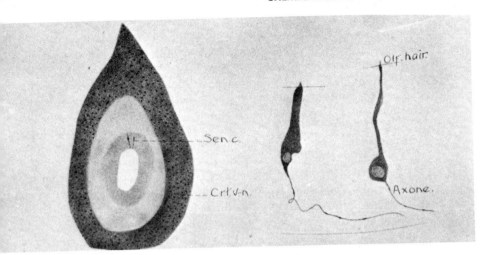

A   B

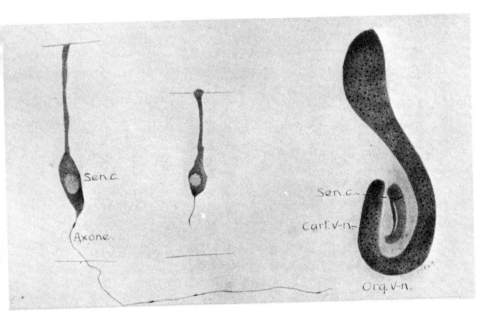

C   D

The oral chemical sensory systems that have been described in some detail are the taste-bud systems that are located on the tongue. The tongue of the cat is pictured in Fig. 12-6. The cat's tongue is extremely mobile and receives a massive motor innervation via the hypoglossal nerve. The mucous membrane covering the tongue consists of a superficial layer of epithelium and a dense layer of connective tissue, the lamina propria. The mucous membrane of the anterior dorsal surface of the tongue forms a multitude of small excrescences called the lingual papillae (Fig. 12-6). The tongue of the cat has several functions: It is used in eating both to separate food particles and to aid in their ingestion; it is used extensively in grooming the body hair; and it is a sensory surface of exceptional diversity and sensitivity. The sensory systems of the tongue are supplied by fibers from the trigeminal ganglion via the lingual nerve, the petrous ganglion of the glossopharyngeal nerve, and the geniculate ganglion of the facial nerve. All three of these ganglia also supply nonchemoreceptive sensory systems. The trigeminal ganglion, for instance, supplies sensory fibers to the tongue via the lingual nerve that are responsive to thermal and mechanical stimulation (Zotterman, 1936).

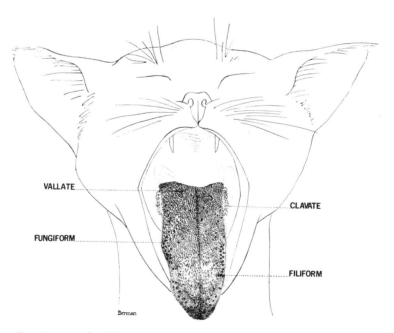

VALLATE

CLAVATE

FUNGIFORM

FILIFORM

Berman

Fig. 12-6. Cat. The different types of papillae found on the cat's tongue. (Artwork by M. Berman)

The chemoreceptive end organs of the tongue that have been described are known as taste buds. The taste buds are contained within the epithelial layer of the lingual mucous membranes and in stained section appear as pale, oval bodies in the darker-stained epithelium. The taste buds extend from the basement lamina, through the superficial epithelium almost to the surface of the tongue. The epithelium over each taste bud is pierced by a small opening, the outer taste pore, which leads into a pitlike excavation and the inner taste pore (Fig. 12-7). Taste buds are specialized chemoreceptor end organs composed of a number of modified epithelial cells, the chemoreceptor or taste cells, that are innervated by nerve fibers. Slender, rod-shaped chemoreceptor cells are oriented perpendicular to the surface and are packed like orange wedges to form a taste bud. From the free surface of the taste cell short microvilli, called taste hairs, project freely through the inner taste pore into the lumen of the pit. Taste buds of the cat tongue have not been described with electron microscopic techniques. Although Murray and Murray (1970) describe different cell types in rabbit taste buds, Scalzi (1967) and Andres (1970) believe that these different types represent chemoreceptor cells in different stages of development and degeneration (Fig. 12-7). It is known that there is a constant turnover of taste bud cells (Beidler and Smallman, 1965), which are formed from epithelial cells.

Taste buds are contained within the epithelial layer of the lingual papillae. Some of the papillae of the cat's tongue are illustrated in Fig. 12-6. Covering most of the central region of the tongue are the filiform papillae. The surface epithelium of these papillae is very thick and keratinized and forms sharp hooks on the tops of the papillae that give the cat's tongue its extremely abrasive texture. The size and shape of the filiform papillae vary with their location. Filiform papillae apparently do not contain taste buds.

On the back of the tongue are located three types of papillae. The vallate or circumvallate papillae are located farthest back and are arranged in a "V" with the point directed toward the gullet. The vallate papillae usually number four to six in the cat (Becker, 1908; Musterle, 1904). The vallate papillae are sunk into the surface of the mucous membrane and each is surrounded by a deep circular trench. The ducts of specialized secretory glands empty into the bottom of the trench (Oppel, 1900). The dorsal surface of the vallate papilla is fairly smooth, but often contains a central depression in which is located a small secondary papilla. Taste buds are located on the sides of the vallate papillae and are most numerous at the base of the papillae. According to Tuckerman (1890), there are about six hundred taste buds in the epithelium of the cat's vallate papillae. These taste buds degenerate if the glossopharyngeal nerve is cut (Vintschgau and Honigschmied, 1876).

The foliate papillae are leaflike outpocketings of the lingual mucosa located on the back lateral margin of the tongue (Gmelin, 1892). According to Becker (1908), they may be absent on one or both sides of the cat tongue. In the dog each foliate papilla consists of a number of smaller papillae arranged like the petals of a flower. Each small papilla of a foliate papilla is separated from one another by a crypt. Most of the taste buds are located on the sides of the papillae facing the crypts, although some have been observed on the surface of the papillae. The taste buds of the foliate papillae are innervated by the glossopharyngeal nerves.

Also found at the back of the cat's tongue on the sides are large clavate papillae (Sonntag, 1923). Clavate papillae are found only in a few species of small Felidae (Sonntag, 1923). They contain no taste buds, and their function is not known.

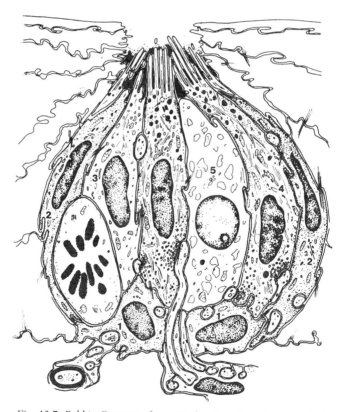

Fig. 12-7. Rabbit. Drawing of a vertical section through a taste bud from the foliate papilla. The different cell types, labeled from one to five are believed to represent different stages in the evolution of a taste cell. (Andres, 1970)

CHEMORECEPTORS OF THE FUNGIFORM PAPILLAE

On the front part of the tongue, taste buds are located on what are known as "fungiform papillae." Fungiform papillae are found most densely on the front edge of the tongue, on the smooth anterior tip, and on the sides of the tongue bordering the filiform papillae (Fig. 12-6). In addition, there is a large agglomeration of fungiform papillae in the center rear of the tongue in front of the vallate papillae. The sizes and shapes of fungiform papillae depend upon their location. The papillae on the front part of the tongue are usually small (less than 0.5 mm in diameter) and often set flush with the surface of the tongue, so they are hard to visualize. At the extreme anterior edge of the tongue, the papillae are located in a row and are bent over and can be extended. On the rear sides and rear center of the tongue, the fungiform papillae are larger (about one mm in diameter) and often extend several millimeters above the surface of the tongue on stalks.

The fungiform papillae are mushroom-shaped papillae covered by a thin layer of epithelium. The blood in the vessels beneath the epidermis gives the fungiform papillae a rose color in the living state. The connective-tissue core of a fungiform papilla forms small, secondary papillae upon which taste buds may be found. The taste buds are situated on the dorsal surface of the fungiform papillae and penetrate the thickness of the epithelium to rest upon the secondary papillae. Each fungiform papilla usually contains more than one taste bud (Kamada, 1957).

These taste buds are innervated by fibers from cells in the small (about eighteen hundred cells) geniculate ganglion (Buskirk, 1945) of the facial nerve (Fig. 12-8). About eight hundred to nine hundred fibers (Bruesch, 1944) take origin from cells located primarily in the ventral regions of this ganglion, travel in the facial canal with the motor fibers of the facial nerve to the middle-ear cavity where they branch off as the chorda tympani, which then joins with trigeminal sensory fibers in the lingual nerve to be distributed to the tongue. The chorda tympani is a mixed nerve containing about 1,955 myelinated and unmyelinated fibers of both efferent and afferent origin (Bruesch, 1944; Foley, 1945). The myelinated fibers of the cat's chorda tympani range in diameter from about 1.5 to 10 microns with a modal diameter of about 5 microns (Fig. 12-9). Chorda tympani fibers apparently supply all of the afferent innervation of the fungiform taste buds since the taste buds degenerate if the chorda tympani is severed (Olmstead, 1922).

Nerve fibers enter the fungiform papilla at the base and form bundles of nerve fibers that go to a taste bud. These fibers surround the outside of the taste bud or enter the taste bud to innervate taste cells. Fibers entering the bud are termed "intragemmal fibers" and those ending in the epithelium around the taste bud are called "perigemmal fibers." The innervation of a single fungiform papilla taste bud has been studied in some detail in the rat

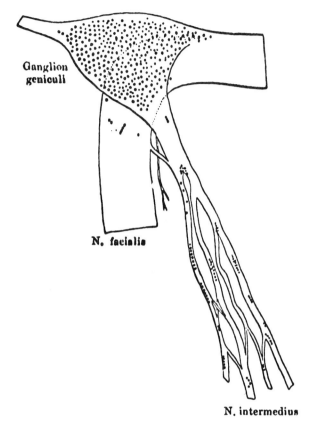

N. intermedius

Fig. 12-8. Ground squirrel. The geniculate ganglion
contains the cell bodies of the neurons that innervate the
taste buds on the fungiform papilla. (Weigner, 1905)

by Beidler (1969). In one rat fungiform papilla 54 fibers were seen to enter
the single taste bud. These fibers (mostly unmyelinated) formed 206
branches that made 220 contacts with the 59 taste cells of the taste bud.

NEUROPHYSIOLOGY OF FUNGIFORM CHEMORECEPTORS

Electrical recordings of single unit activity have been taken from cat chorda
tympani fibers (Zotterman, 1935; Pfaffmann, 1941; Cohen et al., 1955;
Nagaki et al., 1964) and from cat geniculate ganglion cells (Boudreau et al.,
1971), upon which we shall report in some detail. The geniculate ganglion
cells are of the pseudo-unipolar type (Fig. 12-10). Their central processes go
to the brain via the nervus intermedius (Fig. 12-8) and their peripheral

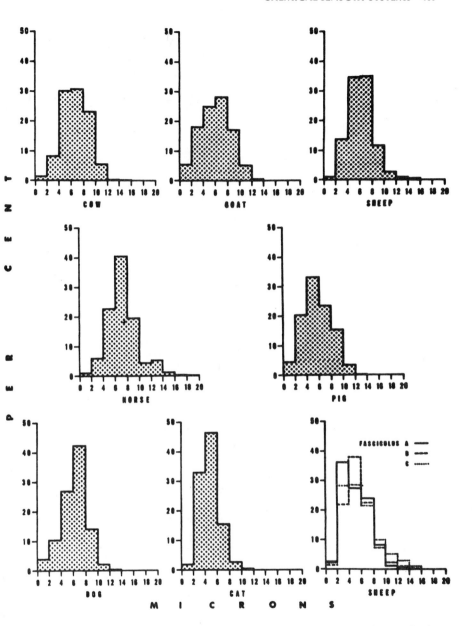

Fig. 12-9. Mammals. Histograms of fiber-diameter distribution of myelinated fibers in chorda tympani of various animals. The superimposed histograms of the fasciculi of a sheep illustrate fiber-diameter distribution in each individual fasciculus. (Kitchell, 1963) Reprinted with permission from Zotterman, Y., *Olfaction and Taste*, Vol. 1, © 1963 Pergamon Press Ltd.

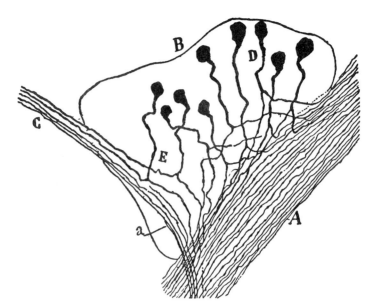

Fig. 12-10. Mouse. Geniculate ganglion cells of the mouse fetus. Golgi stain. A. Trunk of the facial nerve. B. Geniculate ganglion. C. Greater superficial petrosal nerve. D. Sensory cells of the geniculate ganglion that send peripheral fibers over the facial nerve. E. Sensory cells of the geniculate ganglion that send peripheral fibers over the greater superficial petrosal nerve. a. Fibers of central origin. (Ramón y Cajal)

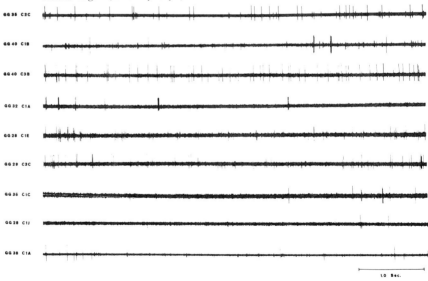

Fig. 12-11. Cat. Examples of the spontaneous activity patterns recorded from nine geniculate ganglion tongue units. (Boudreau et al., 1971)

processes extend to the tongue via the chorda tympani, to the soft palate via the greater superficial petrosal nerve, and to the internal surface of the pinna via the posterior auricular nerve (Rhinehart, 1918).

Geniculate ganglion cells responsive to sensory stimulation of the tongue have been designated "tongue units" and their properties have been investigated by Boudreau *et al.* (1971). The majority of tongue units studied exhibited a low rate of spontaneous activity (Fig. 12-11). Counts of the spontaneous rates for seventy-seven tongue units revealed that most units discharged fewer than forty spikes per 10 seconds with a modal value less than twelve spikes per 10-second period. The interspike interval histograms of the spontaneous activity were extraordinarily complex (Fig. 12-12). Although some histograms were unimodal, most were multimodal. As can be seen in Fig. 12-11, the spontaneous spike activity appears irregularly and, in some units, the spikes are emitted in small bursts. The occurrence of bursting is responsible for the short interval peak in some of the ISI histograms. The ISI histograms shown in Fig. 12-12 are the most complicated examples of spontaneous activity yet reported in a peripheral sensory system.

By electrically stimulating the surface of the cat's tongue, it was possible to excite most tongue units. When the current was lowered to near threshold values, spikes were only elicited when the stimulating probe was on certain papillae. In most cases electrical stimulation of only fungiform papillae was successful in eliciting spike discharge, but in a few cases electrical stimulation of filiform papillae, and in one case of a clavate papilla, excited tongue units. Most tongue units could be discharged by the electrical stimulation of more than one papilla. The fungiform papilla systems of several geniculate ganglion tongue units are shown in Fig. 12-13. The number of fungiform papillae connected to a single tongue unit ranged from one to as many as 12. Occasionally more than one tongue unit could be discharged by the electrical stimulation of a single fungiform papilla. Miller (1971) has demonstrated with rat chorda tympani fiber recordings that the response of a unit to chemical stimulation of one papilla may be enhanced or suppressed by simultaneous chemical stimulation of other papillae. So there is an indication that not only does one geniculate ganglion cell connect to more than one fungiform papilla, but also that chemical stimulation of these papillae may not be equivalent in effect.

Geniculate ganglion tongue units were also stimulated by a variety of chemical substances applied to the tongue. Fig. 12-14 demonstrates the response profiles for six tongue units stimulated with solutions of NaCl, quinine, citric acid, and a variety of foodstuffs in distilled water. As can be observed, one unit was discharged by none of the substances, whereas the activity of the other units was affected by a variety of substances. Quinine solutions sometimes inhibited spontaneous activity. Most of the food

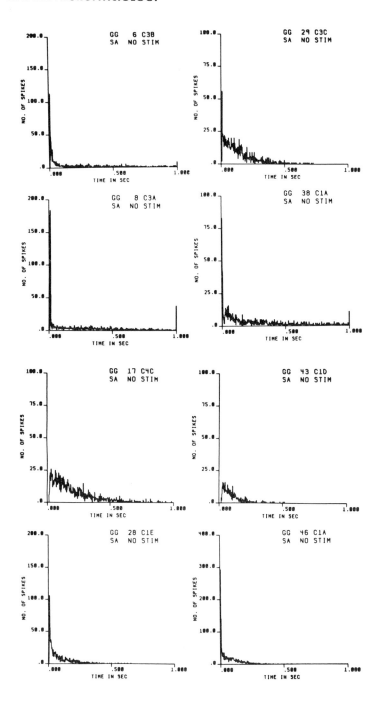

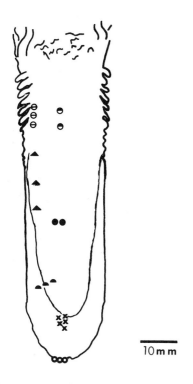

Fig. 12-13. Cat. Examples of the multiple fungiform papilla systems of seven geniculate ganglion tongue units determined by electrical stimulation. The separate symbols denote the fungiform papillae that when electrically stimulated excite a unit. (Boudreau *et al.*, 1971)

10 mm

substances used elicited discharge from the cells except sugar and egg white. Egg yolk and the meats used usually elicited discharge from the cells.

In a later study on geniculate ganglion tongue units, Kruger and Boudreau (1972) investigated their responsiveness to physiological buffer solutions as well as to a variety of salt solutions. Because tongue units had been observed to change their response properties with chemical stimulation, each unit was studied from the unstimulated state so that their responses could be compared. On the basis of quantitative comparisons of discharge to chemical stimuli, two major groups (I and II) of chemoresponsive units were delineated. These two groups of units constituted 71 percent of the thirty-one units studied. Group I units usually exhibited low levels of spontaneous activity, discharged to buffer solutions in the low pH regions, and tended to lose sensitivity to chemical stimulation over time. Group II units tended to discharge to buffer solutions in high pH ranges, exhibited high rates of spontaneous activity, and tended to either maintain responsiveness to chemical stimuli or often increase responsiveness following chemical stimula-

Fig. 12-12. Cat. Interspike interval (ISI) histograms of the spontaneous activity of eight geniculate ganglion tongue units. The last bin is an overflow bin for intervals longer than 1.0 sec. (Boudreau *et al.*, 1971)

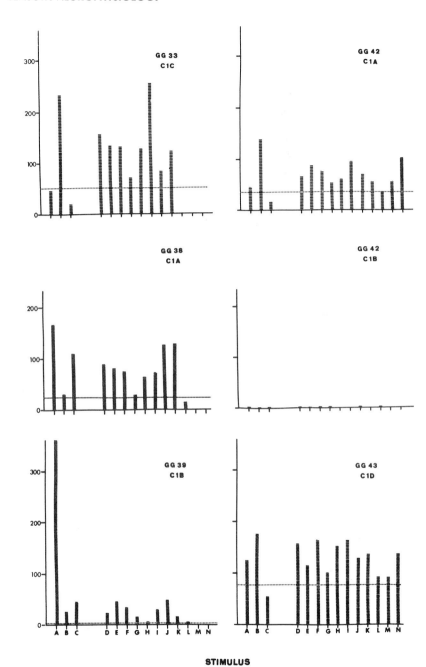

RESPONSE (SPIKES/10 SEC.)

STIMULUS

tion. Some of the response measures used to distinguish members of these two groups are illustrated in Fig. 12-15. As can be seen, some stimuli such as water, citric acid, and quinine discharge units in one group preferentially; others stimulate units from both groups. These two groups of geniculate ganglion units seem to correspond to chorda tympani fiber groups described by Cohen *et al.* (1955) and Nagaki *et al.* (1964). Nagaki *et al.* (1964) have demonstrated that the response of chorda tympani fibers to chemical stimulation is dependent upon the temperature of the chemical solution and upon the particular fiber studied.

THE CAROTID BODY

Coming off the heart is the massive aorta, which supplies the body with oxygenated arterial blood from the left ventricle. The aorta splits into a number of lesser arteries, one of which is the carotid artery. The carotid artery is the main blood supply for the head and neck. Located on different parts of this arterial complex are a number of small chemosensory organs, whereby the nervous system monitors the chemical constitution of the arterial blood. These organs are known as, on the aorta, the aortic bodies (Diamond and Howe, 1956; Paintal and Riley, 1966) and, on the carotid artery, as the carotid body. The anatomy and physiology of the carotid body has recently been reviewed by Biscoe (1971).

The carotid body or carotid glomus is a small (1.0 mm by 1.25 mm) organ located on the arch formed by the branching of the common carotid into the external carotid, the internal carotid, the ascending pharyngeal and the occipital arteries (Fig. 12-16). In the cat the internal carotid artery is quite small and sometimes even closed at its rostral end (Davis and Story, 1943). The carotid body receives a massive supply of blood from an artery branching off the ascending pharyngeal or the occipital artery or their common trunk. This artery divides into a dense honeycomb of smaller blood vessels at the arterial venous junction. De Castro and Rubio (1968) have reported that there are arterial-venous shunts located in the carotid body. The carotid body contains irregular masses of modified epithelial cells closely applied to the endothelium of the blood sinuses. The capillaries surround these small cell agglomerations known as glomeruli (Ross, 1959). Glomeruli are formed primarily by cells of two types, which de Kock (1954) designates

Fig. 12-14. Cat. Response profiles of six geniculate ganglion tongue units to stimulation with different chemical stimuli. The response is indicated by the spikes occurring during the 10 seconds following tongue application of the stimulus. The spontaneous-activity level of each unit is indicated with a dotted line parallel to the abscissa. The following standard stimulus solutions were used: A. 0.1 M citric acid, B. 1.0 M NaCl, C. 0.01 M quinine hydrochloride. The following foods were applied in distilled water solutions: D. pork liver, E. chicken, F. tuna, G. cod, H. milk, I. pork kidney, J. beef heart, L. sucrose, M. egg white, N. egg yolk. (Boudreau *et al.*, 1971)

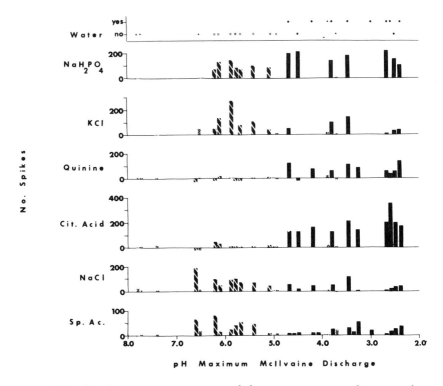

Fig. 12-15. Cat. Figure summarizing some of the response measures from geniculate ganglion tongue units. Each unit is arranged on the abscissa with respect to the pH at which the unit discharged maximally to the McIlvaine buffer series. The spontaneous-activity rate is measured in terms of spikes per 10sec. On the ordinate are response measures (spikes/10 sec) to the different stimuli corrected for the prevailing spontaneous activity level. The negative values indicate rates below spontaneous-activity levels. At the top of the figure are measures indicating whether the unit discharged to deionized water. Group I units are represented by solid bars. Group II units are indicated by cross-hatched bars. Ungrouped units are indicated by checkered bars. Chemical substances used were 1.0 M NaCl, 0.1 M citric acid, 0.01 M quinine hydrochloride, 1.0 M KCl, and 0.5 M NaH2PO4. Not all units were tested with all substances. When a unit was not tested with a particular substance, the space is left blank. (Kruger and Boudreau, 1972)

Type I cells and Type II cells. In each glomerulus, there are 20 to 30 Type I cells and three to six Type II cells (de Kock, 1954). Both of these cell types seem to be involved in chemical monitoring of the blood, even though neither is in direct contact with the capillary blood but rather is separated from it by cells of the sinusoid wall and a layer of fibrous tissue.

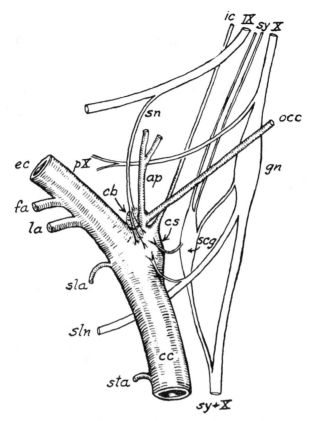

Fig. 12-16. Cat. The left carotid bifurcation and associated nerves, from the outer side. Abbreviations for this figure: ap = ascending pharyngeal artery; cb = carotid body; cc = common carotid artery; cs = carotid sinus; ec = external carotid artery; fa = facial artery; gn = ganglion nodosum; ic = internal carotid artery (obliterated); la = lingual artery; occ = occipital artery; px = pharyngeal branch of X; scg = superior cervical ganglion; sla = superior laryngeal artery· sln = superior laryngeal nerve; sn = "sinus nerve", intercarotid branch of the glossopharyngeal; sta = superior thyroid artery; sy = cervical sympathetic trunk; IX, X = glossopharyngeal and vagus nerves. From Adams, W.E., *The Comparative Morphology of the Carotid Body and Carotid Sinus*, 1958. Courtesy of Charles C. Thomas, Publisher, Springfield, Illinois.

Type I and II cells lie in close proximity to one another, with Type I cells interdigitating with one another. Type II cells envelope small groups of Type I cells with thin cytoplasmic processes (Fig. 12-17). Folded membrane systems can be seen in the Type II cells. The Type I cells may also participate

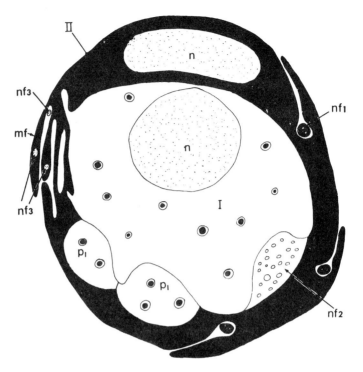

Fig. 12-17. Cat. Layout of Type I (I) and Type II (II) cells of the carotid body and their nerve supply: p1, fingerlike projection of a neighboring Type I cell; n, nucleus; nf1, small nerve fiber carried by Type II cell; nf2, a synaptic bag on the surface of Type I cell; nf3, small nerve fibers carried in a folded membrane system, mf. (de Kock and Dunn, 1968)

in these folded membrane systems, which take up as much as an eighth of the cell's surface (de Kock and Dunn, 1968). Three·different types of nerve endings were observed on Type I and Type II cells by de Kock and Dunn (1968). Two of these nerve-ending types were seen on Type II cells, one of which could be seen in the folded membrane system (Fig. 12-17). In addition to the two types of nerve endings on the Type II cells, a large expanded nerve ending typically occurred on the Type I cell (Fig. 12-17). Details of the nerve endings on the Type I cell and in the folded membrane are presented in Fig. 12-18. When the glossopharyngeal nerve is cut, all nerve endings degenerate except the small nerve fibers in the Type II cell regions other than in the folded membrane complex (de Kock and Dunn, 1968).

In addition to Type I and Type II cells, other cell types have been reported in the carotid body (Adams, 1958; de Kock, 1954). Nerve cells and microganglia (De Castro, 1926) have also been reported in the carotid body.

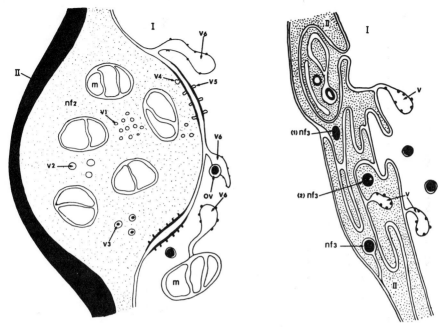

Fig. 12-18. Cat. Left: A synaptic bag (nf2), partly unsheathed by a Type II cell (II), bulges into a Type I cell (I). The bag is filled with mitochondria (m) and vesicles of varying sizes (v1-v5). Vacuoles (v6) in the Type 1 cell "open" into the synaptic cleft region and lie associated with mitochondria and dense-cored vesicles (ov). Right: A folded membrane system within a Type II cell (II), and lying against a Type I cell (I), carrying small nerve fibers (nf3). Two of these (1 and 2) have lost their protecting membrane sheath and lie naked within a granular bed. Vacuoles (v) extend into the cytoplasm of the Type I and Type II cells. (de Kock and Dunn, 1968)

Two nerves innervate the carotid body: the carotid nerve from the glossopharyngeal nerve, and the ganglio-glomerular nerve from the superior cervical ganglion (Gerard and Billingsley, 1923). These nerves also innervate the carotid sinus, a specialized part of the carotid arterial wall containing blood-pressure receptors. The carotid nerve is composed of about six hundred myelinated fibers and about three times as many unmyelinated fibers (Eyzaquirre and Uchizono, 1961). Measurements of the diameters of the fibers of the carotid nerve reveals that the myelinated fibers are mostly of small diameters (Fig. 12-19). In addition to containing afferent fibers, the carotid nerve contains efferent fibers (Biscoe and Sampson, 1968). The ganglio-glomerular nerve contains few myelinated firbers but a large variety of unmyelinated fibers.

The afferent output from the carotid body has been investigated by recording impulse traffic in the carotid nerve. A large number of these fibers that innervate the carotid sinus area (Rees, 1967) are responsive to blood-

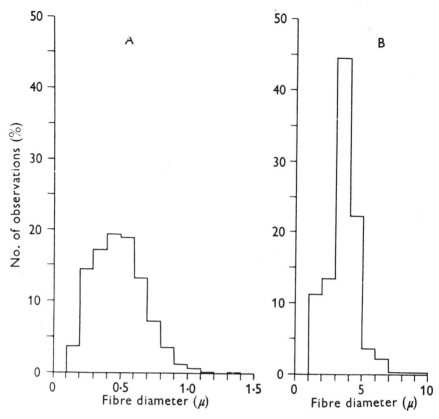

Fig. 12-19. Cat. Diameter distribution curves of fibers in the carotid nerve: A, measurements obtained from 2,037 nonmyelinated fibers analysed from 30 sections made in two nerves. B, measurements from all myelinated fibers (578) from one carotid nerve. (Eyzaguirre and Uchizono, 1961)

pressure changes and not chemical stimuli (Landgren, 1952a, 1952b). Apparently this "baroreceptor" activity can be eliminated by severing the carotid nerve connection with the carotid sinus (Euler *et al.*, 1939). The fiber types observable in the cat's carotid nerve have been investigated by Fidone and Sato (1969). They recorded from both myelinated and unmyelinated fibers as distinguished on the basis of conduction-velocity estimates. The myelinated and unmyelinated fiber groups both contained chemoresponsive and nonchemoresponsive fibers that were responsive to blood pressure. A total of 149 myelinated fibers were isolated. Most of these exhibited irregular spontaneous activity (two to five spikes per second) of the type described by Biscoe and Taylor (1963) and exhibited in interspike interval form in Fig. 12-20. These ISI distributions seem multimodal. Gehrich and Moore (1970) report that there are cyclic variations in fiber discharge that have the same

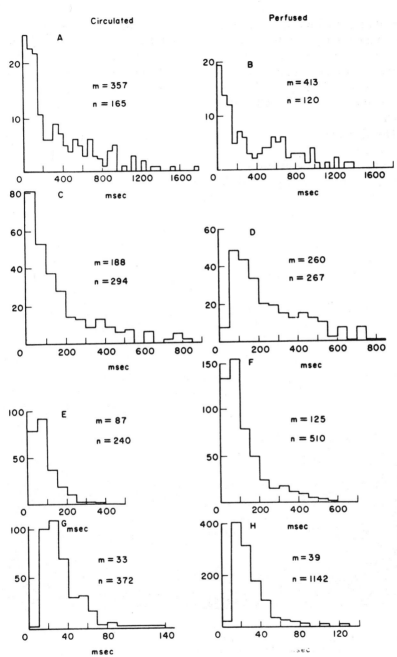

Fig. 12-20. Cat. Interspike interval histograms of spontaneous activity from fibers of normally circulated and artifically perfused cat carotid bodies: Mean interval in msec (m) and number of intervals (n) are shown in each case. (Biscoe and Taylor, 1963)

period as respiration and he art beat. About 5 percent of the chemoresponsive myelinated fibers studied by Fidone and Sato exhibited very regular spontaneous activity, even at low rates (Fig. 12-21). The conduction-velocity estimates of these regular discharging units ranged from seven to 15 meters per second, which puts them in the lower half of the distribution of conduction velocities for all of the chemoresponsive myelinated fibers (Fig. 12-22).

The fifty-two unmyelinated fibers studied by Fidone and Sato in the carotid nerve were classified into three categories: pressure-responsive fibers (15 fibers), chemoresponsive fibers (nine fibers), and the largest group, unresponsive fibers (28 fibers). The fibers in the last group exhibited no spontaneous activity and were unresponsive to the types of chemical and mechanical stimulation used. In their experiment the glossopharyngeal nerve was sectioned centrally and the glomero-ganglular nerve connections with the carotid body were sectioned. The spontaneous-activity rates of the chemoresponsive unmyelinated fibers ranged from zero to five spikes per second. These fibers discharged to the same stimuli that chemoresponsive

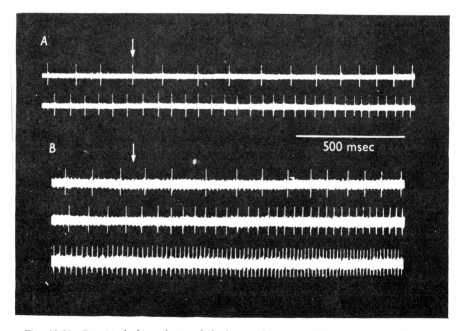

Fig. 12-21. Cat. Marked regularity of discharge of two carotid chemoreceptor A fibers. Conduction velocities, 9 m/sec (A) and 13 m/sec (B). Injections of 10 ug NaCN at arrows; records are continuous in A and B to time of maximum response of each unit. (Fidone and Sato, 1969)

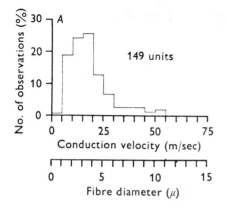

Fig. 12-22. Cat. A, percentage distribution of conduction velocities of 149 carotid chemoreceptor A-fibers. Estimated fiber diameter spectrum from conversion factor of 5.0. (Fidone and Sato, 1969)

myelinated fibers did (NaCN, ACh and acidified saline injections into the carotid artery), but their latencies were longer and their discharge rates lower.

The discharge of carotid chemoresponsive fibers has been reported to be influenced by electrical stimulation of the ganglio-glomerular nerve (Eyzaguirre and Lewin, 1961), raising the possibility that this nerve supplies efferent fibers to the carotid body. Chemoresponsive carotid nerve fibers have been reported to be responsive to a wide variety of chemical substances in the blood. A partial listing of these substances includes oxygen, carbon dioxide, NaCl, DNP, ATP, AMP, ADP, acid, eserine, nicotine, gallamine, and amytal. In some cases the effects of these substances have been interpreted in terms of their hypothesized pharmacological effect on the nerve-receptor synaptic junction (Eyzaguirre and Zapata, 1968). It is more likely that carotid blood chemistry changes have only minimal effect on the measuring instruments themselves but rather interact only at the receptor surfaces. Sensory systems are not only "ruggedized" for operating under extreme environmental conditions, but they are shielded from bodily conditions that might effect their performance. For instance, auditory nerve fibers, sensitive to infinitesimal movements of the stapes and basilar membrane, are apparently insensitive to the shock waves set up throughout the body from arterial pulsations. Vater-Pacini corpuscles are so sensitive to vibrations that they may be discharged by voices, yet they too are rarely reported to discharge to heartbeat. Presumably the chemoresponsive systems of the carotid body are similar to sensory systems elsewhere, and the methods of analysis are probably similar: Divide into neural groups and then determine the stimulus parameters influencing discharge for each group.

BIBLIOGRAPHY

Adal, M.N. and Barker, D. (1962). Intramuscular diameters of afferent nerve fibres in the rectus femoris muscle of the cat. In *Symposium on Muscle Receptors*, (Barker, D., ed.), pp. 249-256. Hong Kong University Press, Hong Kong.

Adams, W.E. (1958). *The Comparative Morphology of the Carotid Body and Carotid Sinus.* C.C. Thomas, Springfield, Ill.

Adamson, J. (1960). *Born Free.* Pantheon Books, New York, N.Y.

– (1961). *Living Free.* Harcourt, Brace and World, Inc., New York, N.Y.

– (1963). *Forever Free.* Harcourt, Brace and World, Inc., New York, N.Y.

– (1969). *The Spotted Sphinx.* Harcourt, Brace and World, Inc., New York, N.Y.

Adrian, E.D. (1928). *The Basis of Sensation.* Christophers, London, England.

Alexander, G. (1901). Zur Anatomie des Ganglion Vestibulare der Saügetiere. *Arch. f. Ohrenheilk.* 51:109-125.

Allison, A.C. (1953). The morphology of the olfactory system in the vertebrates. *Biol. Rev. Cambridge Philo. Soc.* 28:195-244.

– and Warwick, R.T.T. (1949). Quantitative observations on the olfactory system of the rabbit. *Brain* 72:186-197.

Alnaes, E. (1967). Static and dynamic properties of Golgi tendon organs in the anterior tibial and soleus muscles of the cat. *Acta physiol. scand.* 70:176-187.

Alving, B.M. and Cowan, W.M. (1971). Some quantitative observations on the cochlear division of the eighth nerve in the squirrel monkey (Saimiri sciureus). *Brain Res.* 25:229-239.

Andres, K.H. (1966a). Der Feinbau der Regio olfactoria von Makrosmatikern. *Z. Zellforsch.* 69:140-154.

– (1966b). Über die Feinstruktur der Rezeptoren an Sinushaaren. *Z. Zellforsch.* 75:339-365.

– (1969). Der olfaktorische Saum der Katze. *Z. Zellforsch.* 96:250-274.

– (1970). Anatomy and Ultrastructure of the Olfactory Bulb in Fish, Amphibia, Reptiles, Birds and Mammals. In *Taste and Smell in Vertebrates*, (Wolstenholme, G.E. and Knight, J., eds.), pp. 177-196. J. and A. Churchill Co., London.

424

Andrew, B.L. (1954). The sensory innervation of the medial ligament of the knee joint. *J. Physiol.* 123:241-250.

－ and Dodt, E. (1953). The deployment of sensory nerve endings at the knee joint of the cat. *Acta physiol. scand.* 28:287-296.

Ashino, T., Fukase, K., Sekiguchi, S. and Suinaga, T. (1960). On the sensory nerve supply of the upper lip of newborn cat. *Arch. Histol. Jap.* 19:189-202.

Babel, J., Bischoff, A. and Spoendlin, H. (1970). *Ultrastructure of the Peripheral Nervous System and Sense Organs.* Georg Thieme Verlag, Stuttgart.

Ballantyne, J. and Engström, H. (1969). Morphology of the vestibular ganglion cells. *J. Laryngol. Otol.* 83:19-42.

Bang, B.G. and Bang, F.B. (1959). A comparative study of the vertebrate nasal chamber in relation to upper respiratory infections. *Bull. Johns Hopkins Hosp.* 104:107-149.

Barker, D. (1962). The Structure and Distribution of Muscle Receptors. In *Symposium on Muscle Receptors* (Baker, D., ed.), pp 227-240, Hong Kong University Press, Hong Kong.

－ (1963). *Zoology and Medical Research.* University of Durham, Durham.

－ (1967). The Innervation of Mammalian Skeletal Muscle. *In Myotatic, Kinesthetic and Vestibular Mechanisms,* (de Reuck, A.V.S. and Knight, J., eds.), pp. 3-19, Little, Brown and Co., Boston, Mass.

－ and Chin, N.K. (1960). The number and distribution of muscle spindles in certain muscles of the cat. *J. Anat.* 94:473-486.

－ and Cope, M. (1962). The Innervation of Individual Intrafusal Muscle Fibres. In *Symposium on Muscle Receptors,* (Barker, D., ed.), pp. 263-269. Hong Kong University Press, Hong Kong.

－ and Ip, M.C. (1960). The primary and secondary endings of the mammalian muscle spindle. *J. Physiol.* 153:8-10P.

－ (1961). A study of single and tandem types of muscle-spindle in the cat. *Proc. Roy. Soc. Lond.* Series B 154:377-397.

－ (1963). A silver method for demonstrating the innervation of mammalian muscle in teased preparations. *J. Physiol.* 169:73-74P.

－ Ip, M.C. and Adal, M. (1962). A Correlation between the Receptor Population of the Cat's Soleus Muscle and the Afferent Fibre-diameter Spectrum of the Nerve Supplying It. In *Symposium on Muscle Receptors,* (Barker, D., ed.), pp. 257-261. Hong Kong University Press, Hong Kong.

– Stacey, M.J. and Adal, M. (1970). Fusimotor innervation in the cat. *Phil. Trans. Roy. Soc. Lond.* Series B 258:315-346.

Barker, D.J. and Welker, W.I. (1969). Receptive fields of first-order somatic sensory neurons innervating rhinarium in coati and raccoon. *Brain Res.* 14:367-386.

Barker, L.F. (1899). *The Nervous System and its Constituent Neurones.* D. Appleton and Co., New York, N.Y.

Barlow, H.B. (1957). Increment thresholds at low intensities considered as signal/noise discriminations. *J. Physiol.* 136:469-488.

– Fitzhugh, R. and Kuffler, S.W. (1957). Change of organization in receptive fields of cat's retina during dark-adaptation. *J. Physiol.* 137:338-354.

– Hill, R.M. and Levick, W.R. (1964). Retinal ganglion cells responding selectively to direction and speed of image motion in the rabbit. *J. Physiol.* 173:377-407.

– and Levick, W.R. (1969). Changes in the maintained discharge with adaptation level in the cat retina. *J. Physiol.* 202:699-718.

Barnett, C.H., Davies, D.V. and MacConaill, M.A. (1961). *Synovial Joints, Their Structure and Mechanics.* Longmans, Green and Co., London.

Becker, J. (1908). Ueber Zungenpapillen. Ein Beitrag zur phylogenetischen Entwicklung der Geschmacksorgane. *Janaische Zeits. f. Naturwiss.* 36:537-618.

Beddard, F.E. (1902). Observations upon the carpal vibrissae in mammals. *Proc. Zool. Soc. (Lond.)* 1:127-136.

Beidler, L.M. (1960). Physiology of olfaction and gustation. *Ann. Otol. Rhinol. Laryngol.* 69:398-409.

– (1969). Innervation of Rat Fungiform Papilla. In *Olfaction and Taste*, Vol. 3, (Pfafmann, C., ed.), pp. 352-369. The Rockefeller University Press, New York, N.Y.

– and Smallman, R.L. (1965). Renewal of cells within taste buds. *J. cell. Biol.* 27:263-272.

Békésy, G. von (1935). Über akustische Reizung des Vestibularapparatus. *Pflüg. Arch.* 236:59-76.

– (1960). *Experiments in Hearing.* (Trans. and Ed. by E.G. Wever) McGraw-Hill, New York, N.Y.

Bessou, P., Burgess, P.R., Perl, E.R. and Taylor, C.B. (1971). Dynamic properties of mechanoreceptors with unmyelinated (C) fibers. *J. Neurophysiol.* 34:116-131.

–   Emonet-Dénand, F. and Laporte, Y. (1965). Motor fibres innervating extrafusal and intrafusal muscle fibers in the cat. *J. Physiol.* 180:649-672.

–   and Laporte, Y. (1961a). Étude des récepteurs musculaires innervés par les fibres afférentes du groupe III (fibres myelinisées fines), chez le chat. *Arch. ital. Biol.* 99:293-321.

–   (1961b). Some observations on receptors of the soleus muscle innervated by Group III afferent fibres. *J. Physiol.* 55:19P.

_   (1962). Responses from Primary and Secondary Endings of the Same Neuromuscular Spindle of the Tenuissimus Muscle of the Cat. In *Symposium on Muscle Receptors*, (Barker, D., ed.), pp 105-119. Hong Kong University Press, Hong Kong.

–   and Pages, B (1968a). A method of analysing the responses of spindle primary endings to fusinotor stimulation. *J. Physiol.* 196:47-63.

–   and Pages, B (1968b). Frequencygrams of spindle primary endings elicited by stimulation of static and dynamic fusimotor fibres. *J. Physiol.* 196:47-63.

–   and Pages, B. (1969). Spindle secondary ending responses elicited by stimulation of static fusimotor axons. *J. Physiol.* 202:569-584.

–   and Perl, E.R. (1969). Response of cutaneous sensory units with unmyelinated fibers to noxious stimuli. *J. Neurophysiol.* 32:1025-1043.

Bianconi, R. and Van der Meulen, J.P. ((1963). The response to vibration of the end organs of mammalian muscle spindles. *J. Neurophysiol.* 26:177-190.

Biscoe, T.J. (1971). Carotid body: Structure and function. *Physiol. Rev.* 51:437-495.

–   and Sampson. S.R. (1968). Rhythmical and nonrhythmical spontaneous activity recorded from the central cut end of the sinus nerve. *J. Physiol.* 196:327-338.

–   and Taylor, A. (1963). The discharge pattern recorded in chemoreceptor afferent fibres from the cat carotid body with normal circulation and during perfusion. *J. Physiol.* 168:332-344.

Bishop, G.H. and Clare, M.H. (1955). Organization and distribution of fibers in the optic tract of the cat. *J. comp. Neurol.* 103:269-304.

Bishop, P.O., Jeremy, D. and Lance, J.W. (1953). The optic nerve. Properties of a central tract. *J. Physiol.* 121:415-432.

–   Kozak, W. and Vakkur, G.J. (1962). Some quantitative aspects of the cat's eye: Axis and plane of reference, visual field co-ordinates and optics. *J. Physiol.* 163:466-502.

Blevins, C.E. (1963). Innervation of the tensor tympani muscle of the cat. *Amer. J. Anat.* 113:287-301.

‒   (1964). Studies on the innervation of the stapedius muscle of the cat. *Anat. rec.* 149:157-172.

Blinkov, S.M. and Glezer, I.I. (1968). *The Human Brain in Figures and Tables.* Basic Books, Inc., New York, N.Y.

Bloom, W. and Fawcett, D.W. (1968). *A Textbook of Histology,* ninth edition. Saunders Co., Philadelphia, Pa.

Blunt, M.J., Wendell-Smith, C.P. and Baldwin, F. (1965), Glia-nerve fibre relationships in mammalian optic nerve. *J. Anat.* 99:1-11.

Bonnet, R. (1878). Studien uber die Innervation der Haarbalge der Hausthiere. *Morph. Jahr.* 4:331-398.

Boorer, M. (1970). *Wildcats.* Grosset and Dunlap, New York, N.Y.

Borg, G., Diamant, H., Oakley, B., Strom, L. and Zotterman, Y. (1967). A Comparative Study of Neural and Psychophysical Responses to Gustatory Stimuli. In *Olfaction and Taste,* Vol. 2, (Hayashi, T., ed.), pp. 253-264. Pergamon Press, New York, N.Y.

Boudreau, J.C., Bradley, B., Bierer, P., Kruger, S. and Tsuchitani, C. (1971). Single unit recordings from the geniculate ganglion of the facial nerve of the cat. *Exp. Brain Res.* 13:461-488.

‒   and Tsuchitani, C. (1968). Binaural interaction in the cat superior olive S-segment. *J. Neurophysiol.* 3:442-454.

‒   (1970). Cat Superior Olive S-segment Cell Discharge to Tonal Stimulation. In *Contributions to Sensory Physiology,* (Neff, W.D., ed.), pp. 144-213. Academic Press, New York, N.Y.

Boycott, B.B. and Dowling, J.E. (1969). Organization of the primate retina: Light microscopy. *Phil. Trans Roy. Soc. Lond.* Series B 225:109-184.

Boyd, I.A. (1954). The histological structure of the receptors in the knee-joint of the cat correlated with their physiological response. *J. Physiol.* 124:476-488.

‒   (1956). The tennissimus muscle of the cat. *J. Physiol.* 133:35-36P.

– (1962). The structure and innervation of the nuclear bag muscle fibre system and the nuclear chain muscle fibre system in mammalian muscle spindles. *Phil. Trans. Roy. Soc. Lond.* Series B 245:81-136.

Brearley, E.A. and Kenshalo, D.R. (1970). Behavioral measurements of the sensitivity of cat's upper lip to warm and cool stimuli. *J. comp. physiol. Psychol.* 70:1-4.

Bridgman, C. (1968). The structure of tendon organs in the cat: A proposed mechanism for responding to muscle tension. *Anat. Rec.* 162:209-220.

Bridgman, C.F., Shumpert, E.E. and Eldred, E. (1969). Insertions of intrafusal fibers in muscle spindles of the cat and other mammals. *Anat. Rec.* 164:391-401.

Brodal, A. (1969). *Neurological Anatomy in Relation to Clinical Medicine.* Oxford University Press, New York, N.Y.

– and Pompeiano, O. (1957). The vestibular nuclei in the cat. *J. Anat.* 91:438-454.

Brown, A.G. and Hayden, R.E. (1971). The distribution of cutaneous receptors in the rabbit's hind limb and differential electrical stimulation of their axons. *J. Physiol.* 213:495-506.

– and Iggo, A. (1967). A quantitative study of cutaneous receptors and afferent fibres in the cat and rabbit. *J. Physiol.* 193:707-733.

– Iggo, A. and Miller, S. (1967). Myelinated afferent nerve fibers from the skin of the rabbit ear. *Exp. Neurol.* 18:338-349.

Brown, J.E. and Major, D. (1966). Cat retinal ganglion cell dendritic fields. *Exp. Neurol.* 15:70-78.

– and Rojas, J.A. (1965). Rat retinal ganglion cells: Receptive field organization and maintained activity. *J. Neurophysiol.* 28:1073-3090.

Brown, K.T. and Tasaki, K. (1961). Localization of electrical activity in the cat retina by an electrode marking method. *J. Physiol.* 158:281-295.

– and Wiesel, T.N. (1958). Intraretinal recording in the unopened cat eye. *Amer. J. Ophthal.* 46:91-98.

– (1959). Intraretinal recording with micropipette electrodes in the intact cat eye. *J. Physiol.* 149:537-562.

Brown, M.C., Crowe, A. and Matthews, P.B.C. (1965). Observations on the fusimotor fibres of the tibialis posterior muscle of the cat. *J. Physiol.* 177:140-159.

– Engberg, I. and Matthews, P.B.C. (1967). The relative sensitivity to vibration of muscle receptors of the cat. *J. Physiol.* 192:773-800.

– and Matthews, P.B.C. (1966). On the Sub-division of the Efferent Fibres to Muscle Spindles into Static and Dynamic Fusimotor Fibres. In *Control and Innervation of Skeletal Muscle*, (Andrew, B.L., ed.), pp. 18-34. Thomas and Co., Dundee, Scotland.

Bruesch, S.R. (1944). The distribution of myelinated afferent fibers in the branches of the cat's facial nerve. *J. comp. Neurol.* 81:169-191.

– and Arey, L.B. (1942). The number of myelinated and unmyelinated fibers in the optic nerve of vertebrates. *J. comp. Neurol.* 77:631-665.

Burgess, P.R. (1971). *Personal Communication.*

– and Clark, F.J. (1969a). Characteristics of knee joint receptors in the cat. *J. Physiol.* 203:317-335.

– (1969b). Dorsal column projection of fibres from the cat knee joint. *J. Physiol.* 203:301-315.

– and Perl, E.R. (1967). Myelinated afferent fibres responding specifically to noxious stimulation of the skin, *J. Physiol.* 190:541-562.

– Petit, D. and Warren, R.M. (1968). Receptor types in cat hairy skin supplied by myelinated fibers. *J. Neurophysiol.* 31:833-848.

Burns, B.D. (1961). Electrical Recording from the Nervous System. In *Methods in Medical Research*, Vol. 9, (Quastrel, J.A., ed.), pp. 343-380. Year Book Medical Publishers, Chicago, Ill.

Buskirk, C. van (1945). The seventh nerve complex. *J. comp. Neurol.* 82:303-326.

Casey, D.E. and Hahn, J.F. (1970). Thermal effects on response of cat touch corpuscle. *Exp. Neurol.* 28:35-45.

de Castro, F. (1926). Sur la structure et l'innervation de la glande intercarotidienne (glomus caroticum) de l'homme et des mammifères, et sur nouveau système d'innervation autonome du nerf glossopharyngien. *Trav. Lab. Invest. Biol. Univ. Madrid.* 24:365-432.

– (1932). Sympathetic Ganglia, Normal and Pathological. In *Cytology and Cellular Pathology of the Nervous System*, Vol. 1, (Penfield, W., ed.), pp. 317-380. P.B. Hoeber, Inc., New York, N.Y.

–   and Rubio, M. (1968). The Anatomy and Innervation of the Blood Vessels of the Carotid Body and the Role of Chemoreceptive Reactions in the Autoregulation of the Blood Flow. In *Arterial Chemoreceptors*, (Torrance, R.W., ed.), pp. 267-278. Blackwell Scientific Publications, Oxford.

Cauna, N. (1969). The fine morphology of the sensory receptor organs in the auricle of the rat. *J. comp. Neurol.* 136:81-98.

Chandoha, W. (1963). *Walter Chandoha's Book of Kittens and Cats*, Bramhall House, New York, N.Y.

Chang, H.T. (1956). Fibre groups in primary optic pathway of cat. *J. Neurophysiol.* 19:224-231.

Chievitz, J.H. (1889). Untersuchungen über die Area centralis retinae. *Arch. Anat. Physiol. Lpz.* Anat. Abtheil., Suppl., pp. 139-196.

–   (1891). Ueber das Vorkommen der Area centralis retinae in den vier hoheren Wirbelthierklassen. *Arch. f. Anat. u. Physiol.* 15:311-334.

Clark, G.M. and Dunlop, C.W. (1969). Poststimulus-time response patterns in the nuclei of the cat superior olivary complex. *Exp. Neurol.* 23:266-290.

Clark, S.L. (1926). Nissl granules of primary afferent neurons. *J. comp. Neurol.* 41:423-451.

Clark, W.E. le Gros (1957). Inquiries into the anatomical basis of olfactory discrimination. *Proc. Roy. Soc. Lond.* Series B 146:299-319.

Cleland, B.G. and Enroth-Cugell, C. (1968). Quantitative aspects of sensitivity and summation in the cat retina. *J. Physiol.* 198:17-38.

–   and Enroth-Cugell, C. (1970). Quantitative aspects of gain and latency in the cat retina. *J. Physiol.* 206:73-91.

Cohen, L.A. (1955). Activity of knee joint proprioceptors recorded from posterior articular nerve. *Yale J. Biol. Med.* 28:225-232.

Cohen, M.J., Hagiwara, S. and Zotterman, Y. (1955). The response spectrum of taste fibers in the cat: A single fiber analysis. *Acta physiol. scand.* 33:316-332.

Colbert, E.H. (1969). *Evolution of the Vertebrates*, Second Edition. John Wiley and Sons, New York, N.Y.

Colby, E.D. (1970). Induced estrus and timed pregnancies in cats. *Lab. Anim. Care* 20:1075-1080.

Cooper, S. (1960). Muscle Spindles and Other Muscle Receptors. In *The Structure and Function of Muscle*, Vol. 1, (Bourne, G.H., ed.), pp. 381-420. Academic Press, New York, N.Y.

‒   (1961). The responses of the primary and secondary endings of muscle spindles with intact motor innervation during applied stretch. *Quart. J. exp. Physiol.* 46:389-398.

Copenhaver, W.H. and Johnson, P.D. (1958). *Bailey's Textbook of Histology*, Fourteenth Edition. Williams and Wilkins Co., Baltimore.

Coronios, J.D. (1933). Development of behavior in the fetal cat. *Genetic Psychol. Mono. Child Behav., Anim. Behav., Comp. Psychol.* 14:283-386.

Creed, R.F.S. (1958). The histology of mammalian skin, with special reference to the dog and cat. *Vet. Rec.* 70:171-175.

Creutzfeldt, O.D., Sakmann, B., Scheich, H. and Korn, A. (1970). Sensitivity distribution and spatial summation within receptive field center of retinal on-center ganglion cells and transfer function of the retina. *J. Neurophysiol.* 33:654-671.

Crevel, H. van and Verhaart, W.J.C. (1963). The rate of secondary degeneration in the central nervous system. II. The optic nerve of the cat. *J. Anat.* 97:451-464.

Crouch, J.E. (1969). *Text-Atlas of Cat Anatomy*. Lea and Febiger, Philadelphia, Pa.

Crowe, A. and Matthews, P.B.C. (1964a). The effects of stimulation of static and dynamic fusimotor fibres on the response to stretching of the primary endings of muscle spindles. *J. Physiol.* 174:109-131.

‒   (1964b). Further studies of static and dynamic fusimotor fibres. *J. Physiol.* 174:132-151.

Danforth, C.H. (1925a). Studies on hair with special reference to hypertrichosis. *Arch. Derm. Syphil.* 11:637-653.

‒   (1925b). Hair in its relation to questions of homology and phylogeny. *Amer. J. Anat.* 36:47-68.

Darian-Smith, I., Mutton, P. and Proctor, R. (1965). Functional organization of tactile cutaneous afferents within the semilunar ganglion and trigeminal spinal tract of the cat. *J. Neurophysiol.* 28:682-694.

Darwin, C. (1896). *Animals and Plants Under Domestication*. Vol. 1, pp. 45-50. D. Appleton and Co., New York, N.Y.

Davis, D.D. and Story, H.E. (1943). Carotid circulation in the domestic cat. Chicago Field Museum of Natural History. *Zool. Series* 28:5-47.

Davison, A. (1947). *Mammalian Anatomy*. (Revised by F. Stromsten). Blakiston Co., Philadelphia, Pa.

Dawes, J.D.K. (1952). The course of the nasal airstreams. *J. Laryngol. Otol.* 66:583-593.

Dawson, W.W. (1962). Chemical stimulation of the peripheral trigeminal nerve. *Nature* 196:341-345.

Deaver, J.B. (1900). *Surgical Anatomy*. Vol. 2. Blakiston Co., Philadelphia, Pa.

Denis, A. (1964). *Cats of the World*. Houghton Mifflin Co., Boston, Mass.

Diamond, J. and Howe, A. (1956). Chemoreceptor activity in the aortic bodies of the cat. *J. Physiol.* 134:319-326.

Dogiel, A.S. (1897). Der Bau der Spinalganglien des Menschen und der Säugetiere. *Anat. Anz. 12:140-152.*

  −   (1908). Der Bau der Spinalganglien des Menschen und der Säugetiere. Gustav Fischer, Jena.

Dohlman, G. (1941). The role of the perilymph in vestibular reactions. *Arch. Ohr. Nas. u. Kehlk. Heilk.* 150:25-30.

Dominis, J. and Edey, M. (1968). *The Cats of Africa.*Time-Life Books, New York, N.Y.

Donner, K.O. and Willmer, E.N. (1950). An analysis of the response from single visual-purple-dependent elements in the retina of the cat. *J. Physiol.* 111:160-173.

Donovan, A. (1966). The postnatal development of the cat retina. *Exp. Eye Res.* 5:249-254.

  −   (1967). The nerve fibre composition of the cat optic nerve. *J. Anat.* 101:1-11.

Dorst, J. and Dandelot, P. (1970). *A Field Guide to the Larger Mammals of Africa*. Houghton Mifflin Co., Boston, Mass.

Dowben, R.M. and Rose, J.E. (1953). A metal filled microelectrode. *Science* 188:22.

Dowling, J.E. (1965). Foveal receptors of the monkey retina: Fine structure. *Science* 147:57-59.

— (1970). Organization of vertebrate retinas. *Invest. Ophthal.* 9:655-680.

— and Boycott, B.B. (1965). Neural Connections of the Retina: Fine Structure of the Inner Plexiform Layer. In *Cold Spring Harbor Symposium on Quantitative Biology,* Vol. 30, Sensory Receptors, pp. 393-402. Cold Spring Harbor Lab. of Quantitative Biology, Cold Spring Harbor, Long Island, N.Y.

— (1966). Organization of the primate retina: Electron microscopy. *Proc. Roy. Soc.* (Lond.) Series B. 166:80-111.

— Brown, J.E. and Major, D. (1966). Synapses of horizontal cells in rabbit and cat retinas. 153:1639-1641.

DuBois, F.S. and Foley, J.O. (1936). Experimental studies on the vagus and the spinal accessory nerves in the cat. *Anat. Rec.* 64:285-307.

— (1937). Quantitative studies of the vagus nerve in the cat. II. The ratio of jugular to nodose fibers. *J. comp. Neurol.* 67:69-87.

Duncan, D. and Keyser, L.L. (1938). Further determinations of the numbers of fibers and cells in the dorsal roots and ganglia of the cat. *J. comp. Neurol.* 68:479-490.

Dusser de Barenne, J.G. (1934). The Labyrinthine and Postural Mechanisms. In *Handbook of General Experimental Psychology,* (Murchison, C., ed.), pp. 204-246. Clark University Press, Worcester, Mass.

Eberhard, T. (1954). Food habits of Pennsylvania house cats. *J. Wildlife Mgt.* 18:284-286.

Eccles, J.C. (1957). *The Physiology of Nerve Cells.* Johns Hopkins Press, Baltimore, Md.

— (1964). *The Physiology of Synapses.* Springer-Verlag, Berlin.

Ehrenbrand, F. and Witteman, G. (1970). Ueber synaptische Structuren im Ganglion vestibulare der Maus. *Anat. Anz.* 126:300-308.

Ekholm, J. (1967). Postnatal changes in cutaneous reflexes and in the discharge pattern of cutaneous and articular sense organs. *Acta physiol. scand.* Suppl. 297.

Engström, H. (1967). The ultrastructure of the sensory cells of the cochlea. *J. Laryngol. Otol.* 81:687-715.

— Ades, H. and Andersson, A. (1966). *Structural Pattern of the Organ of Corti.* Olmquist and Wiksell, Stockholm.

– Ades, H. and Hawkins, J. (1965). The Vestibular Sensory Cells and their Innervation. In *Symposia Biologica Hungarica*, (Szentagothai, J., ed.). pp. 21-41. Akademiai Kiado, Budapest.

Erulker, S.D., Butler, R.A. and Gerstein, G.L. (1968). Excitation and inhibition in cochlear nucleus. II. Frequency modulated tones. *J. Neurophysiol.* 131:537-548.

Euler, U.S. von, Liljestrand, G. and Zotterman, Y. (1939). The excitation mechanism of the chemoreceptors of the carotid body. *Skand. Arch. f. Physiol.* 83:132-152.

Evans, E.F. (1970). Narrow 'tuning' of the responses of cochlear nerve fibres emanating from the exposed basilar membrane. *J. Physiol.* 208:75-76P.

Ewer, R.F. (1968). *Ethology of Mammals.* Plenum Press, New York, N.Y.

Eyzaguirre, C. and Lewin, J. (1961). The effect of sympathetic stimulation on carotid nerve activity. *J. Physiol.* 159:251-267.

– and Uchizono, K. (1961). Observations on the fibre content of nerves reaching the carotid body of the cat. *J. Physiol.* 159:268-281.

– and Zapata, P. (1968). A Discussion of Possible Transmitter or Generator Substances in Carotid Body Chemoreceptors. In *Arterial Chemoreceptors*, (Torrance, R.W., ed.), pp. 213-251. Blackwell Scientific Publications, Oxford.

Fernand, V.S.V. (1970). The afferent innervation of two infrahyoid muscles of the cat. *J. Physiol.* 208:757-771.

Fernández, C. (1951). The innervation of the cochlea (guinea pig). *Laryngoscope* 61:1152-1172.

– and Goldberg, J.M. (1971). Physiology of first-order afferents innervating the semicircular canals of the squirrel monkey. II. The response to sinusoidal stimulation and the dynamics of the peripheral vestibular system. *J. Neurophysiol.* 34:661-675.

– and Karapas, F. (1967). The course and termination of the stria of Monakow and Held in the cat. *J. comp. Neurol.* 131:371-386.

– and Valentinuzzi, M. (1968). A study on the biophysical characteristics of the cat labyrinth. *Acta oto-laryngol.* 65:293-310.

Fex, J. (1962). Auditory activity in centrifugal and centripetal cochlear fibers in cat, a study of a feedback system. *Acta physiol. scand.* Suppl. 189.

Fidone, S.J. and Sato, A. (1969). A study of chemoreceptor and baroreceptor A- and C-fibres in the cat carotid nerve. *J. Physiol.* 205:527-548.

Fidel-Osipova, S.I., Yemets, G.L. and Burichenko, A.V. (1961). Electrophysiological and histomorphological characteristics of the joint capsule receptors. *Fyzyol. Zh.* 7:197-205.

Fitzgerald, M.J.T. and Alexander, R.W. (1969). The intramuscular ganglia of the cat's tongue. *J. Anat.* 105:27-46.

– and Lavelle, S.M. (1966). Response of murine cutaneous nerves to skin painting with methylcholanthrene. *Anat. Rec.* 154:617-634.

Fitzgerald, O. (1940). Discharges from the sensory organs of the cat's vibrissae and the modification in their activity by ions. *J. Physiol.* 98:163-178.

Foley, J.O. (1945). The sensory and motor axons of the chorda tympani. *Proc. Soc. Exp. Biol. Med.* 60:262-267.

– (1947). Functional components of the greater superficial petrosal nerve. *Proc. Soc. Exper. Biol. Med.* 64:158-162.

– (1960). A quantitative study of the functional components of the facial nerve. *Am. J. Anat.* 107:237-244.

– and DuBois, F.S. (1934). An experimental study of the rootlets of the vagus nerve in the cat. *J. comp. Neurol.* 60:137-159.

– (1937). Quantitative studies of the vagus nerve in the cat. I. The ratio of sensory to motor fibers. *J. comp. Neurol.* 67:49-67.

– (1943). An experimental study of the facial nerve. *J. comp. Neurol.* 79:79-101.

– Pepper, H.R. and Kessler, W.H. (1946). The ratio of nerve fibers to nerve cells in the geniculate ganglion. *J. comp. Neurol.* 85:141-148.

– and Sackett, W.W. (1950). On the number of cells and fibers in the glossopharyngeal nerve of the cat. *Anat. Rec.* 106:303 (Abstract).

Forbush, E.H. (1916). *The Domestic Cat. Bird Killer, Mouser and Destroyer of Wildlife. Means of Utilizing and Controlling It. Economic Biology Bull. No. 2, Massachusetts State Board of Agriculture, Boston, Mass.*

Frank, K. and Becker, M.C. (1964). Microelectrodes for Recording and Stimulation. *In Physical Techniques in Biological Research*, Vol. 5, (Nastuk, W.L., ed.), pp. 22-87. Academic Press, New York, N.Y.

Frankova, H. (1968). Comparison of the occurrence and variability of joint receptors in Rhesus monkey and man. *Folia Morph.* 16:83-92.

Freeman, M.A.R. and Wyke, B. (1967). The innervation of the knee joint. An anatomical and histological study in the cat. *J. Anat.* 101:505-532.

Freeman, W.J. (1963). The Electrical Activity of a Primary Sensory Cortex: Analysis of EEG Waves. In *International Review of Neurobiology*, Vol. 5, (Pfeiffer, C.C. and Smythies, J.R., eds.), pp. 53-119. Academic Press, New York, N.Y.

Frei, O. (1928). Bau and Leistung der Ballen unserer Haussäugetiere. *Jahrb. f. morph. u. mikrosk. Anat.* Abt. 1 Gegenbauers morph. Jahrb. 59:253-291.

Fritz, F. (1909). Über einen Sinnesapparat am Unterarm der Katze nebst Bemerkungen über den Bau des Sinusbalges. *Z. f. wissenschaf. Zoologie* 92:291-305.

Frost, H.M. (1960). Introduction to joint biomechanics. *Henry Ford Hosp. Med. Bull.* 8:415-432.

Fukada, Y. (1971). Receptive field organization of cat optic nerve fibers with special reference to conduction velocity. *Vision Res.* 11:209-226.

–   Motokawa, K, Norton, A.C. and Tasaki, K. (1966). Functional significance of conduction velocity in the transfer of flicker information in the optic nerve of the cat. *J. Neurophysiol.* 29:698-714.

Fuster, J.M., Herz, A. and Creutzfeldt, O.D. (1965). Interval analysis of cell discharge in spontaneous and optically modulated activity in the visual system. *Arch. ital. Biol.* 103:159-177.

Gacek, R.R. (1960). Efferent Component of the Vestibular Nerve. In *Neural Mechanisms of the Auditory and Vestibular Systems*, (Rasmussen, G.L. and Windle, W., eds.), pp. 276-284. C.C. Thomas, Springfield, Ill.

–   (1961). The macula neglecta in the feline species. *J. comp. Neurol.* 116:317-323.

–   (1969). The course and central termination of first order neurons supplying vestibular endorgans in the cat. *Acta oto-laryng.* Suppl. 254.

–   (1970). *Personal Communication.*

–   Nomura, Y. and Balogh, K. (1965). Acetylcholinesterase activity in the efferent fibers of the statoacoustic nerve. *Acta oto-laryng.* 59:541-553.

–   and Rasmussen, G.L. (1961). Fiber analysis of the stato-acoustic nerve of guinea pig, cat and monkey. *Anat. Rec.* 139:455-463.

Galambos, R. and Davis, H. (1948). Action potentials from single auditory-nerve fibers? *Science* 108:513.

–   Schwartzkopf, J. and Rupert, A. (1959). Microelectrode study of superior olivary nuclei. *Amer. J. Physiol.* 197:527-536.

Gallego, A. (1965). Connexions transversales au niveau des couches plexiformes de la retine. *Actual Neurophysiol.* 6:5-27.

Gardner, E.D. (1944). The distribution and termination of nerves in the knee joint of the cat. *J. comp. Neurol.* 80:11-32.

Gasser, H.S. (1956). Olfactory nerve fibers. *J. gen. Physiol.* 39:473-496.

Gehrich, J.L. and Moore, G.P. (1970). Cyclic variations in carotid body chemoreceptor activity. *Physiologist* 13:203.

Gerard, M.W. and Billingsley, P.R. (1923). The innervation of the carotid body. *Anat. Rec.* 25:391-400.

Gerstein, G.L., Butler, R.A. and Erulkar, S.D. (1968). Excitation and inhibition in cochlear nucleus. I. Tone-burst stimulation. *J. Neurophysiol.* 131:526-536.

Gesteland, R.C., Howland, B., Lettvin, J.Y. and Pitts, W.H. (1959). Comments on microelectrodes. *Proc. IRE* 47:1856-1862.

–   Lettvin, J.Y. and Pitts, W.H. (1965). Chemical transmission in the nose of the frog. *J. Physiol.* 181:525-559.

–   and Rojas, A. (1963). Odor Specificities of the Frog's Olfactory Receptors. In *Proceedings of the First International Symposium on Olfaction and Taste*, (Zotterman, Y., ed.), pp. 19-34. Pergamon Press, New York, N.Y.

Gilbert, S.G. (1968). *Pictorial Anatomy of the Cat*. University of Washington Press, Seattle, Wash.

Gmelin, D. (1892). Zur Morphologie der Papilla vallata und foliata. *Arch. f. mikros. Anat. u. Entwicklung.* 40:1-28.

Goglia, G. (1965). La morfologia ed il significato funzionale dei corpuscali de Pacini intercalati. *Quand. Anat. Pratica* 21:1-16.

Goldberg, J.M., Smith, F.D. and Adrian, H.O. (1963). Response of single units of the superior olivary complex of the cat to acoustic stimuli: Laterality of afferent projections. *Anat. Rec.* 145:232 (Abstract).

–   and Fernández, C. (1971a). Physiology of first-order afferents innervating the semicircular canals of the squirrel monkey: I. The resting discharge and the response to constant angular accelerations. *J. Neurophysiol.* 34:635-660.

— (1971b). Physiology of first-order afferents innervating the semicircular canals of the squirrel monkey. III. Variations among units in their discharge properties. *J. Neurophysiol.* 34:676-684.

Goldstein, J.L. and Kiang, N.Y-S. (1968). Neural correlates of the aural combination tone 2f1-f2. *Proc. IEEE* 56:981-992.

Granit, R. (1944). Stimulus intensity in relation to excitation and pre- and post-excitatory inhibition in isolated elements of mammalian retinae. *J. Physiol.* 103:103-118.

— (1962). Neurophysiology of the Retina. In *The Eye*, Vol. 2, (Davison, H., ed.), pp. 575-691. Academic Press, New York, N.Y.

— (1970). *The Basis of Motor Control.* Academic Press, New York, N.Y.

— Kellerth, J.O. and Williams, T.D. (1964a). Intracellular aspects of stimulating motoneurones by muscle stretch. *J. Physiol.* 174:435-452.

— (1964b). 'Adjacent' and 'remote' post-synaptic inhibition in motoneurones stimulated by muscle stretch. *J. Physiol.* 174:453-472.

Gray, J. (1968). *Animal Locomotion.* W.W. Norton and Co., New York, N.Y.

Gray, J.A.B. (1959). Initiation of Impulses at Receptors. In *Handbook of Physiology, Section 1:* Neurophysiology, Vol. 1, (Field, J., ed.), pp. 123-146. Waverly Press, Baltimore, Md.

— (1959b). Mechanical into electrical energy in certain mechanoreceptors. *Prog. Biophys. Biophys. Chem.* 9:285-324.

Gray, P.R. (1966). A statistical analysis of electrophysiological data from auditory fibers in the cat. Techn. Report No. 451. Mass. Inst. Tech., Res. Lab. Elect., Cambridge Mass.

Green, J.D. (1958). A simple microelectrode for recording from the central nervous system. *Nature* 182:962.

Groen, J.J., Lowenstein, O. and Vendrik, A.J.H. (1952). The mechanical analysis of the responses from the end-organs of the horizontal semicircular canal in the isolated elasmobranch labyrinth. *J. Physiol.* 117:329-346.

Guggisberg, C.A.W. (1962). *Simba.* Bailey Brothers and Swinfen, London.

Guinan, J.J. (1968). Firing Patterns and Locations of Single Auditory neurons in the Brain stem (Superior Olivary Complex) of Anesthetized Cats. Ph.D. Dissertation, Mass. Inst. Tech., Cambridge, Mass.

– Norris, B.E. and Swift, S.H. (1967). A paucity of unit responses in the accessory superior olive of barbiturate anesthetized cats. *J. Acoust. Soc. Amer.* 41:1585 (Abstract).

– and Peake, W.T. (1967). Middle-ear characteristics of anesthetized cats. *J. Acoust. Soc. Amer.* 41:1237-1261.

Gylek, F. (1912). Untersuchungen über das Planum nasale der Hauscarnivoren und de Befeuchtungsmodus an demselben. *Anat. Anz.* 40:449-463.

Ha, H. (1970). Axonal bifurcation in the dorsal root ganglion of the cat: a light and electron microscopic study. *J. comp. Neurol.* 140:227-240.

Hahn, J.F. (1971). Stimulus-response relationships in first-order sensory fibres from cat vibrissae. *J. Physiol.* 213:215-226.

Halata, Z. (1970). Zu den Nervenendigungen (Merkelsche Endigungen) in der haarlosen Nasenhaut der Katze. *Z. Zellforsch.* 106:51-60.

Hall, J.L. (1965). Binaural interaction in the accessory superior olivary nucleus of the cat. *J. Acoust. Soc. Amer.* 37:814-823.

Hall, V.E. and Pierce, G.N. (1934). Litter size, birth weight and growth to weaning in the cat. *Anat. Rec.* 60:111-124.

Harmon, W.W. (1963). *Principles of the Statistical Theory of Communication.* McGraw-Hill Book Co., New York, N.Y.

Harrison, J.M. and Feldman, M.L. (1970). Anatomical Aspects of the Cochlear Nucleus and Superior Olivary Complex. In *Contributions to Sensory Physiology,* Vol. 4, (Neff, W.D., ed.), pp. 95-142. Academic Press, New York, N.Y.

– and Irving, R. (1965). The anterior ventral cochlear nucleus. *J. comp. Neurol.* 124:15-42.

– and Irving, R. (1966). Ascending connections of the anterior ventral cochlear nucleus in the rat. *J. comp. Neurol.* 126:51-64.

Hartline, H.K. (1938). The response of single optic nerve fibers of the vertebrate eye to illumination of the retina. *Amer. J. Physiol.* 121:400-415.

Hartridge, H. and Yamada, K. (1922). Accommodation and other optical properties of the eye of the cat. *Brit. J. Ophthal.* 6:481-492.

Heiss, W.-D. and Bornschein, H. (1966). Multimodale Intervalhistogramme der Daueraktivität von retinalen Neuronen der Katze. *Kybernetik* 3:187-191.

Held, H. (1893). Die centrale Gehörleitung. *Arch. Anat. Physiol. anat. Abtheil.* 201-248.

Helmholtz, H.L.F. (1873). *The Mechanisms of the Ossicles of the Ear and Membrana Tympani.* (Trans by A.H. Buck and N. Smith). William Wood and Co., New York, N.Y.

Henkind, P. (1966). The retinal vascular system of the domestic cat. *Exp. Eye Res.* 5:10-20.

Henriques, B.L. and Sperling, A.L. (1966). Marking of sited cells after electrophysiologic study. *J. appl. Physiol.* 21:1247-1250.

Hensel, H. (1952). Afferente Impulse aus den Kältereceptoren der äusseren Haut. *Pflüg. Arch.* 256:195-211.

– and Boman, K.K.A. (1960). Afferent impulses in cutaneous sensory nerves in human subjects. *J. Neurophysiol.* 23:564-578.

– and Huopaniemi, T. (1969). Static and dynamic properties of warm fibres in the infraorbital nerve. *Pflüg. Arch.* 309:1-10.

– and Kenshalo, D.R. (1969). Warm receptors in the nasal region of cats. *J. Physiol.* 204:99-112.

– and Wurster, R.D. (1970). Static properties of cold receptors in nasal area of cats. *J. Neurophysiol.* 33:271-275.

Herxheimer, A. (1960). The Autonomic Innervation of the Skin. In *Advances in Biology of Skin*, Vol. 1, Cutaneous Innervation, (Montagna, W., ed.), pp. 63-73. Pergamon Press, New York, N.Y.

Herz, A. von, Creutzfeldt, O.D. and Fuster, J. (1964). Statistische Eigenshaften der Neuronaktivität im ascendierenden visuellen System. *Kybernetik* 2:61-71.

Hess, A. (1970). Vertebrate slow muscle fibers. *Physiol. Rev.* 50:40-62.

Hildebrand, M. (1960). How animals run. *Sci. Amer.* 202:148-157.

Hill, J.P. and Tribe, M. (1924). The early development of the cat (Felis domestica). *Quart. J. Microsc. Sci.* 68:513-602.

Hnik, P., Beránek, L. and Zelená, I. (1963). Sensory outflow from chronically tenatomized muscles. *Physiol. bohemoslov.* 12:23-29.

Hofer, H. (1914). Das Haar der Katze, seine Gruppenstellung und die Entwicklung der Beihaare. *Arch. f. mikros. Anat.* 85:220-278

Hoffman, H.H. and Kuntz, A. (1957). Vagus nerve components. *Anat. Rec.* 127:551-567.

Holmes, F. and Davenport, H. (1940). Cells and fibers in spinal nerves. *J. comp. Neurol.* 73:1-5.

Honrubia, F.M. and Elliott, J.H. (1969). Horizontal cell of the mammalian retina. *Arch. Ophthal.* 82:98-104.

–   and Elliott, J.H. (1970). Dendritic fields of the retinal ganglion cells in the cat. *Arch. Ophthal.* 84:221-223.

Hornocker, M.G. (1969). Winter territoriality in mountain lions. *J. Wildl. Mgmt.* 33:457-464.

Howe, H.A. (1935). The reaction of the cochlear nerve to destruction of its end organs: A study on deaf albino cats. *J. comp. Neurol.* 62:73-79.

Hromada, J. and Poláček, P. (1958). A contribution to the morphology of encapsulated nerve endings in the joint capsule and in the periarticular tissue. *Acta anat.* 33:187-202.

Hubbs, E.L. (1951). Food habits of feral house cats. *Calif. Fish Game* 37:177-189.

Hubel, D. (1957). Tungsten microelectrode for recording from single units. *Science* 125:549-550.

Hughes, G.W. and Maffei, L. (1965). On the origin of the dark discharge of retinal ganglion cells. *Arch. ital. Biol.* 103:45-59.

Hunt, C.C. (1954). Relation of function to diameter in afferent fibers of muscle nerves. *J. gen. Physiol.* 38:177-131.

–   (1961). On the nature of vibration receptors in the hind limb of the cat. *J. Physiol.* 155:175-186.

–   and McIntyre, A.K. (1960a). Properties of cutaneous touch receptors in cat. *J. Physiol.* 153:88-98.

–   and McIntyre, A.K. (1960b). An analysis of fibre diameter and receptor characteristics of myelinated cutaneous afferent fibres in cat. *J. Physiol.* 153:99-112.

Hursh, J.B. (1939). Conduction velocity and diameter of nerve fibres. *Amer. J. Physiol.* 127:131-139.

Igarashi, M. (1965). Redefinition of the macula neglecta in mammals. *J. comp. Neurol.* 125:287-294.

Iggo, A. (1958). The electrophysiological identification of single nerve fibres, with particular reference to the slowest-conducting vagal afferent fibres in the cat. *J. Physiol.* 142:110-126.

—   (1960). Cutaneous mechanoreceptors with afferent C fibres. *J. Physiol.* 152:337-353.

—   (1966a). Cutaneous Receptors with a High Sensitivity to Mechanical Displacement. In *Touch, Heat and Pain*, (deReuck, A.V.S. and Knight, J., eds.), pp. 237-256. Little, Brown and Co., Boston, Mass.

—   (1966b). Physiology of visceral afferent systems. *Acta neuroveg.* 28:121-134.

—   (1968). Electrophysiological and Histological Studies of Cutaneous Mechanoreceptors. In *The Skin Senses*, (Kenshalo, D.R., ed.), pp. 84-111. C.C. Thomas, Springfield, Ill.

—   (1969). Cutaneous thermoreceptors in primates and subprimates. *J. Physiol.* 200:403-430.

—   (1970). Somesthetic Sensory Mechanisms. In *Dukes' Physiology of Domestic Animals*, (Swenson, M.J., ed.), pp. 947-990. Cornell University Press, Ithaca, N.Y.

—   and Muir, A.R. (1969). The structure and function of a slowly adapting touch corpuscle in hairy skin. *J. Physiol.* 200:763-796.

Ishii, D. and Balogh, K. (1968). Distribution of efferent nerve endings in the organ of Corti. Their graphic reconstruction in cochleae by localization of acetylcholinesterase activity. *Acta oto-laryng.* 66:282-288.

Iurato, S. (1964). Fibre efferenti dirette crociate alle cellule acoustishe dell'organo del Corti. *Monit. Zool. Ital.* Suppl. 72:62-63.

—   (1967). *Submicroscopic Structure of the Inner Ear.* Pergamon Press, New York, N.Y.

Jänig, W. (1971). The afferent innervation of the central pad of the cat's hind foot. *Brain Res.* 28:203-216.

—   Schmidt, R.F. and Zimmermann, M. (1968). Single unit responses and the total afferent outflow from the cat's foot pad upon mechanical stimulation. *Exp. Brain Res.* 6:100-115.

Jansen, J. and Rudjard, T. (1964). On the silent period and Golgi tendon organs of the soleus muscle of the cat. *Acta physiol. scand.* 62:364-379.

Jansen, J.K.S. (1967). On the Functional Properties of Stretch Receptors of Mammalian Skeletal Muscles. In *Myotatic, Kinesthetic and Vestibular Mechanisms*, (deReuck, A.V.S. and Knight, J., eds.), pp. 20-39. Little, Brown and Co., Boston, Mass.

Jayne, H. (1898). *Mammalian Anatomy*. J.B. Lippincott Co., Philadelphia, Pa.

Johnstone, B.M. and Boyle, A.J.F. (1967). Basilar membrane vibration examined with the Mossbauer technique. *Science* 158:389-390.

Jones, K.L. (1937). Cell fiber ratios in the vagus nerve. *J. comp. Neurol.* 67:469-482.

Kamada, S. (1955). On the innervation, especially sensory innervation of mucous membrane of the oral cavity of cat. *Arch. Hist. Jap.* 8:243-260.

Kasprzak, H., Tapper, D.N. and Craig, P.H. (1970). Functional development of the tactile pad receptor system. *Exp. Neurol.* 26:439-446.

Katsuki, Y., Suga, N., and Kanno, Y. (1962). Neural mechanism of the peripheral and central auditory system in monkeys. *J. Acoust. Soc. Amer.* 34:1396-1410.

Keen, J.A. (1939). A note on the comparative size of the cochlear canal in mammals. *J. Anat.* 73:592-597.

Kennedy, J.L. and Smith, K.U. (1935). Visual thresholds of real movement in the cat. *J. gen. Psychol.* 46:470-476.

Kenshalo, D.R. (1964). The temperature sensitivity of furred skin of cats. *J. Physiol.* 172:439-448.

– Duncan, D.G. and Weymark, C. (1967). Thresholds for thermal stimulation of the inner thigh, footpad and face of cats. *J. comp. physiol. Psychol.* 63:133-138.

Kiang, N.Y-S. (1965). Stimulus coding in the auditory nerve and cochlear nucleus. *Acta oto-laryng.* 59:186-200.

– (1968). A survey of recent developments in the study of auditory physiology. *Ann. Otol. Rhinol. Laryngol.* 77:656-675.

– (1970). Comments in Discussion. In *Symposium on Sensorineural Hearing Loss*, (Wolstenholm, G.E.W. and Knight, J., eds.), p. 272. J. and A. Churchill, London.

– Baer, T., Marr, E.M. and Demont, D. (1969). Discharge rates of single auditory-nerve fibers as function of tone level. *J. Acoust. Soc. Amer.* 46:106 (Abstract).

–   and Goldstein, M.H. (1962). Temporal coding of neural responses to acoustic stimuli. *IRE Trans.* IT-8: 113-119.

–   Marr, E.M. and Demont, D. (1967). Sensitivity of auditory-nerve fibers to tonal stimuli. *J. Acoust. Soc. Amer.* 42:1206 (Abstract).

–   Moxon, E.C. and Levine, R.A. (1970). Auditory-nerve Activity in Cats with Normal and Abnormal Cochleas. In *Symposium on Sensorineural Hearing Loss,* (Wolstenholm, G.E.W. and Knight, J., eds.), pp. 241-268. J. and A. Churchill, London.

–   Pfeiffer, R.R., Warr, W.B. and Backus, A.S.N. (1965a). Stimulus coding in the cochlear nucleus. *Ann. Otol. Rhinol. Laryngol.* 74:463-485.

–   Sachs, M.B. and Peake, W.T. (1967). Shapes of tuning curves for single auditory-nerve fibers. *J. Acoust. Amer.* 42:1341-1342.

–   Watanabe, T., Thomas, E.C. and Clark, L.F. (1962). Stimulus coding in the cat's auditory nerve. *Ann. Otol. Rhinol. Laryngol.* 71:1009-1026.

–   (1965b). *Discharge Patterns of Single Fibers in the Cat's Auditory Nerve.* Res. Mono. No. 35, M.I.T. Press, Cambridge, Mass.

Kitchell, R.L. (1963). Comparative Anatomical and Physiological Studies of Gustatory Mechanisms. In *olfaction and taste,* Vol. 1, (Zotterman, Y., ed.), pp. 235-255. Pergamon Press, New York, N.Y.

Koch, S.L. (1916). The structure of the third, fourth, fifth, sixth, ninth, eleventh and twelfth cranial nerves. *J. comp. Neurol.* 26:541-552.

DeKock, L.L. (1954). The intra-glomerular tissues of the carotid body. *Acta anat.* 21:101-116.

–   and Dunn, A.E.G. (1966). An electron microscope study of the carotid body. *Acta anat.* 64:163-178.

–   (1968). Electron-microscopic Investigation of the Nerve Endings in Carotid Body. In *Arterial Chemoreceptors,* (Torrance, R.W., ed.), pp. 179-187. Blackwell Scientific Publications, Oxford.

Koenig, H.E., Tokad, Y. and Kesavan, H.K. (1967). *Analysis of Discrete Physical Systems.* McGraw-Hill Book Co., New York, N.Y.

Koeber, K.C., Pfeiffer, R.R., Warr, W.B. and Kiang, N.Y-S. (1966). Spontaneous spike discharges from single units in the cochlear nucleus after destruction of the cochlea. *Exp. Neurol.* 16:119-130.

Kramer, B. (1970). Anti-litter campaign: Groups seek to curb fecundity of felines. Wall Street Journal, Vol. 176, No. 106, Nov. 27.

Kruger, S. and Boudreau, J.C. (1972). Response of cat geniculate ganglion tongue cells to some chemical stimuli. *Brain Res.*

Ksjunin, P. (1901). Ueber das elastische Gewebe des Haarbalgs der Sinushaare nebst Bemerkungen über die Blutgefässe der Haarpapille. *Arch. f. mikros. Anat.* 57:128-150.

Kuffler, S.W. (1953). Discharge patterns and functional organization of mammalian retina. *J. Neurophysiol.* 16:37-68.

–   Fitzhugh, R. and Barlow, H.B. (1957). Maintained activity in the cat's retina in light and darkness. *J. gen. Physiol.* 40:683-702.

Kuntz, A. and Hamilton, J.W. (1938). Afferent innervation of the skin. *Anat. Rec.* 71:387-400.

Landgren, S. (1952a). The baroceptor activity in the carotid sinus nerve and the distensibility of the sinus wall. *Acta physiol. scand.* 26:35-56.

–   (1952b). On the excitation mechanism of the carotid baroceptors. *Acta physiol. scand.* 26:1-34.

Langworthy, O.R. (1929). A Correlated Study of the Development of Reflex Activity in Fetal and young Kittens and the Myelinization of Tracts in the Nervous System. In *Contributions to Embryology*, Vol. 20, pp. 127-172. Carnegie Institute of Washington, Washington, D.C.

Larsell, O. (1919). Studies on the nervus terminalis: mammals. *J. comp. Anat.* 30:3-68.

–   and Fenton, R.A. (1928). The embryology and neurohistology of sphenopalatine ganglion connections; a contribution to the study of otalgia. *Laryngoscope* 38:371-389.

Lauruschkus, G. (1942). Über Riechfeldgrosse und Riechfeldkoeffizient bei einigen Hunderassen und der Katze. *Arch. Tierheilk.* 77:473-497.

Leicester, J. and Stone, J. (1967). Ganglion, amacrine and horizontal cells of the cat's retina. *Vision Res.* 7:695-705.

Lenhossék, M.V. (1894). Die Nervenendigungen in der Riechschleimhaut. In *Beiträge zur Histologie des Nervensystems und der Sinnesorgane.* pp. 71-78. J.F. Bergmann, Wiesbaden.

Lennox, M. (1958). Single fiber responses to electrical stimulation in the cat's optic tract. *J. Neurophysiol.* 21:62-69.

Lessing, D. (1967). *Particularly Cats.* Simon and Schuster, Inc., New York, N.Y.

Leyhausen, P. (1963). The communal organization of solitary mammals. *Symp. Zool. Soc. Lond.* No. 13-14, pp. 249-263.

Lindblom, U. and Tapper, D.N. (1966). Integration of impulse activity in a peripheral sensory unit. *Exp. Neurol.* 15:63-69.

Lindeman, H. (1969). Studies on the Morphology of the Sensory Regions of the Vestibular Apparatus. *Adv. Anat. Embry. Cell Biol.* Vol. 42.

Lochte, T. (1934). Untersuchungen über die Unterscheidungsmerkmale der Deckhaare der Haustiere. *Deut. Z. f. d. ges. Gerichtl. Med.* 23:267-280.

Loewenstein, W.R. (Editor) (1971). *Handbook of Sensory Physiology, Vol. 1. Principles of Receptor Physiology.* Springer-Verlag, New York, N.Y.

– (1971). Mechano-electric Transduction in the Pacinian Corpuscle. Initiation of Sensory Impulses in Mechanoreceptors. In *Handbook of Sensory Physiology,* Vol. 1, (Loewenstein, W.R., ed.), pp. 269-290. Springer-Verlag, Berlin.

Longley, W.H. (1910). Factors which influence the maturation of the egg and ovulation of the domestic cat. *Science* 31:465-466.

Lorente de Nó, R. (1926). Études sur l'anatomie et la physiologie du labyrinthe de l'oreille et du VIII nerf. *Trav. Lab. Invest. Biol. Univ. Madrid* 24:53-153.

– (1933a). Anatomy of the eighth nerve. The central projection of the nerve endings of the internal ear. *Laryngoscope* 43:1-38.

– (1933b). Anatomy of the eigth nerve. III. General plan of structure of the primary cochlear nuclei. *Laryngoscope* 43:327-350.

De Lorenzo, A.J. (1957). Electron microscopic observations of the olfactory mucosa and olfactory nerve. *J. Biophys. Biochem. Cytol.* 3:839-850.

– (1963). Studies on the Ultrastructure and Histophysiology of Cell Membranes, Nerve Fibres and Synaptic Junctions in Chemoreceptors. In *Olfaction and Taste,* Vol. 1, (Zotterman, Y., ed.), pp. 5-18. Pergamon Press, New York, N.Y.

– (1970). The Olfactory Neuron and the Blood-brain Barrier. In *Taste and Smell in Vertebrates,* (Wolstenholme, G.E. and Knight, J., eds.), pp. 151-176. J. and A. Churchill Co., London.

Lowenstein, O. and Sand, A. (1940). The mechanism of the semicircular canal. A study of the responses of single-fibre preparations to angular accelerations and to rotation at constant speed. *Proc. Roy. Soc. Lond.* Series B 129:256-275.

Lundberg, A. and Winsbury, G. (1960). Selective adequate activation of large afferents from muscle spindles and Golgi tendon organs. *Acta physiol. scand.* 49:155-164.

Lynn, B. (1969). The nature and location of certain phasic mechanoreceptors in the cat's foot. *J. Physiol.* 201:765-773.

MacConaill, M.A. (1966). The geometry and algebra of articular kinematics. *Biomed. Eng.* 1:205-211.

McCabe, J.S. and Low, F.N. (1969). The subarachnoid angle: An area of transition in peripheral nerve. *Anat. Rec.* 164:15-34.

McCotter, R.E. (1913). The nervus terminalis in the adult dog and cat. *J. comp. Neurol.* 23:145-152.

McElvain, S.M., Bright, R.D. and Johnson, P.R. (1941). The constituents of the volatile oil of catnip. I. Nepetalic acid, nepetalactone and related compounds. *J. Amer. Chem. Soc.* 63:58563.

— Walters, P.M. and Bright, R.D. (1942). The constituents of the volatile oil of catnip. II. The neutral components, nepetalic anhydride. *J. Amer. Chem. Soc.* 64:1828-1831.

McMurry, F. and Sperry, C. (1941). Food of feral house cats in Oklahoma, a progress report. *J. Mammalogy* 22:185-190.

Malinovský, L. (1966a). The variability of encapsulated corpuscles in the upper lip and tongue of the domestic cat (Felis ocreata L., F. domestica). *Folia Morph.* 14:175-191.

— (1966b). Variability of sensory corpuscles in the skin of the nose and in the area of sulcus labii maxillaris of the domestic cat. *Folia Morph.* 14:417-429.

— (1966c). Variability of sensory nerve endings in foot pads of a domestic cat. *Acta anat.* 64:82-106.

— (1967). Some problems connected with the evaluation of skin receptors and their classification. *Folia Morph.* 15:18-25.

— (1970). Ein Beitrag zur Entwicklung einfacher sensibler Körperchen bei der Hauskatze (Felis silvestris, F. catus L.). *Acta anat.* 76:220-235.

– and Matonoha, P. (1968). Sensory corpuscles in the upper lip of some artiodactyla. *Folia Morph.* 16:422-431.

Manolson, F. (1970). *My Cat's in Love or How to Survive Your Feline's Sex Life, Pregnancy and Kittening.* St. Martin's Press, New York, N.Y.

Manter, J.T. (1938). The dynamics of quadrupedal walking. *J. exp. Biol.* 15:422-430.

Marey, M. (1894). Des mouvements que certains animaux exécutent pour retomber sur leurs, pieds, lorsqu'ils sont precipités d'un lien élevé. *Comptes Rendus des Seances de L'Academie de Sciences.* 119:714-717.

Marg, E. (1964). A rugged, reliable and sterilizable microelectrode for recording single units from the brain. *Nature* 202:601-603.

Martens, H.R. and Allen, D.R. (1969). *Introduction to Systems Theory.* C.E. Merrill Publishing Co., Columbus, Ohio.

Martin, P.S. and Wright, H.E. (1967). *Pleistocene Extinctions.* Yale University Press, New Haven, Conn.

Matheson, C. (1944). The domestic cat as a factor in urban ecology. *J. Anim. ecol.* 13:130-133.

Matthew, W.D. (1910). The phylogeny of the Felidae. *N.Y. Bull. Amer. Mus. Nat. Hist.* 28:289-316.

Matthews, B.H.C. (1933). Nerve endings in mammalian muscle. *J. Physiol.* 78:1-53.

Matthews, P.B.C. (1963). The response of de-efferented muscle spindle receptors to stretching at different velocities. *J. Physiol.* 168:660-678.

– (1964). Muscle spindles and their motor control. *Physiol. Rev.* 44:219-288.

– and Stein, R.B. (1969). The regularity of primary and secondary muscle spindle afferent discharges. *J. Physiol.* 202:59-82.

Maturana, H.R. and Frenk, S. (1963). Directional movement and horizontal edge detectors in the pigeon retina. *Science* 142:977-979.

Mead, L.C. (1942). Visual brightness discrimination in the cat as a function of illumination. *J. genet. Psychol.* 60:223-257.

Mei, N. (1970). Disposition anatomique et propriétés électrophysiologiques des neurones sensitifs vagaux chez le chat. *Exp. Brain Res.* 11:465-479.

Meikle, T.H. and Sprague, J.M. (1964). The Neural Organization of the Visual Pathways in the Cat. In *International Review of Neurobiology*, Vol. 6, (Pfeiffer, C.P. and Smythies, J.R., eds.), pp. 149-184. Academic Press, New York, N.Y.

Mello, N.K. and Peterson, N.J. (1964). Behavioral evidence for color discrimination in cat. *J. Neurophysiol.* 27:323-333.

Menner, E. (1929). Untersuchungen über die Retina mit besonderen Berucksichtigung der äusseren Körnerschicht. *Z. vergl. Physiol.* 8:761-827.

Merkel, F. (1875). Tastzellen und Tastkörperchen bei den Hausthieren und beim Menschen. *Arch. mikros. Anat.* 11:636-652.

Merriam, J.C. and Stock, C. (1932). The Felidae of Rancho La Brea. Publication No. 422, Carnegie Institute of Washington, Washington, D.C.

Michael, R.P. (1961). Observations upon the sexual behavior of the domestic cat (Felis catus L.) under laboratory conditions. *Behavior* 18:1-24.

Miller, I.J. (1971). Peripheral interactions among single papilla inputs to gustatory nerve fibers. *J. gen. Physiol.* 57:1-25.

Miller, J.D., Watson, C.S. and Covell, W.P. (1963). Deafening effects of noise on the cat. *Acta oto-laryng.* Suppl. 176.

Miller, S., Taylor, D.A. and Weddell, G. (1962). Extracellular single fibre recording technique for peripheral nerves without section of nerve or incision of perineurium. *Nature* 196:1215.

Missotten, L. (1965). *The Ultrastructure of the Retina.* Arscia, Uitgaven, N.V.

Mivart, G. (1881). *The Cat.* John Murray, London.

Moelk, M. (1944). Vocalizing in the house-cat; a phonetic and functional study. *Amer. J. Psychol.* 57:184-205.

Molnar, C.E. and Pfeiffer, R.R. (1968). Interpretation of spontaneous spike discharge patterns of neurons in the cochlear nucleus. *Proc. IEEE* 56:993-1004.

Montagna, W. (1962). The Pilary System. In *The Structure and Function of Skin*, (Bourne, G.H., ed.), pp. 174-219. Academic Press, New York, N.Y.

Montandon, P., Gacek, R.R. and Kimura, B. (1970). Crista neglecta in the cat and human. *Ann. Otol. Rhinol. Laryngol.* 79:105-112.

Moore, G.P., Perkel, D.H. and Segundo, J.P. (1966). Statistical analysis and functional interpretation of neuronal spike data. *Ann. Rev. Physiol.* 28:493-522.

Morest, D.K. (1968). The collateral system of the medial nucleus of the trapezoid body of the cat, its neuronal architecture and relation to the olivocochlear bundle. *Brain Res.* 9:288-311.

Moulton, D.G. and Beidler, L.M. (1967). Structure and function in the peripheral olfactory system. *Physiol. Rev.* 47:1-52.

Moushegian, G., Rupert, A. and Whitcomb, M.A. (1964a). Medial superior-olivary unit response patterns to monaural and binaural clicks. *J. Acoust. Soc. Amer.* 36:196-202.

– Rupert, A. and Whitcomb, M.A. (1964b). Brain stem neuronal response patterns to monaural and binaural tones. *J. Neurophysiol.* 27:1174-1191.

Moxon, E.C. and Kiang, N.Y-S. (1967). Discharge rates of auditory-nerve fibers in response to electric and acoustic stimuli. *J. Acoust. Soc. Amer.* 42:1206 (Abstract).

Müller, A. (1955). Quantitätive Untersuchungen am Riechepithel des Hundes. Z. *Zellforsch.* 41:335-350.

Munger, B.L. (1971). Patterns of Organization of Peripheral Sensory Receptors. In *Handbook of Sensory Physiology,* Vol. 1, (Loewenstein, W.R., ed.), pp. 523-556. Springer-Verlag, New York, N.Y.

Murray, R.G. and Murray, A. (1970). The Anatomy and Ultrastructure of Taste Endings. In *Taste and smell in Vertebrates,* (Wolstenholme, G.E.W. and Knight, J;, eds.), pp. 3-30. J. and A. Churchill, London.

Musterle, F. (1904). Zur Anatomie der unwallten Zungenpapillen der Katze und des Hundes. *Arch. f. Wissensch. u. Prakt. Thierh.* 30:141-161.

Mykytowycz, R. (1970). The Roles of Skin Glands in Mammalian Communication. In *Advances in Chemoreception,* Vol. 1, (Johnston, J., Moulton, D. and Turk, A., eds.), pp. 327-360. Meredith Co., New York, N.Y.

Nagaki, J., Yamashita, S. and Sato, M. (1964). Neural response of cat to taste stimuli of varying temperatures. *Jap. J. Physiol.* 14:67-89.

Nauta, W.J.H. and Ebbesson, S.O.E. (1970). *Contemporary Research Methods in Neuroanatomy.* Springer-Verlag, New York, N.Y.

– and Gygax, P.A. (1954). Silver impregnation of degenerating axons in the central nervous system. *Stain Tech.* 29:91-93.

Negus, V.E. (1956). The organ of Jacobson. *J. Anat.* 90:515-519.

– (1958). *The Comparative Anatomy and Physiology of the Nose and Paranasal Sinuses.* E. and S. Livingstone, Ltd., London.

Niijima, A. (1969). Afferent discharges from osmoreceptors in the liver of the guinea pig. *Science* 166:1519-1520.

Nilsson, B.Y. (1969a). Hair discs and Pacinian corpuscles functionally associated with the carpal tactile hairs in the cat. *Acta physiol. scand.* 77:417-428.

– (1969b). Structure and function of the tactile hair receptors on the cat's foreleg. *Acta physiol. scand.* 77:396-416.

Noback, C.R. (1951). Morphology and phylogeny of hair. *Ann. N.Y. Acad. Sci.* 53:476-492.

Ochs, S. (1965). *Elements of Neurophysiology.* John Wiley and Sons, New York, N.Y.

O'Connell, R.J. and Mozell, M.M. (1969). Quantitative stimulation of frog olfactory receptors. *J. Neurophysiol.* 32:51-63.

Ogawa, T., Bishop, P.O. and Levick, W.R. (1966). Temporal characteristics of responses to photic stimulation by single ganglion cells in the unopened eye of the cat. *Neurophysiol.* 29:1-30.

Olmsted, J.M.D. (1922). Taste fibers and the chorda tympani nerve. *J. comp. Neurol.* 34:337-341.

Oppel, A. (1900). *Lehrbuch der Vergleichenden Mikroskopischen Anatomie der Wirbeltiere.* Gustav Fisher, Jena.

Ortiz-Picon, J. (1955). The neuroglia of the sensory ganglia. *Anat. Rec.* 121:513-529.

Osen, K.K. (1969a). Cytoarchitecture of the cochlear nuclei in the cat. *J. comp. Neurol.* 136:453-484.

– (1969b). The intrinsic organization of the cochlear nuclei in the cat. *Acta oto-laryng.* 67:352-359.

– (1970a). Afferent and Efferent Connections of Three Well-defined Cell Types of the Cat Cochlear Nuclei. In *Excitatory Synaptic Mechanisms.* (Andersen, P. and Jansen, J.K.S., eds.), pp. 295-300. Universitetsforlaget, Oslo.

– (1970b). Course and termination of the primary afferents in the cochlear nuclei of the cat. An experimental anatomical study. *Arch. ital. Biol.* 108:21-51.

– and Roth, K. (1969). Histochemical localization of cholinesterases in the cochlear nuclei of the cat, with notes on the origin of acetylcholinesterase positive afferents and the superior olive. *Brain Res.* 16:165-185.

Ottoson, D. (1956). Analysis of the electrical activity of the olfactory epithelium. *Acta physiol. scand.* Suppl. 122.

Overbasch, J.F.A. (1927). Experimentel-anatomische Onderzoekingen ober de Projectie der Retina in het centrale Zenuwstelsel. Inaug. Dissert. Paris, Amsterdam. As cited by Meikle and Sprague (1964).

Ozeki, M. and Sato, M. (1965). Changes in the membrane potential and the membrane conductance associated with a sustained compression of the non-myelinated nerve terminal in Pacinian corpuscles. *J. Physiol.* 180:186-208.

Paintal, A.S. (1960). Functional analysis of group III afferent fibres of mammalian muscles. *J. Physiol.* 152:250-270.

— (1967). A comparison of the nerve impulses of mammalian non-medullated nerve fibres with those of the smallest diameter medullated fibres. *J. Physiol.* 193:523-533.

— and Riley, R.L. (1966). Responses of aortic chemoreceptors. *J. appl. Physiol.* 21:543-548.

Papez, J.W. (1929). *Comparative Neurology.* Thomas Y. Crowell Co., New York, N.Y.

— (1930). Superior olivary nucleus, its fiber connections. *A.M.A. Arch. Neurol. Psychiat.* 24:1-20.

Parakkal, P. (1970). Morphogenesis of the hair follicle during catagen. *Z. Zellforsch.* 107:174-186.

Perkel, D.H. and Bullock, T.H. (1968). Neural coding. *Neurosci. Res. Prog. Bull.* 6:221-348.

— Gerstein, G.L. and Moore, G.P. (1967a). Neuronal spike trains and stochastic point processes. I. The single spike train. *Biophys. J.* 7:391-418.

— (1967b). Neuronal spike trains and stochastic point processes. II. Simultaneous spike trains. *Biophys. J.* 7:419-440.

Petit, D. and Burgess, P.R. (1968). Dorsal column projection of receptors in cat hairy skin supplied by myelinated fibers. *J. Neurophysiol.* 31:849-855.

Pfaffman, C. (1941). Gustatory afferent impulses. *J. cell. comp. Physiol.* 17:243-258.

Pfeiffer, R.R. (1966a). Anteroventral cochlear nucleus: Wave forms of extracellularly recorded spike potentials. *Science* 154:667-668.

– (1966b). Classification of response patterns of spike discharges for units in the cochlear nucleus: Tone-burst stimulation. *Exp. Brain Res.* 1:220-235.

– and Kiang, N.Y-S. (1965). Spike discharge patterns of spontaneous and continuously stimulated activity in the cochlear nucleus of anesthetized cats. *Biophys. J.* 5:301-316.

Pick, J. (1970). *The Autonomic Nervous System.* J.B. Lippincott Co., Philadelphia, Pa.

Pineda, A., Maxwell, D.S. and Kruger, L. (1967). The fine structure of neurons and satellite cells in the trigeminal ganglion of cat and monkey. *Amer. J. Anat.* 121:461-488.

Pinkus, F. (1905). Über Hautsinnesorgane neben dem menschlicher Haar (Haarscheiben) und ihre vergleichend-anatomische Bedeutung. *Arch. mikros. Anat.* 65:121-179.

– (1927). Die Haarscheibe. In *Judassohn's Handbuch der Haut- und Geschlechts-Krankheiten.* Vol. 1, Part 1. Springer, Berlin.

Pocock, R.I. (1907). On English Domestic Cats. In *Proceedings of the Zoological Society of London,* pp. 143-168. Longmans, Green and Co., London.

– (1914a). On the Facial Vibrissae of Mammalia. In *Proceedings of the Zoological Society of London,* pp. 889-912. Longmans, Green and Co., London.

– (1914b). On the Feet and Other External Features of the Canidae and Ursidae. In *Proceedings of the Zoological Society of London,* pp. 913-941. Longmans, Green and Co., London.

– (1917). The classification of existing Felidae. *Ann. Mag. Nat. Hist.* 20:330-350.

– (1939). *The Fauna of British India, Including Ceylon and Burma. Mammalia,* Vol. 1. Taylor and Francis, Ltd., London.

– (1951). *Catalogue of the Genus Felis.* Jarrold and Sons, Ltd., Norwich.

Polácek, P. (1961). Differences in the structure and variability of encapsulated nerve endings in the joints of some species of mammals. *Acta anat.* 47:112-124.

– (1963). Die Nervenversorgung des Huft- und Kniegelenkes und ihre Besonderheiten. *Anat. Anz.* 112:243-256.

– (1965). Differences in the structure and variability of spray-like nerve endings in the joints of some mammals. *Acta anat.* 62:568-583.

—   (1966). *Receptors of the Joints*. Lékařská Fakulta University J.E. Purkyně, Brno.

—   (1968). Über die strukturellen Unterschiede der Rezeptorenreihen in der Vaginalwand der Katze und ihre mogliche funktionelle Bedeutung. *Z. mikr. Anat. Forsch.* 78:1-34.

—   and Halata, Z. (1970). Development of simple encapsulated corpuscles in the nasolabial region of the cat. *Folia Morph.* 18:359-368.

—   Malinovský, L., Sklenská, A. and Novotný, V. (1969). Zur Frage der Determination der sensiblen Nervenfasern. *Sbornik védeckých praci Lekařska fakulty KU v Hradci Králóve* 12:417-426.

—   and Peregrin, J. (1968). Contribution to the relationship between the structure and the function of the sensory nerve endings. *Scripta medica* 41:265-274.

Polyak, S. (1941). *The Retina*. University of Chicago Press, Chicago, Ill.

Poulos, D.A. and Lende, R.A. (1970a). Response of trigeminal ganglion neurons to thermal stimulation of oral-facial regions. I. Steady-state response. *J. Neurophysiol.* 33:508-517.

—   (1970b). Response of trigeminal ganglion neurons to thermal stimulation of oral-facial regions. II. Temperature change response. *J. Neurophysiol.* 33:518-526.

Powell, T.P.S. and Cowan, W.M. (1962). An experimental study of the projection of the cochlea. *J. Anat.* 96:269-284.

Pratt, L. (1969). A histochemical study of the course and distribution of the efferent vestibular fibers to the maculae of the saccule and utricle. *Laryngoscope* 79:1515-1545.

Pubols, B.H., Welker, W.I. and Johnson, J.I. (1965). Somatic sensory representation of forelimb in dorsal root fibers of raccoon, coatimundi and cat. *J. Neurophysiol.* 28:312-341.

Quilliam, T.A. (1968). Non-auditory vibration receptors. *Internat. Audiology* 7:311-321.

Ralls, K. (1971). Mammalian scent marking. *Science* 171:443-449.

Ramón-Moliner, E. (1968). The Morphology of Dendrites. In *The Structure and Function of Nervous Tissue*, Vol. 1, (Bourne, G.H., ed.), pp. 205-226. Academic Press, New York, N.Y.

Ramón y Cajal, S. (1902). Textura del lobulo olfativo accesorio. *Trab. Lab. Invest. Biol. Univ. Madrid* 1:141-150.

— (1904). *Textura del Sistema Nervioso de Hombre y de los Vertebredos.* Nicolas Moya, Madrid.

— (1907). Die Struktur der sensiblen Ganglien des Menschen und der Tiere. *Ergebn. d. Anat. u. Entwick.* 16:177-215.

— (1909). *Histologie du Système Nerveux de L'homme et des Vertébrés.* Consejo Sup. de Invest. Cient., Inst. Ramón y Cajal, Madrid. 1952 reprint.

— (1928). *Degeneration and Regeneration of the Nervous System.* (1952 translation of *Estudios Sobre la Degeneracion y Regeneracion del Systema Nervioso*). Translated and edited by R.M. May. Hafner Publishing Co., New York, N.Y.

— (1933). La rétine des vertébrés. *Trab. Lab. Invest. Biol. Univ. Madrid* Suppl. 28.

— (1954). *Neuron Theory or Reticular Theory?* (Translated by W.U. Purkiss and C.A. Fox). Consejo Sup. de Invest. Cient., Inst. Ramón y Cajal, Madrid.

— (1960). *Studies on Vertebrate Neurogenesis.* (Translated and edited by L. Girth). C.C. Thomas, Springfield, Ill.

Ranson, S.W. (1909). Alterations in the spinal ganglion cells following neurotomy. *J. comp. Neurol. Psychiat.* 19:125-153.

Rassmussen, A.T. (1943). *Outlines of Neuroanatomy,* third edition. Brown Publishing Co., Dubuque, Iowa.

Rasmussen, G.L. (1946). The olivary peduncle and other fiber projections of the superior olivary complex. *J. comp. Neurol.* 84:141-219.

— (1953). Further observations of the efferent cochlear bundle. *J. comp. Neurol.* 99:61-74.

— (1960). Efferent Fibers of the Cochlear Nerve and Cochlear Nucleus. In *Neural Mechanisms of the Auditory and Vestibular Systems,* (Rasmussen, G.L. and Windle, W., eds.), pp. 105-115. C.C. Thomas, Springfield, Ill.

— (1967). Efferent Connections of the Cochlear Nucleus. In *Sensorineural Hearing Processes and Disorders,* (Graham, A.B., ed.), pp. 61-75. Little, Brown and Co., Boston, Mass.

— and Gacek, R.R. (1958). Concerning the question of an efferent fiber component of the vestibular nerve of the cat. *Anat. Rec.* 130:361-362.

Read, E.A. (1908). Contribution to the knowledge of the olfactory apparatus in dog, cat and man. *Amer. J. Anat.* 8:17-47.

Rees, P.M. (1967). Observations on the fine structure and distribution of presumptive baroreceptor nerves at the carotid sinus. *J. comp. Neurol.* 131:517-548.

Reighard, J. and Jennings, H.S. (1929). *Anatomy of the Cat*, second edition. Henry Holt and Co., New York, N.Y.

Retzius, M.G. (1884). *Morphologisch-Histologische Studien II. Das Gehörorgan der Reptilien, der Vögel und der Säugetiere.* Samson and Wallin, Stockholm.

Reza, F.M. (1961). *An Introduction to Information Theory.* McGraw-Hill Book Co., New York, N.Y.

Rhinehart, D.A. (1918). The nervus facialis of the albino mouse. *J. comp. Neurol.* 30:81-125.

Roberts, T.D. (1967). *Neurophysiology of Postural Mechanisms.* Plenum Press, New York, N.Y.

Robinson, R. (1971). *Genetics for Cat Breeders.* Pergamon Press, New York, N.Y.

Rodieck, R.W. (1967a). Maintained activity of cat retinal ganglion cells. *J. Neurophysiol.* 30:1043-1071.

- (1967b). Receptive fields in the cat's retina: a new type. *Science* 157:90-91.

- Kiang, N.Y.-S. and Gerstein, G.L. (1962). Some quantitative methods for the study of spontaneous activity of single neurons. *Biophys. J.* 2:351-368.

- and Smith, P.S. (1966). Slow dark discharge rhythms of cat retinal ganglion cells. *J. Neurophysiol.* 29:942-953.

- and Stone, J. (1965). Response of cat retinal ganglion cells to moving visual patterns. *J. Neurophysiol.* 28:819-832.

Romer, A.S. (1966). *Vertebrate Paleontology, Third Edition.* University of Chicago Press, Chicago, Ill.

- (1970). *The Vertebrate Body.* W.B. Saunders Co., Philadelphia, Pa.

Ronnefeld, U. (1969). Verbreitung und Lebensweise afrikanischer Feloida (Felidae et Hyanidae). *Säugetierkdl. Mitt.* 17:285-350.

Rose, J.E., Galambos, R. and Hughes, J.R. (1959). Microelectrode studies of the cochlear nuclei of the cat. *Bull. Johns Hopkins Hosp.* 104:211-251.

Rosenblatt, J.S. (1965). Effects of Experience on Sexual Behavior in Male Cats. In *Sex and Behavior*, (Beach, F., ed.), pp. 416-439. John Wiley and Sons, New York, N.Y.

   – and Aronson, L.R. (1958). The decline of sexual behavior in male cats after castration with special reference to the role of prior sexual experience. *Behaviour* 12:285-338.

   Rosenblueth, A. and Bard, P. (1932). The innervation and functions of the nictitating membrane in the cat. *Amer. J. Physiol.* 100:537-544.

   Rosenthal, F., Woodbury, J.W. and Patton, H.D. (1966). Dipole characteristics of pyramidal cell activity in cat precruciate cortex. *J. Neurophysiol.* 29:612-625.

   Ross, L.L. (1959). Electron microscopic observations of the carotid body of the cat. *J. Biophys. Biochem. Cytol.* 6:253-262.

   Rossi, G. and Cortesiana, G. (1965). The efferent cochlear and vestibular system in Lepus cuniculus L. *Acta anat.* 60:362-381.

   Ruffini, A. (1905). Les Expansions Nerveuses de la Peau chez l'Homme et Quelques autres Mammiféres. In *Revue Générale de Histologie*, Vol. 1, (Reanut, J. and Regaud, Cl., eds.), pp. 421-540. A. Storck and Cie, Lyon-Paris.

   Rupert, A., Moushegian, G. and Whitcomb, M.A. (1965). Superior-olivary response patterns to monaural and binaural clicks. *J. Acoust. Soc. Amer.* 39:1069-1076.

   Rushton, W.A.H. (1949). The structure responsible for action potential spikes in the cat's retina. *Nature* 164:743-744.

   – (1950). Giant ganglion cells in the cat's retina. *J. Physiol.* 111:26-27P.

   Sachs, M.B. and Kiang, N.Y-S. (1968). Two-tone inhibition in auditory-nerve fibers. *J. Acoust. Soc. Amer.* 43:1120-1128.

   Saito, H., Shimahara, T. and Fukada, Y. (1970). Four types of responses to light and dark spot stimuli in the cat optic nerve. *Tohoku J. exp. Med.* 102:127-133.

   Sakmann, B. and Creutzfeldt, O.D. (1969). Scotopic and mesopic light adaptation in the cat's retina. *Pflüg. Arch.* 313:168-185.

   Sando, I. (1965). The anatomical interrelationships of the cochlear nerve fibers. *Acta oto-laryng.* 59:417-436.

   Sasaoka, S. (1939a). Über das Kaliber den Markhaltigen Nervenfasern im Gelenkäst. *Jap. J. Med. Sci. (Anat.), Trans. Abstr.* 7:315-322.

   – (1939b). Characteristika in den Kaliberverhaltnissen der Markscheide bei den Muskel-, Haut- und Gelenkästen. *Jap. J. Med. Sci. (Anat.), Trans. Abstr.* 7:323-342.

   Sato, M. (1961). Response of Pacinian corpuscles to sinusoidal vibration. *J. Physiol.* 159:391-409.

Scalzi, H.A. (1967). The cytoarchitecture of gustatory receptors from the rabbit foliate papillae. Z. Zellforsch. 80:413-435.

— and Price, H.M. (1971).The arrangement and sensory innervation of the intrafusal fibers in the feline muscle spindle. J. Ultrastruct. Res. 36:375-390.

Schaller, G.B. (1967). The Deer and the Tiger—a Study of Wildlife in India. University of Chicago Press, Chicago, Ill.

Scharf, J.H. (1950a). Die markhaltigen Ganglienzellen und ihre Beziehungen zu den myeloganestischen Theorien. Jahr. f. morph. u. mikr. Anat. 91:187-252.

— (1950b). Untersuchungen an markhaltigen Ganglienzellen in der Wirbeltierreihe und beim Menschen. Anat. Anz. Supp. 97:207-213.

— (1958). Handbuch der Mikroskopischen Anatomie des Menschen, Vol. 4, Part 3, Nerven System Dritter Teil Sensible Ganglien. Springer-Verlag, Berlin.

Schmiedberger, G. (1932). Über die Bedeutung der Schnurrhaare bei Katzen. Z. vergl. Physiol. 17:387-407.

Schmidt, R. and Creutzfeldt, O.D. (1968). Veranderungen von Spontanaktivität und Reizantwort retinaler und geniculärer Neurone der Katze bei fraktionierter Injektion von Pentobarbital-Na. Pflüg. Arch. 300:129-147.

Schmidt, W. (1957). Uber das Schwellgewebe in der Nasenhöhle der Katze. Z. Anat. Entwicklungsges. 120:124-128.

Schneirla, T.C., Rosenblatt, J.S. and Tobach, E. (1963). Maternal Behavior in the Cat. In Maternal Behavior in Mammals, (Rheingold, H.L., ed.), pp. 122-168. John Wiley and Sons, New York, N.Y.

Schuknecht, H.F. (1960). Neuroanatomical Correlates of Auditory Sensitivity and Pitch Discrimination in the Cat. In Neural Mechanisms of the Auditory and Vestibular Systems, (Rasmussen, G.L. and Windle, W., eds.), pp. 76-90. C.C. Thomas, Springfield, Ill.

— and Sutton, S. (1953). Hearing losses after experimental lesions in basal coil of cochlea. Arch. Otolaryng. 57:129-146.

— and Woellner, R.C. (1953). Hearing losses following partial section of the cochlear nerve. Laryngoscope 113:441-465.

Schultze, M. (1856). Über die Endigungsweise des Geruchsnerven und der Epithelialgebilde der Nasenschleimhaut. Monatsber. Deut. Akad. Wiss. Berlin 21:504-515.

— (1866). Zur Anatomie und Physiologie der Retina. Arch. mikr. Anat. Entw. Mech. 2:175-286.

Schwartz, M. (1970). *Information Transmission, Modulation and Noise.* McGraw-Hill Book Co., New York, N.Y.

Scott, P.P. (1968). The Special Features of Nutrition of Cats, with Observations on Wild Felidae Nutrition in the London Zoo. In *Symposium of the Zoological Society of London,* No. 21, (Crawford, M.A., ed.), pp. 21-36. Academic Press, New York, N.Y.

Sechzer, J.A. and Brown, J.L. (1964). Color discrimination in the cat. *Science* 144:427-429.

Sekiguchi, S. (1960). On the nerve supply of the outer genitals in tomcat. *Arch. Hist. Jap.* 18:611-634.

Shantha, T.R. and Bourne, G.H. (1968). The Perineural Epithelium—A New Concept. In *The Structure and Function of Nervous Tissue,* Vol. 1, (Bourne, G.H., ed.), pp. 379-459. Academic Press, New York, N.Y.

Shehata, R. (1970). Pacinian corpuscles in bladder wall and outside ureter of the cat. *Acta anat.* 77:139-143.

Shibuya, T. and Tucker, D. (1967). Si¬gle Unit Responses of Olfactory Receptors in Vultures. In *Olfaction and Taste,* Vol. 2, (Hayashi, T., ed.), pp. 219-234. Pergamon Press, Oxford.

Shkolnik-Yarros, E.G. (1971). Neurons of the cat's retina. *Vision Res.* 11:7-26.

Silver, S. (1970). Digital voice communication. *Elec. World* 84:27-30.

Simmons, F.B. and Linehan, J.A. (1968). Observations on a single auditory nerve fiber over a six-week period. *J. Neurophysiol.* 31:799-805.

Simpson, F. (1903). *The Book of the Cat.* Cassell and Co., New York, N.Y.

Sitwell, N. (1970). Leopard skin coats look better on leopards. *Animals* 13:352-363.

Sjöstrand, F.S. (1959). Fine structure of cytoplasm: The organization of membrane layers. *Rev. Mod. Phys.* 31:301-318.

Sklenská, A. (1965). Sensory nerve endings in joint capsules of domestic and wild rabbit. *Folia Morph.* 13:372-383.

— (1968). Joint receptors in certain eventoed ungulates (Artiodactyla) and their comparison with those in rodents (Rodentia) and in lagomorphs (Lagomorpha). *Folia Morph.* 16:74-82.

— (1969). Über Unterscheide in Häufigkeit, Verteilung und Struktur der Rezeptoren in einigen grossen Gelenken der Extremitäten von Wirbeltieren. *Z. mikr. anat. Forsch.* 80:249-259.

Skoglund, S. (1956). Anatomical and physiological studies of knee joint innervation in the cat. *Acta physiol. scand.* Suppl. 124.

Smith, C.A. (1956). Microscopic structure of the utricle. *Ann. Otol.* 65:450-469.

— and Rasmussen, G.L. (1965). Nerve Endings in the Maculae and Cristae of the Chinchilla Vestibule, with a Special Reference to the Efferents. In *Role of the Vestibular Organs in the Exploration of Space.* N.A.S.A. SP-152. National Aeronautics and Space Admin., Washington, D.C.

Smith, C.M. (1963). Neuromuscular pharmacology: Drugs and muscle spindles. *Ann. Rev. Pharm.* 3:223-242.

Smith, K.R. (1970). The ultrastructure of the human Haarscheibe and Merkel cell. *J. Invest. Dermatol.* 54:150-159.

Smith, K.U. (1936). Visual discrimination in the cat. IV. The visual acuity of the cat in relation to stimulus distance. *J. genet. Psychol.* 49:297-313.

— (1938). Visual discrimination in the cat. VI. The relation between pattern vision and visual acuity and the optic projection centers of the nervous system. *J. genet. Psychol.* 53:271272.

Smith, L.S. (1971). Editorial. *Cat Fancy* 14:2.

Sonntag, C.F. (1923). The comparative anatomy of the tongues of the mammalia. *Proc. Zool. Soc. Lond.* 9:129-153.

Spinelli, D.N. (1967). Receptive field organization of ganglion cells in the cat's retina. *Exp. Neurol.* 19:291-315.

Spoendlin, H. (1966). *The Organization of the Cochlear Receptor. Adv. Oto-Rhino-Laryngol.* Vol. 13.

— (1968). Ultrastructure and Peripheral Innervation Pattern of the Receptor in Relation to the First Coding of the Acoustic Message. In *Hearing Mechanisms in Vertebrates,* (deReuck, A.V.S. and Knight, J., eds.), pp. 89-125. Little, Brown and Co., Boston, Mass.

— (1969). Innervation patterns in the organ of Corti of the cat. *Acta oto-laryng.* 67:239-254.

— (1970). Structural Basis of Peripheral Frequency Analysis. In *Frequency Analysis and Periodicity Detection in Hearing,* (Plomp, R. and Smoorenburg, G.F., eds.), pp. 2-40. A.W. Sijthoff, Leiden, The Netherlands.

— and Gacek, R.R. (1963). Electromicroscopic study of the efferent and afferent innervation of the organ of Corti. *Ann. Otol. Rhinol. Laryngol.* 72:660-686.

Stacey, M.J. (1969). Free nerve endings in skeletal muscles of the cat. *J. Anat.* 105:231-254.

Steinhausen, W. (1931). Über den Nachweis der Bewegung der Cupula in der intakten Bogengangsampullen des Labyrinthes bei der natürlichen rotatorischen und calorischen Reizung. *Pflüg. Arch.* 228:322-328.

– (1933). Über die Funktion der Cupula in den Bogengangsampullen des Labyrinthes. *Z. Hals- Nas- Ohrheilk.* 34:201-209.

Stevens, S.S. and Davis, H. (1938). *Hearing, its Psychology and Physiology.* John Wiley and Sons, New York, N.Y.

Stone, J. (1965). A quantitative analysis of the distribution of ganglion cells in the cat's retina. *J. comp. Neurol.* 124:337-352.

– (1966). The naso-temporal division of the cat's retina. *J. comp. Neurol.* 126:585-600.

– and Fabian, M. (1966). Specialized receptive fields of the cat's retina. *Science* 152:1277-1279.

– (1968). Summing properties of cat's retinal ganglion cell. *Vision Res.* 8:1023-1040.

Stopp, P.E. and Whitfield, I.C. (1963). The influence of microelectrodes on neuronal discharge patterns in the auditory system. *J. Physiol.* 167:169-180.

Stotler, W.A. (1953). An experimental study of the cells and connections of the superior olivary complex of the cat. *J. comp. Neurol.* 98:401-431.

Streeter, G.L. (1906). On the development of the membranous labyrinth and the acoustic and facial nerves in the human embryo. *Amer. J. Anat.* 6:139-165.

Strickland, J.H. (1958). The Microscopic Anatomy of the Skin and External Ear of Felis Domesticus. M.S. Dissertation. College of Veterinary Medicine, Michigan State University.

– and Calhoun, M.L. (1960). The microscoptic anatomy of the external ear of Felis domesticus. *Amer. J. Vet. Res.* 21:845-850.

– (1963). The integumentary system of the cat. *Amer. J. Vet. Res.* 24:1018-1029.

Stuart, D., Mosher, C, Gerlach, R. and Reinking, R. (1970). Selective activation of Ia afferents by transient muscle stretch. *Exp. Brain Res.* 10:477-487.

Sunderland, S. and Roche, A.F. (1958). Axon-myelin relationships in peripheral nerve fibers. *Acta anat.* 33:1-37.

Taber, E. (1961). The cytoarchitecture of the brain stem of the cat. I. Brain stem nuclei of the cat. *J. comp. Neurol.* 116:27-70.

Talbot, W.H., Darian-Smith, I., Kornhuber, H.H. and Mountcastle, V.B. (1968). The sense of flutter vibration: Comparison of human capacity with response patterns of mechanoreceptive afferents from the monkey hand. *J. Neurophysiol.* 31:301-334.

Tapper, D. (1965). Stimulus-response relationships in the cutaneous slowly-adapting mechanoreceptor in hairy skin of the cat. *Exp. Neurol.* 13:364-385.

−   (1970). Behavioral evaluation of the tactile pad receptor system in hairy skin of the cat. *Exp. Neurol.* 26:447-459.

Tasaki, I. (1959). Conduction of Nerve Impulse. In *Handbook of Physiology, Section 1: Neurophysiology*, Vol. 1, (Field, J., ed.), pp. 75-122. Waverly Press, Baltimore, Md.

Tembrock, G. (1970). Bioakustische Untersuchungen an Säugetieren des Berliner Tierparkes. *Milu* 3:78-96.

Thenius, E. (1967). Zur Phylogenie der Feliden Z. *Zool. Syst. Evolutionforsch.* 5:129-143.

Thieulin, G. (1927). Recherches sur le Globe Oculaire et sur la Vision der Chien et du Chat Thèse Vétérinaire, Ecole Nationale Vétérinaire D'Alfort, Danzig, Paris.

Thomas, R.C. and Wilson, V.J. (1966). Marking single neurons by staining with intracellular recording microelectrodes. *Science* 151:1538-1539.

Thorn, F. (1970). Detection of luminance differences by the cat. *J. comp. physiol. Psychol.* 70:326-334.

Tokuyasu, K. and Yamada, E. (1959). Fine structure of the retina studied with electron microscope. IV. Morphogenesis of outer segments of retinal rods. *J. Biophys. Biochem. Cytol.* 6:225-230.

Tonndorf, J. and Khanna, S.M. (1970). The role of the tympanic membrane in middle ear transmission. *Ann. Otol. Rhinol. Laryngol.* 79:743-753.

Tsuchitani, C. and Boudreau, J.C. (1964). Wave activity in the superior olivary complex of the cat. *J. Neurophysiol.* 27:814-827.

−   (1966). Single unit analysis of cat superior olive S-segment with tonal stimuli. *J. Neurophysiol.* 29:684-697.

—   (1967). Encoding of stimulus frequency and intensity by cat superior olive S-segment cells. *J. Acoust. Soc. amer.* 42:794-805.

—   (1969). Stimulus level of dichotically presented tones and cat superior olive S-segment cell discharge. *J. Acoust. Soc. Amer.* 46:979-988.

Tucker, D. (1963). Olfactory, Vomeronasal and Trigeminal Receptor Responses to Odorants. In *Olfaction and Taste*, Vol. 1, (Zotterman, Y., ed.), pp. 45-69. Pergamon Press, New York, N.Y.

Tuckerman, F. (1890). On the gustatory organs of the mammalia. *Boston Soc. Nat. Hist. Proc.* 24:470-482.

—   (1892). Further observations on the gustatory organs of the mammalia. *J. Morph.* 7:69-94.

Uyama, Y. (1934). Regionäre Verschiedenheiten der Horizontalzellen mit besonderen Berücksichtigungen ihrer Verbreitung und Anordnung in der Netzhaut. *Graefs Arch. Ophthal.* 132:10-19.

Vakkur, G.J. and Bishop, P.O. (1963). The schematic eye in the cat. *Vision Res.* 3:357-381.

—   and Kozak, W. (1963. Visual optics in the cat, including posterior nodal distance and retinal landmarks. *Vision Res.* 3:289-314.

Van Horn, R.N. (1970). Vibrissae structure in the Rhesus monkey. *Folia primat.* 13:241-285.

Van Noort, J. (1969). *The Structure and Connections of the Inferior Colliculus.* Van Gorcum and Co., Leiden.

Vintschgau, M.V. and Honigschmied, J. (1876). Nervus glossopharyngeus und Schmeckbecher. *Arch. ges. Physiol.* 14:443-448.

Voit, M. (1907). Zur Frage der Verästelung des Nervus acousticus bei den Säugetieren. *Anat. Anz.* 31:635-640.

Voneida, T.H. and Robinson, J.S. (1970). Effect of brain bisection on capacity for cross comparison of patterned visual input. *Exp. Neurol.* 26:60-71.

DeVries, H. (1950). The mechanics of the labyrinth otoliths. *Acta oto-laryng.* 38:262-273.

Walker, E.P. (1964). *Mammals of the World*, Vol. 11, pp. 1268-1282. The Johns Hopkins University Press, Baltimore, Md.

Walker, W. (1967). *A Study of the Cat*. W.B. Saunders Co., Philadelphia, Pa.

Walls, G.L. (1942). *The Vertebrate Eye and its Adaptive Radiation*. Cranbrook Press, Bloomfield Hills, Mich.

Warr, W.B. (1966). Fiber degeneration following lesions in the anterior ventral cochlear nucleus of the cat. *Exp. Neurol.* 14:453-474.

—   (1969). Fiber degeneration following lesions in the posteroventral cochlear nucleus of the cat. *Exp. Neurol.* 23:140-155.

Warrington, W.B. and Griffith, F. (1904). On the cells of the spinal ganglia and on the relationship of their histological structure to the axonal distribution. *Brain* 27:297-326.

Weddell, G. and Pallie, W. (1955). Studies on the innervation of skin. II. The number, size and distribution of hairs, hair follicles and orifices from which the hairs emerge in the rabbit ear. *J. Anat.* 89:175-188.

—   and Palmer, E. (1955a). Studies on the innervation of skin. I. The origin, course and number of sensory nerves supplying the rabbit ear. *J. Anat.* 89:162-174.

—   (1955b). Nerve endings in mammalian skin. *Biol. Rev.* 30:159-195.

—   Taylor, D.A. and Williams, C.M. (1955c). Studies on the innervation of skin. III. The patterned arrangement of the spinal sensory nerves to the rabbit ear. *J. Anat.* 89:317-342.

Weigner, K. (1905). Über den Verlauf des Nervus intermedius. *Anatomische Hefte.* 29:7-157.

Werblin, F.S. and Dowling, J.E. (1969). Organization of the retina of the mudpuppy, Necturus maculosus. II. Intracellular recording. *J. Neurophysiol.* 32:339-355.

Werner, C.F. (1940). *Des Labyrinth*. George Thieme, Leipzig.

Werner, G. and Mountcastle, V.B. (1965). Neural activity in mechanoreceptive cutaneous afferents: Stimulus-response relations, Weber functions, and information transmission. *J. Neurophysiol.* 28:359-397.

Wersäll, J. (1956). Studies on the structure and innervation of the sensory epithelium of the cristae ampullares in the guinea pig. *Acta oto-laryng.* Suppl. 126.

Wever, E.G. (1964). The Physiology of the Peripheral Hearing Mechanism. In *Neurological Aspects of Auditory and Vestibular Disorders*, (Fields, W.S. and Alford, B.R., eds.), pp. 24-50. C.C. Thomas, Springfield, Ill.

—   (1965). Structure and function of the lizard ear. *J. Aud. Res.* 5:331-371.

—   and Lawrence, M. (1954). *Physiological Acoustics.* Princeton University Press, Princeton, N.J.

—   and Smith, K.R. (1948). The middle ear in sound conduction. *Arch. Otolaryng.* 48:19-35.

Wheeler, A., Cristie, D., Cohen, E., Jarman, C. and Lanworn, B. (1970). *Animals of the World.* Hamlyn Publishing Group, Ltd., London.

Wiederhold, M.L. (1970). Variations in the effects of electric stimulation of the crossed olivocochlear bundle on cat single auditory-nerve fiber responses to tone bursts. *J. Acoust. Soc. Amer.* 48:966-977.

—   and Kiang, N.Y-S. (1970). Effects of electric stimulation on the crossed olivocochlear bundle on single auditory-nerve fibers in the cat. *J. Acoust. Soc. Amer.* 48:950-965.

Wiener, F.M., Pfeiffer, R.R. and Backus, A.S.N. (1965). On the sound pressure transformation by the head and auditory meatus of the cat. *Acta oto-laryng.* 61:255-269.

Wiesel, T.H. (1960). Receptive fields of ganglion cells in the cat's retina. *J. Physiol.* 153:583-594.

Wilson, C. and Weston, E. (1946). *The Cats of Wildcat Hill.* Duell, Sloan and Pierce, New York, N.Y.

Wilson, J.G. (1907). The nerves and nerve-endings in the membrana tympani. *J. comp. Neurol. Psychol.* 17:459-469.

Windle, W.F. (1926). The distribution and probable significance of unmyelinated nerve fibers in the trigeminal nerve of the cat. *J. comp. Neurol.* 41:453-477.

—   (1931). The sensory components of the spinal accessory nerve. *J. comp. Neurol.* 53:115-127.

Winters, R.W. and Walter, J.W. (1970). Transient and steady state stimulus-response relations for cat retinal ganglion cells. *Vision Res.* 10:461-477.

Wolff, D. (1936). The ganglion spirale cochleae. *Amer. J. Anat.* 60:55-77.

Wynne-Edwards, V.C. (1962). *Animal dispersion in Relation to Social Behavior.* Oliver and Boyd, Ltd., Edinburgh.

Young, S.P. (1958). *The Bobcat of North America*. The Stockpole Co., Harrisburg, Pa.

—   and Goldman, E.A. (1964). *The Puma*. Dover Publications, New York, N.Y. (A republication of the work first published in 1946 by the American Wildlife Institute.)

Zeuner, F.E. (1950). The cat. *Oryx* 1:65-71.

—   (1963). *A History of Domesticated Animals*. Harper and Row, New York, N.Y.

Zotterman, Y. (1935). Action potentials in the glossopharyngeal nerve and in the chorda tympani. *Skand. Arch. Physiol.* 72:73-77.

—   (1936). Specific action potentials in the lingual nerve of the cat. *Scand. Arch. Physiol.* 75:105-120.

—   (1939). Touch, pain and tickling: An electrophysiological investigation on cutaneous nerves. *J. Physiol.* 95:1-28.

Zucker, E. and Welker, W.I. (1969). Coding of somatic sensory input by vibrissae neurons in the rat's trigeminal ganglion. *Brain Res.* 12:138-156.

Zurn, J. (1902). Vergleichende histologische Untersuchungen über die Retina und die Area centralis retinae der Haussäugethiere. *Arch. Anat. Physiol. Anat. Abth.* Suppl. 99-144.

INDEX